T0313229

Economic Evaluation of Cancer Drugs

Using Clinical Trial and Real-World Data

Chapman & Hall/CRC Biostatistics Series

Recently Published Titles

Bayesian Methods for Repeated Measures
Lyle D. Broemeling

Modern Adaptive Randomized Clinical Trials
Statistical and Practical Aspects
Oleksandr Sverdlov

Medical Product Safety Evaluation
Biological Models and Statistical Methods
Jie Chen, Joseph Heyse, Tze Leung Lai

Statistical Methods for Survival Trial Design
With Applications to Cancer Clinical Trials Using R
Jianrong Wu

Bayesian Applications in Pharmaceutical Development
Satrajit Roychoudhury, Soumi Lahiri

Platform Trials in Drug Development
Umbrella Trials and Basket Trials
Zoran Antonjevic and Robert Beckman

Innovative Strategies, Statistical Solutions and Simulations for Modern Clinical Trials
Mark Chang, John Balser, Robin Bliss and Jim Roach

Cost-effectiveness Analysis of Medical Treatments
A Statistical Decision Theory Approach
Elias Moreno, Francisco Jose Vazquez-Polo and Miguel Angel Negrin-Hernandez

Analysis of Incidence Rates
Peter Cummings

Mixture Modelling for Medical and Health Sciences
Shu-Kay Ng, Liming Xiang, Kelvin Kai Wing Yau

Economic Evaluation of Cancer Drugs
Using Clinical Trial and Real-World Data
Iftekhar Khan, Ralph Crott, Zahid Bashir

Economic Evaluation of Cancer Drugs

Using Clinical Trial and Real-World Data

Iftekhar Khan,
Ralph Crott, and Zahid Bashir

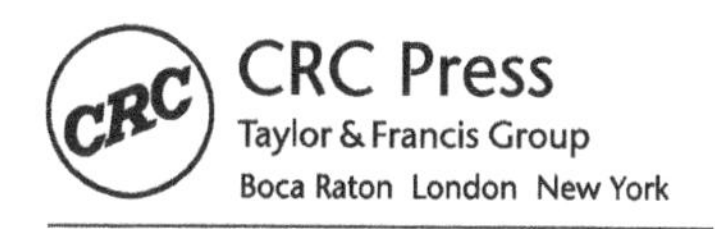

CRC Press is an imprint of the
Taylor & Francis Group, an **informa** business
A CHAPMAN & HALL BOOK

CRC Press
Taylor & Francis Group
6000 Broken Sound Parkway NW, Suite 300
Boca Raton, FL 33487-2742

Printed on acid-free paper

International Standard Book Number-13: 978-1-498-76130-7 (Hardback)

Visit the Taylor & Francis Web site at
http://www.taylorandfrancis.com

and the CRC Press Web site at
http://www.crcpress.com

These are our works, these works our souls display

Behold our works, when we have passed away

For Suhailah, Yohanis, Hanzalah, my father, and all those affected by cancer

For Jon and Fiona, my children

For Saima, Hassan, and Hibba

Contents

Preface

The cost of cancer care has increased hugely and put pressure on health-care systems around the world. An important part of this cost is the cost of cancer medicines. Economic evaluation of cancer drugs is an extremely important area that affects health policy and access to cancer treatment. The economic evaluation of cancer drugs can involve careful trial design, robust economic modeling, and sound statistical analysis and research methodology, drawing together the disciplines of medical statistics, clinical research, and economics.

Several books already exist that address theoretical or practical aspects of cost-effectiveness analysis. However, no unified text on the cost-effectiveness of cancer medicines is currently available. This book attempts to deal with the matter within a practical framework, focusing on key concepts and drawing on the experiences of health technology appraisals (HTA) of cancer drugs – either approved or rejected by government reimbursement agencies (the payers). This book also offers an insight into how health economic evaluation of cancer interventions has been carried out in practice, with many examples throughout, where data are collected in clinical trials or in real-world settings.

This book is not just about performing cost-effectiveness analyses of cancer drugs using clinical trial and real-world data, but also emphasizes the strategic importance of economic evaluation through the drug development process. It also offers guidance and advice on the complex factors at play before, during, and after an economic evaluation for a cancer intervention. In addition, this book bridges the gap between industry (pharmaceutical) applications of economic evaluation and what students may learn on university courses. The book is suitable for statisticians, health economists, cancer researchers, oncologists, and anyone with an interest in the cost-effectiveness of interventions for cancer using clinical trial and/or real-world data. It would also be a valuable book for a postgraduate course in health economics.

We candidly admit that our objectives have been set high when structuring this book. Economic evaluation covers several disciplines and addressing all of these has been challenging. We hope that the material in this book is suitable for a range of researchers of varying abilities, so that some will find the entire book useful whereas, for others, particular chapters will be useful. As a student textbook, this book can be complemented by additional reading material suggested in the bibliography.

Iftekhar Khan
Centre for Statistics in Medicine, University of Oxford
Ralph Crott
Consultant Health Economist, Belgium
Zahid Bashir
Clinical Consultant in Cancer Trials

Acknowledgments

We would like to gratefully acknowledge helpful reviews by Dr. Noan-Min Chau from the Licensing Division of UK Medicines and Health Regulator Agency (MHRA) and also Tarita Murray-Thomas from the Clinical Practice Research Data Link (CPRD) within the MHRA. Their comments have resulted in a much-improved text. We also acknowledge the reviews by Dr. Suhailah Khan and Uzma Ikramullah for proofreading parts of the text. We graciously acknowledge the National Institute for Health and Care Excellence (NICE), which has made available to the public such excellent material, as demonstrated in this book. Finally, we would like to thank the anonymous reviewers of earlier chapters. Their comments have been extremely helpful enabling us to deliver a much-improved text.

About the Authors

Dr. Iftekhar Khan is a medical statistician and health economist by qualification and training. Dr. Khan has extensive experience in cancer trials in industry, academia, and regulatory environments, spanning over 18 years. He was formerly associate professor in Medical Statistics and Methodology at King's College, London, and lead statistician at UCL CRUK Cancer Trials Centre and Oxford University's Center for Statistics in Medicine. Professor Khan is also a Senior Research Fellow in Health Economics at the University of Warwick and a Senior Statistical Assessor within the Licensing Division of the UK Medicine and Health Regulation Agency where he regularly evaluates oncologic and other drugs and devices for licensing.

Dr. Ralph Crott is a former professor in Pharmacoeconomics at the University of Montreal in Quebec, Canada and former head of the EORTC Health Economics Unit (Brussels, Belgium) and former senior health economist at the Belgian HTA organization (KCE). Dr. Crott has been active in economic evaluation of new medical technology since 1984. He also held research and/or teaching positions at York University in the United Kingdom and the Catholic University of Louvain, Belgium. He received his PhD in applied economics at the Catholic University of Louvain (UCL, Belgium) and holds additional masters degrees in econometrics (Flemish University of Brussels (VUB, Belgium), biostatistics (Limburg University, Belgium), public health with a major in clinical research (Catholic University of Louvain, Belgium), and technology assessment (Aston University, United Kingdom).

Dr. Zahid Bashir has over twelve years of experience working in the pharmaceutical industry, specifically in medical affairs and oncology drug development, where he is involved in the design and execution of oncological clinical trials and development of reimbursement dossiers for HTA submission. Dr. Bashir also has extensive clinical experience in teaching oncology and haematology in the UK NHS hospital.

Acronyms and Abbreviations

ACD	advanced consultation document
AE	adverse events
AEMPS	Agencia Española de Medicamentos y Productos Sanitarios
AFT	accelerated failure time
AHRQ	Agency for Healthcare Research and Quality
AIC	Akaike Information Criterion
ALK	anaplastic lymphoma kinase
ASCO	American Society of Clinical Oncology
ASMR	medical improvement score
ATC	average total cost
AUC	area under the curve
BB	beta binomial
BEV	bevacizumab
BIM	budget impact model
BNF	British National Formulary
BRCA	breast cancer gene
BSC	best supportive care
CADTH	Canadian Agency for Drugs and Technologies in Health
CAP	chemotherapy for advanced prostate cancer
CCG	clinical commissioning group
CCyR	complete cytogenic response
CDF	Cancer Drug Fund
CDR	Common Drug Review
CE	cost-effectiveness
CEA	cost-effectiveness analysis
CEAC	cost-effectiveness acceptability curve
CEESP	Commission d'Évaluation Économique et de Santé Publique
CESP	Comité Economique des Produits de Santé
CHEERS	Consolidated Health Economic Evaluation Reporting
chemo-RT	chemoradiotherapy
CI	confidence interval
CMA	cost minimization analysis
CML	chronic myeloid leukemia
CMS	Center for Medicare Services
CPRD	Clinical Practice Research Datalink
CPT	current procedural terminology
CR	complete response
CRA	clinical research associate
CRC	colorectal cancer

CRF	case report form
CRUK	Cancer Research UK
CSM	condition-specific measures
CSRI	client services receipt inventory
CT	computed (axial) tomography
CUA	cost-utility analysis
CV	cabozanitib and vandetanib
DALY	disability-adjusted life-years
DAPA	dementia and physical activity
DCF	data collection form
DES	discrete event simulation
DFS	disease-free survival
DICE	discretely integrated condition event
DLBCL	diffuse large B-cell lymphoma
DMC	data monitoring committee
DoR	duration of response
DRG	diagnostic-related group
EAMS	early access to medicine
ECOG	Eastern Cooperative Oncology Group
eCRF	electronic case report form (CRF)
EFS	event-free survival
EGFR	epidermal growth factor receptor
EHR	electronic health records
EINB	expected incremental net benefit
EMA	European Medicines Agency
ENB	expected net benefit
ENMB	expected net monetary benefit
ENBS	expected net benefit of sampling
EoL	end-of-life
EORTC	European Organization for Research and Treatment of Cancer
ERG	evidence review group
ESMO	European Society of Medical Oncology
EUnetHTA	European Network of Health Technology assessment
EVPI	expected value of perfect information
EVPPI	expected value of partially perfect information
EVSI	expected value of sample information
FACT	Functional Assessment of Cancer Therapy
FDA	Food and Drug Administration
FDAAA	FDA Amendments Act
FDG-PET	2-fluoro-2-deoxyglucose positron emission tomography
FISH	fluorescence in situ hybridization
GCP	Good Clinical Practice
GDP	gross domestic product
GDPR	General Data Protection Regulation

GLM	general / generalized linear model
GLOBOCAN	Global Cancer Observatory Database
HAS	Haute Autorité de Santé
HCCor	half-cycle correction
HCC	hepatocellular carcinoma
HEAP	health economic analysis plan
HES	Hospital Episode Statistics
HR	hazard ratio
HRQoL	health-related quality of life
HTA	health technology assessment
HUI	health utility index
ICD	international classification of diseases
ICD-O	international classification of diseases for oncology
ICER	incremental cost-effectiveness ratio
ICERev	Institute for Clinical and Economic Review
IDMC	independent data monitoring committee
INB	incremental net benefit
INFORMED	Information Exchange and Data Transformation
INMB	incremental net monetary benefit
IPCW	inverse probability-of-censoring weighting
IQWiG	Institute for Quality and Efficiency
irRC	immune-related response criteria
ISPOR	International Society of Pharmacoeconomics and Outcomes Research
ITC	indirect treatment comparison
ITT	intention-to-treat
IV	instrumental variable
IV	intravenous
KM	Kaplan-Meier
LCS	lung cancer scale
LMG	life-month gained (as unit)
LOCF	last observation carried forward
LSmean	least squares mean
LT	liver transplantation
LYG	life-years gained
MAMS	multi-arm, multi-stage
MAR	missing at random
MCAR	missing completely at random
MCID	minimum clinical important difference
MCO	managed care organization
MDS	myelodysplastic syndrome
MDT	multidisciplinary team
MED	minimum effective dose
MHRA	Medicines and Healthcare products Regulatory Agency
MI	multiple imputation

mITT	modified ITT
MLM	multilevel models
MM	multiple myeloma
MMR	major molecular response
MNAR	missing not at random
MPFS	Medicare Physician Fee Schedule
MRD	minimal residual disease
MSM	marginal structural model
MTA	multiple technology appraisal
MTC	mixed treatment comparison
MTD	maximum tolerated dose
NBM	negative binomial model
NCCN	National Comprehensive Cancer Network
NCI	National Cancer Institute
NCLA	National Lung Cancer Audit
NCR	National Cancer Registry
NCRS	National Cancer Registration Service
NHB	net health benefit
NHS	National Health Service
NICE	National Institute of Health and Care Excellence
NIHR	National Institute for Health Research
NMA	network meta-analysis
NMB	net monetary benefit
NPV	net present value
NSCLC	non-small-cell lung cancer/carcinoma
OCS	ovarian cancer-specific
QD	once daily
OLE	open label extension
OLS	ordinary least square
ORR	objective response rate
ORR	overall response rate
OS	overall survival
PAE	potential adverse event
PAS	patient-access scheme
PBAC	Pharmaceutical Benefits Advisory Committee
PBM	preference-based measures
PBS	Pharmaceutical Benefits Scheme
pCODR	pan-Canadian Oncology Drug Review
pCR	pathological complete response
PCS	prostate cancer subscale
PD	progressive disease
PFS	progression-free survival
PFS1	progression-free survival 1
PH	proportional hazards
PIM	promising innovative medicine

PP	post-progression
PP	per protocol
PRCT	pragmatic RCT
PPRS	Pharmaceutical Price Regulation Scheme
PPS	post-progression survival
PR	partial response
PS	propensity score
PSA	probabilistic sensitivity analysis
PSM	propensity score model
PSSRU	Personal Social Services Research Unit
QALY	quality-adjusted life-year
QLQ	Quality of Life Questionnaire
QoL	quality of life
QTWiST	Quality of Time Spent Without Symptoms of Disease and Toxicity
RBRVS	resource-based relative value system
RCC	renal cell cancer
RCT	random clinical trial
REC	research ethics committees
RECIST	Response Evaluation Criteria in Solid Tumors
RFA	radiofrequency ablation
RP	Royston-Parmar
RPSFTM	rank-preserving structural failure time model
RT	radiotherapy (see chemo-RT)
RWD	real-world data
RWE	real-world evidence
SACT	systemic anti-cancer therapy
SAPs	statistical analysis plan
SBRT	stereotactic body radiation therapy
SD	stable disease
STDev	standard deviation
SDiff	standardized difference
SE	standard error
SG	standard gamble
SMC	Scottish Medicines Consortium
SNM	structural nested model
SNNM	structural nested mean model
SNS	Sistema Nacional de Salud
SR	surgical resection
STA	single technology appraisal
TA	technology appraisal
TACE	transarterial chemoembolization
TEAE	treatment emergent adverse events
THIN	The Health Improvement Network
TKI	tyrosine kinase inhibitor

TOI	Trial Outcome Index
TPS	tumor proportion score
TSD	technical support document
TTBT	time to next treatment
TTF	time-to-treatment failure
TTO	time trade-off
TTP	time to progression
UCLH	University College London Hospitals Foundation Trust
VAS	visual analog scale
VBP	value-based pricing
VOI	value of information
VSI	value of sample information
WHO	World Health Organization
WTP	willingness to pay
YLL	years of life lost
ZIN	Zorginstituut Nederland

1

Introduction to Cancer

1.1 Cancer

The term 'carcinoma' is derived from the Greek word 'karkinos,' meaning crab. Hippocrates associated cancer with the shape of a crab, because of the way it spreads through the body and its persistent nature (Long, 1999).

Cancer is prevalent worldwide and impacts not only millions of people but also their families, carers, health systems, and even employers. Cancer impacts people's physical, cognitive, and functional ability as well as their health-related quality of life (HRQoL) and economic well-being. The National Cancer Institute's *Dictionary of Cancer Terms* (NCI, 2015) defines cancer as:

> A term for diseases in which abnormal cells divide without control and can invade nearby tissues. Cancer cells can also spread to other parts of the body through the blood and lymph systems. There are several main types of cancer. Carcinoma is cancer that begins in the skin or in tissues that line or cover internal organs. Sarcoma is cancer that begins in bone, cartilage, fat, muscle, blood vessels, or other connective or supportive tissue. Leukaemia is cancer that starts in blood-forming tissue, such as the bone marrow and causes large numbers of abnormal blood cells to be produced and enter the blood. Lymphoma and multiple myelomas are cancers that begin in the cells of the immune system. Central nervous system cancers are cancers that begin in the tissues of the brain and spinal cord.

1.2 Epidemiology of Cancer

An estimated 14.1 million new cases of cancer occurred across the world in 2018. The four most common types of cancers are lung, female breast, colorectal, and prostate cancer (Bray et al., 2018). According to the Global Cancer Incidence, Mortality and Prevalence study (GLOBOCAN) (Bray et al., 2018), prostate cancer is the most commonly diagnosed cancer among males from

87 countries, especially in North and South America and northern, western, and southern Europe. Lung cancer is the most commonly diagnosed cancer among males in eastern Europe. Among females, breast cancer is the most common cancer in North America, Europe, and Oceania. Breast and cervical cancers are the most frequently diagnosed cancers in Latin America and the Caribbean, Africa, and most of Asia. However, the most common female cancers in Asia also include lung, liver, and thyroid.

Due to more screening, earlier detection, and improved treatment, cancer mortality rates are either plateauing or decreasing, particularly in the high-income regions.

Table 1.1 summarizes the types of cancers and some key symptoms and features, along with the common clinical and economic outcomes collected in clinical cancer research.

These endpoints will be discussed in more detail in Chapter 2. For indolent malignancies with long survival, other endpoints such as cytogenetic response and minimal residual disease are used to assess the effectiveness of new drugs, particularly in earlier lines of treatment. Surrogate endpoints are also discussed in more detail in Chapter 2. For a single cancer type, there are likely to be further subtypes (e.g. adenocarcinoma) for which some treatments might work better for patients belonging to this subpopulation.

1.2.1 Cancer Trends

Mortality rates in several developing and low-income regions are increasing for some of these cancers due to increases in smoking, excess body weight, and physical inactivity. In 2011, there were nearly 8 million cancer-related deaths. All cancers, taken together, are now a leading cause of disease-related death worldwide, responsible for about 14% of the total of 55 million deaths from all causes in 2011. Cancer incidence in the UK is reported to have increased between 1993 and 2015 especially for females (Figure 1.1).

On the other hand, cancer incidence appears to be decreasing globally for many cancers in the United States, Europe, and other high-income countries. In low- to middle-income countries, the trend for cancers is unclear. Liver cancer, however, is reported to be increasing globally. Table 1.2 provides a summary of mortality trends for different cancer types between the years 2000 and 2019 (Hashim, 2016).

Example 1.1: Lung Cancer

Lung cancer is one of the leading causes of cancer-related deaths in the world and accounts for nearly 1.4 million deaths per year worldwide, with a yearly incidence of over 41,000 in the UK alone (Cancer Research UK [CRUK] Statistics, 2012). More than 8 out of 10 lung cancer cases occur in people aged 60 and over. Rates of lung cancer in Scotland are among the highest in the world, owing to the high prevalence of smoking.

TABLE 1.1

Examples of Some Common Cancers Regarding Clinical and Economic Outcomes

Cancer	Tumor Type	Common Symptoms	Key Features	Clinical Outcomes	Key Economic Outcomes
Lung cancer	Solid	Cough, blood in sputum, pain, weight loss	Short survival, diagnosed late	PFS, OS[a]	– Cost of treatment – Radiotherapy – Biomarker testing – Palliative Care – Quality of Life – Nursing visits – GP visits – Hospital visits – Physiotherapy aids/equipment – family support – childcare costs
Melanoma	Solid	Changing mole, mass, symptoms due to distant disease spread	Aggressive	PFS, OS	
Diffuse large B cell lymphoma	Solid	Enlarged lymph nodes, pain, weight loss, fever, night sweats, local symptoms due to enlarged mass e.g. intestinal obstruction	Aggressive lymphoma, short survival without treatment	PFS, OS	
Chronic myeloid leukemia	Blood	Incidental diagnosis on routine blood tests, fatigue, bone pain, weight loss, sweats	Indolent	Cytogenetic response	
Glioblastoma	Solid	Headache, vomiting, neurologic symptoms	Aggressive, short survival	PFS, OS	
Colorectal carcinoma	Solid	Blood in stools, pain, mass in abdomen, unexplained changes in bowel habits	Aggressive, short survival time	PFS, OS	
Hepatocellular carcinoma	Solid	Nonspecific symptoms due to underlying liver disease, mass in abdomen	Aggressive, short survival time		
Gastric cancer	Solid	Mass in abdomen, pain, weight loss, vomiting, blood in vomit, symptoms due to obstruction	Aggressive, short survival time	PFS, OS	

[a] *Note*: OS: overall survival; PFS: progression-free survival.

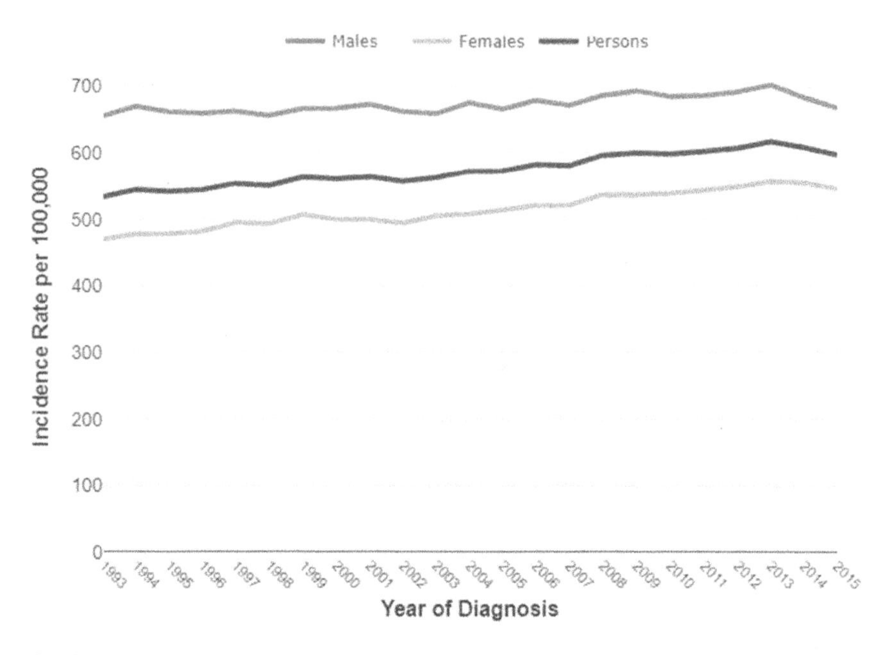

FIGURE 1.1
All cancers excluding non-melanoma skin cancer, European age-standardized incidence rates, UK, 1993–2015.

Source: CRUK Cancer Statistics.

TABLE 1.2

Summary of Countries by Cancer Type Showing Where Deaths from Each Type of Cancer are Increasing/Decreasing

Cancer	Increasing[a]	Decreasing
All	Brazil, Cuba, Latvia, Moldova, Serbia, and Malaysia	Decreasing for other countries
Stomach cancer	Not increasing in any country	Decreasing for all countries
Colorectal cancer	Latin America, Asia, South Africa, Romania, Malaysia, Kuwait, and Latvia	Decreasing for other countries
Liver cancer	North America, Asia, and Latin America	Decreasing for other countries
Lung cancer	Women: most countries: North America, Spain, Belgium, and Denmark Men: Venezuela, Moldova, Malaysia, Serbia, Bulgaria, Portugal, and Romania	Decreasing for: Ireland, Asian countries, Lithuania, and some Latin American countries
Breast cancer	Japan/Korea, Malaysia, Philippines, South Africa, and Latin America	Decreasing for other countries
Uterine cancer	Puerto Rico, Malaysia, and Philippines	Decreasing for other countries
Prostate cancer	Malaysia, Latvia, Serbia, Moldova, Ukraine, Belarus, USSR, and Korea	Decreasing for other countries

[a] *Note:* See Hashim et al. (2016) for list of country studies.

Lung cancer incidence in a given country is directly linked with the level of tobacco smoking in that country. Lung cancer-related deaths occur approximately two to three decades after the widespread uptake of smoking in any given country, with mortality trends approximating the incidence trends. Among males, lung cancer mortality rates have peaked and are now decreasing in many developed countries, reflecting the uptake and subsequent decline in male smoking prevalence. Lung cancer incidence in women lagged behind that in males because women began smoking later.

In countries with the earliest uptake of smoking among women (e.g. US, UK, and Australia), lung cancer mortality rates have peaked, whereas they continue to climb in countries where women began smoking later. Lung cancer is often diagnosed later in life, frequently with aggressive disease progression leading to high mortality rates for this cancer. In the 1950s, for every 1 lung cancer case diagnosed in women in the UK, there were 6 in men. That ratio is now 3 cases in women for every 4 in men. The lowest lung cancer rates in the world for men and women are in Northern, Western, and Middle African countries and South-Central Asia; but this will also change if the current trends in the uptake of smoking persist (Jemal et al., 2011; Toms, 2004; CRUK Statistics, 2012).

1.3 Prognostic Factors Associated with Cancer Outcomes

Prognostic factors are known or unknown factors that may be related to either an increased or decreased chance (risk) of a (cancer-related) outcome such as death (overall survival), disease progression, or any other outcome of interest, including surrogate outcomes (Chapter 2). The relationship between prognostic factors and cancer outcomes can influence the value of cancer treatments. For example, if the survival benefit for patients with a poor prognosis, defined by, say, an Eastern Cooperative Oncology Group (ECOG) performance status of 3 or 4, is lower (in general, higher values of ECOG suggest the patient has a worse prognosis) compared to patients with better prognoses (e.g. ECOG of 0 to 1), then ECOG would be considered an important prognostic factor. The survival benefit may be greater in lower ECOG patients (because patients might be relatively healthier or fitter for, say, surgery or chemotherapy). Consequently, the treatment might be more cost-effective for patients who are ECOG (0–1) compared to ECOG (2–3). Therefore, prognostic factors play an important role in trial design considerations from *both* a clinical and a health economic perspective.

One example of this is the use of a biomarker, a chemical test conducted to determine the genetic disposition of a patient. The result of the test could be related to a higher or lower clinical benefit. For example, the epidermal growth factor receptor (EGFR) is one type of marker that a patient might have. Patients with a known biomarker status (e.g. EGFR +ve for the drug

Erlotinib, used to treat lung cancer patients) are reported to have longer survival than those who are EGFR –ve. Despite the costs of the biomarker test and other health resource use, including the cost of the drug, the targeted treatment might still therefore offer greater value (be more cost-effective) for future patients who test EGFR +ve.

Risk factors may not act independently but may be additive or multiplicative in nature. That is, higher survival rates associated with ECOG status might also depend on the ages of patients. It may be that better ECOG status and age (younger patients might be relatively fitter) are associated with higher survival rates compared to the survival rates of those who are older and have poorer ECOG status. Hence treatment benefit may be dependent on a combination of factors. These are called interactions. Such interactions can play an important role in subgroup analyses from both a clinical and health economic perspective.

Several risk factors common to different cancer types have been reported. Some of these factors include age, genetic disposition (e.g. biomarker status), smoking, lifestyle (e.g. insufficient physical activity, alcohol, diet), obesity, and infections. These factors are associated with a high proportion of cancers worldwide but may also vary by region or country. Smoking, in particular, is the single most preventable cause of cancer death in the world; around a third of tobacco-caused deaths are due to cancer. Excessive alcohol consumption is reported to be associated with 13% of cancer-related deaths (Ferlay et al., 2010).

1.4 Economic Burden of Cancer

1.4.1 Health Expenditure

The constraint on healthcare resources, particularly during times of economic turmoil and instability, may result in governments taking a hard look at all public expenditure, including the medicine budget. Policymakers have a limited budget from which to decide how healthcare resources are provided for its citizens. What this means in practice is that the 'payers' (i.e. governments or health insurance providers who contribute toward the cost of healthcare provision for their citizens or customers) are likely to be more selective and choose with greater care from the healthcare options (i.e. new treatments) available to patients (due to budget constraints). Just like most individuals cannot have all the things they want, either because they do not have sufficient resources (e.g. money, time), healthcare systems also have similar constraints when trying to meet the demands of its consumers (patients).

Figure 1.2 shows the worldwide healthcare annual expenditure between 2000 and 2013 as a percentage of gross domestic product (GDP) as reported by the World Health Organization (WHO). It shows that health expenditure as a

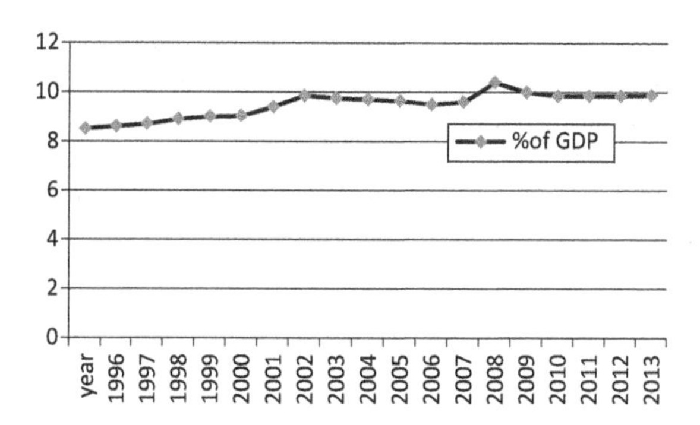

FIGURE 1.2
Health expenditure as a fraction of GDP between 1996 and 2014.

Source: https ://da ta.wo rldba nk.or g/ind icato r/SH. XPD.C HEX.G D.ZS.

percentage of GDP has generally increased over the past 20 years, although with some cyclical variation. Hence, the expenditure on health relative to available resources (GDP) is increasing at a significant rate. An examination of similar graphs per country shows an increasing expenditure trend for developed and mid-sized undeveloped countries (WHO Report, 2014).

1.4.2 Healthcare Expenditure on Drugs

The economic burden of treating cancer is high worldwide. Cancer has the most devastating economic impact in the world compared to other diseases. The exact worldwide economic costs of cancer are unknown but are estimated to be at least US $895 billion. With a growing and aging population, prevention efforts are critical for reducing new cancer cases, human suffering, and economic costs. Since 1995, the cost of cancer drugs has increased by an average of 10% annually (NCI, 2016). The largest economic burden for cancer patients is often related to the direct cost of cancer treatment, namely treatment drugs, and the costs to treat associated toxicities.

In 2014, the cost of every new cancer drug approved in the US exceeded $120,000 per year of treatment. An American Society of Clinical Oncology (ASCO) statement highlighted that in the decade from 2010 to 2020, between $125 billion and $158 billion will have been spent on cancer care (Lowell et al., 2015). Drug cost is a major (but not the only) cost component associated with treating cancer. Other costs include the costs of treating side effects, surgery, or radiotherapy, all of which can be significant. Given that one in three people will be diagnosed with cancer in their lifetime, the future cost of cancer treatment and care is likely to be a serious economic burden.

In the UK, the annual economic burden of cancer is estimated to be £15 billion. The National Health Service (NHS) increased its budget for cancer drugs from £200 million in 2013 to an expected £340 million in 2015 (NHS Statistics, 2015), a 70% increase in the so-called Cancer Drug Fund (CDF, NHS Statistics 2013, 2014). This represents the cost of cancer drugs alone.

The CDF was set up in 2011 by the UK government to make funds available for paying for cancer drugs. It was changed in 2016 as its form had become economically unsustainable. One critical change was an explicit reference to cost-effectiveness (CE) and resolving its uncertainty, which underlines the importance of the costs of treating cancer:

> Managed access agreements between NHS England and pharmaceutical companies, setting out the terms of a drug's entry into the CDF and the means by which data will be collected to resolve any uncertainty relating to a drug's clinical and *cost-effectiveness*. (NHS Statistics 2013, 2014)

One objective of government health departments is the desire to optimize the use of cancer drugs by a combination of negotiated price reductions (of drugs) and improved clinical effectiveness. Some cancer drugs were removed from the CDF list due to their lack of cost-effectiveness. The National Institute of Health and Care Excellence (NICE), the UK body that publishes guidelines on the value of new health technologies, has defined acceptable cost-effectiveness thresholds as high as £50,000 per quality-adjusted life-year (QALY). A QALY (see Section 1.6.1.8) is a composite measure of the length of life and the quality of life experienced during this period. Hence, a survival time of 1 year in perfect quality of life is 1 QALY, but if the quality of life was scored at 0.5 (using a 0 to 1 scale, 0 being death and 1 being full health), the QALY would be 0.5 (6 months). In 2016 the CDF underwent a review of which one key objective was to ensure cancer drugs (in fact all drugs) offer strong value for money (Cohen, 2017).

As an example, in the UK the total annual cost of treating lung cancer in 2012 was about £3 billion (20% of cancer costs) – the yearly average cost per patient was £9,071. This was comparable to £2,756 for bowel cancer, £1,584 for prostate cancer and £1,076 for breast cancer (ACS, 2016). Therefore, the costs associated with treating and managing lung cancer can be three times higher compared to the other types of cancer. In the US, the mean *monthly* cost of treating lung cancer patients was estimated at £1,669 (no active treatment) and £5,814 for chemoradiotherapy (exchange rate of £1 = $1.61).

Example 1.2 Costs and QALYs Reported in Some Published Cost-Utility Studies

Table 1.3 shows the key results from 47 published cost-effectiveness analyses in a lung cancer setting. About 20% did not report QALYs. Of the 80% that did report the cost per QALY (36 out of 47), only 13 out of 36 (36%) reported this to be below £30,000 (see Chapter 2 on ICERs).

TABLE 1.3
Published Costs and QALYs in Lung Cancer

Treatment	Cost (£)	QALY	Cost/QALY (£)	Year	Source (See Bibliography)
Paclitaxel	28,210	0.53	53,227	2011	Goulart et al.
	27,902	0.923	30,230	2010	Brown et al.
	21,967	NR	NR	2000	Berthelot et al.
	24,216	NR	NR	2000	Berthelot et al.
	26,228	NR	NR	2000	Berthelot et al.
	33,685	0.4513	74,639	2009	Klein, R.
Gemcitabine	27,837	0.934	29,804	2010	Brown et al.
	27,401	0.966	28,365	2010	Brown et al.
	18,129	NR	NR	2000	Berthelot et al.
	47,876	1.96	24,427	2013	Wang et al.
	38,859	0.4676	83,102	2009	Klein, R.
Vinorelbine	23,516	0.888	26,482	2010	Brown et al.
	16,678	NR	NR	2000	Berthelot et al.
	17,482	NR	NR	2000	Berthelot et al.
	6,901	NR	NR	2010	Maniadakis
Docetaxel	4,129	0.1606	25,712	2012	Thongprasert et al.
	13,956	0.206	67,748	2010	Lewis et al.
	27,409	0.42	65,260	2010	Asukai et al.
	24,798	0.225	110,215	2008	Araujo et al.
	24,904	0.42	59,296	2008	Carlson
	11,622	0.42	27,672	2011	Vergnenge et al.
	20,903	NR	NR	2011	Cromwell et al.
Pemetrexed	5,791	0.1715	33,767	2012	Thongprasert et al.
	29,387	0.52	56,514	2010	Asukai et al.
	27,764	0.241	115,205	2008	Araujo et al.
	37,119	0.41	90,533	2008	Carlson
	14,239	0.41	34,729	2011	Vergnenge et al.
	17,455	0.97	17,995	2010	Greenhalgh et al.
	41,731	0.5016	83,195	2009	Klein, R.
	8,905	0.41	21,720	2012	Fragoulakis
Gefitinib	3,973	0.1745	22,766	2012	Thongprasert et al.
	NR	1.111	NR	2010	Brown et al.
	19,787	0.79	250,47	2013	Zhu
	7,704	0.79	9,752	2013	Zhu
	28,471	0.91	31,287	2012	Gilberto de Lima Lopez
	8,980	0.2881	31,170	2010	Ontario Health
	10,536	0.3188	33,048	2010	Ontario Health
Erlotinib	13,730	0.238	57,689	2010	Lewis et al.
	22,439	0.25	89,756	2008	Araujo et al.

(Continued)

TABLE 1.3 (CONTINUED)

Published Costs and QALYs in Lung Cancer

Treatment	Cost (£)	QALY	Cost/QALY (£)	Year	Source (See Bibliography)
	23,567	0.42	56,112	2008	Carlson
	5,286	0.1745	30,292	2012	Thongprasert et al.
	25,546	1.4	18,247	2013	Wang et al.
	23,503	0.51	46,085	2012	Chouaid et al.
	12,909	0.33	39,119	2013	Chouaid
	8,104	0.42	19,296	2012	Fragoulakis
	22,744	NR	NR	2011	Cromwell
	7,488	NR	NR	2010	Bradbury et al.

In the UK, the cost-effectiveness threshold is set to between £20,000 and £30,000. The data in Table 1.3 shows the difficulties and challenges involved in finding cost-effective lung cancer drugs. The variation in costs and QALYs in Table 1.3 may be due to any number of factors, including variations in populations, geography, clinical trial design (e.g. patient follow-up), how costs were collected, and so forth. We will discuss these aspects in later chapters.

1.5 Treatments for Cancer

Common approaches for treating cancer (solid tumors) include (i) surgery, followed by (ii) chemotherapy, and (iii) radiotherapy (though not necessarily in that order). Despite treatment with chemotherapy, cancer recurrence is not uncommon. Recent novel chemotherapy (e.g. immunotherapy) treatments use the body's immune system to fight and kill cancer cells. Although some of these drugs have proved to be cost-effective, others have not (see later in Chapter 10 for examples). For blood cancers (e.g. leukemia), surgery is not an option and chemotherapy is often the first choice of treatment.

An example of treatment options for a patient diagnosed with non-small-cell lung cancer (NSCLC) in the UK is shown in Figure 1.3. Often, a particular treatment may be used for several different tumor types, often resulting in similar side effects across tumors, with a marked impact on HRQoL.

HRQoL and patient-reported outcomes are a central part of economic evaluation. (HRQoL will be discussed more fully in Chapter 3.)

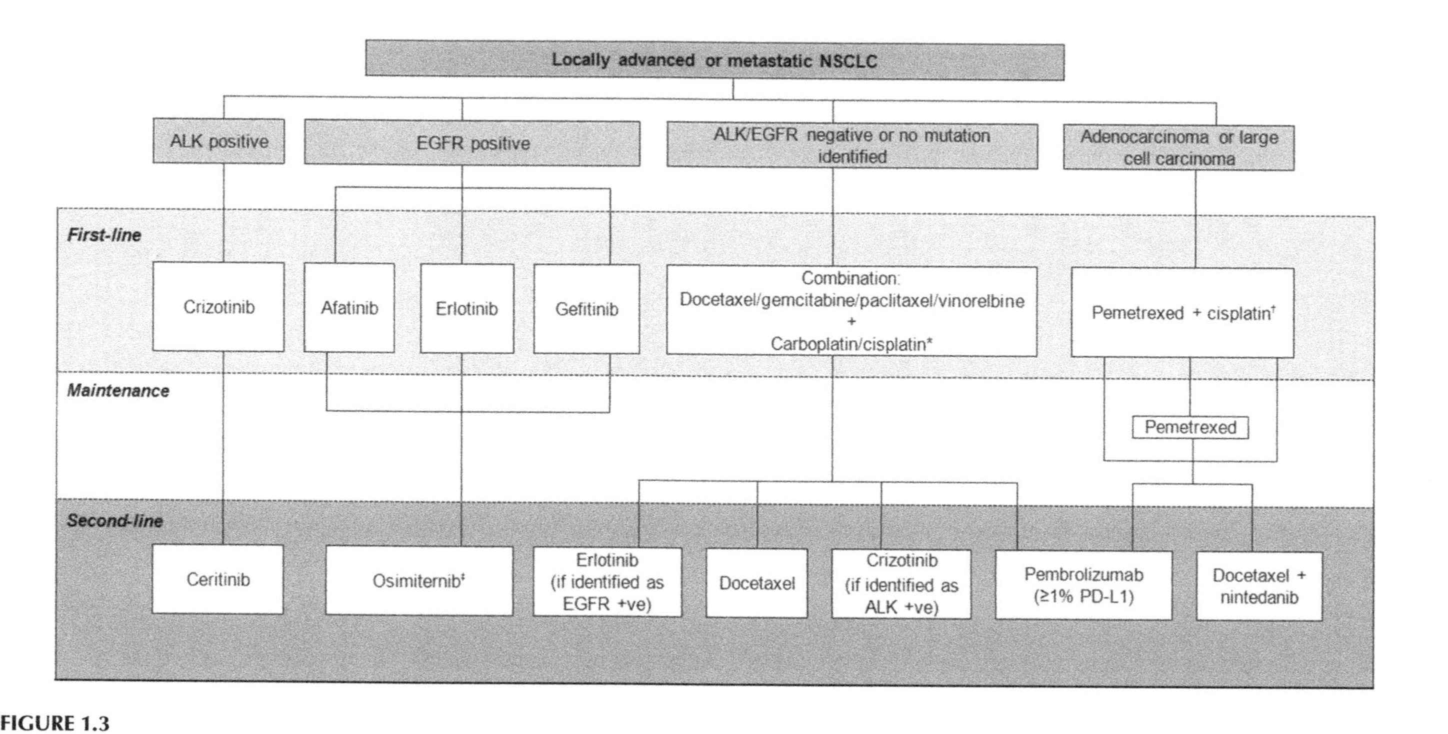

FIGURE 1.3
Example of common treatment options for NSCLC: advanced or metastatic NSCLC treatment pathway based on NICE guidance CG121.

1.6 Important Economic Concepts for Cost-Effectiveness of Cancer Interventions

Economic evaluation is the process of systematic identification, measurement, and evaluation of the inputs and outcomes of two (or more) alternative activities (health interventions) and their subsequent comparative analysis (Drummond, 2002, 2015). Economic evaluation in the context of cancer involves assessing the value of various cancer treatments, often through a metric that combines the quantity (length) of life and the quality of life experienced during that time, called a QALY. This is particularly valuable when some expensive cancer drugs demonstrate modest or small improvements in survival (e.g. 1 or 2 weeks). In later chapters of this book, we will discuss the importance of HRQoL for economic evaluation in a cancer context.

Concerns have been raised as to whether healthcare should be considered an economic good (Morris et al., 2012; Santerre & Neun, 2000). Some think these concerns are unfounded because, ultimately, healthcare resource is finite and scarce. There is a limited supply of doctors, nurses, and healthcare staff, so it is unlikely that any healthcare system in the world can achieve a level of spending on the health of its citizens that would meet all their healthcare needs. In some cases, access to cancer treatments might be more readily available in one region of a country and not in another, creating regional equity issues (Chamberlain et al., 2015). It is reported, using real-world data from registries, that women and those living in economically deprived areas have less access to cancer treatment compared to other groups (Chamberlain et al., 2015). Some have controversially argued that we can achieve healthcare for most individuals by *not* treating criminals, smokers, and alcoholics, whereas others have argued that healthcare is a basic human right and that it is not appropriate to treat it like an 'economic good,' as if it were any consumer good or service (Morris et al., 2015). We will leave these questions to the economic philosophers and policymakers because they involve complicated judgments, which need not concern us here.

1.6.1 Economics, Health Economics, Economic Evaluation, and Pharmacoeconomics

Economics is the science of scarcity and choice. Health economics is related to the supply and demand for healthcare. Although health itself is not an economic good, healthcare resource *is* an economic good. Healthcare resource refers to items such as hospital beds, treatments, drugs, surgeries, GP time, and so on. These resources usually have costs associated with them. For example, a visit to the doctor might be valued at £100 for one hour. Government institutions might make decisions at the national level on how the total healthcare demand and supply can be met for a given budget constraint.

However, what is usually of concern in the pharmaceuticals context for comparing new treatments is pharmacoeconomics. Pharmacoeconomics uses certain principles of health economics for making policy decisions on the supply and demand for medicines – particularly in clinical trials. The methods (analysis techniques) used in pharmacoeconomics involve the description and analysis of the costs of drug therapy to healthcare systems and society. It identifies, measures, and compares the costs and consequences of pharmaceutical products and services (Rascati, 2009). The process of using these methods is called 'economic evaluation.' Economic evaluation applies mathematical and statistical methods to compare the costs and consequences of alternative healthcare options (Drummond 2002, 2005).

The term pharmacoeconomics might be considered as nothing more than a generic term for economic evaluation of medical interventions (specifically drugs). Rather than the cumbersome 'economic evaluation of drugs,' pharmacoeconomics is a simpler term. However, pharmacoeconomics might also address questions on affordability (and not just efficiency) of a new drug, using budget impact models (BIMs). A BIM measures the net cumulative cost of a particular treatment for a given number of patients in a specific population. This is accomplished by implementing comparative cost-determination analyses for competing scenarios, both including and excluding the product of interest (Sullivan et al., 2014).

For over a decade, economic evaluation has become an increasingly important component of clinical trials. The number of Phase III clinical trials with a health economic component has also increased substantially. In particular, submissions to reimbursement authorities – e.g. government-led subgroups that assess the evidence for the 'value' a new treatment offers, such as the Scottish Medicines Consortium (SMC) and the National Institute for Clinical Health Excellence (NICE) in the UK, have also increased by more than 45% over the same period.

In this book, we consider economic evaluation in the context of pharmacoeconomics, i.e. evaluating the costs and benefits of treatments from clinical trials where data are collected prospectively in the trial. However, we also extend this to determining costs and effects outside a controlled clinical or experimental setting (in the real world). Economic evaluation uses various techniques to assess the value of pharmaceutical interventions and health strategies. In short, the terms 'pharmacoeconomics,' 'cost-effectiveness,' and 'economic evaluation' may be used interchangeably when describing approaches to estimate the economic value of new cancer interventions.

1.6.1.1 Value

When it comes to healthcare, the average person has no idea about the price for surgery or a treatment plan, especially when healthcare is considered to be 'free of charge,' such as with the NHS in the UK. We might all be aware of the price of diamonds or footballs, and most of us can value them (in relative terms), or at least we are likely to put the price of diamonds higher than that of footballs. Consequently, people may pay a premium price for diamonds and similar goods. However, it is likely that, in a severe drought, someone could well exchange diamonds for a cup of water (due to its scarcity).

Health products (or services) are not items we can buy 'off the shelf.' Therefore, it is harder to value and subsequently put a price on them. This is true whether the health item is a new treatment or something as complex as surgery. Some economists have suggested that the problem of value could be determined by how much one was prepared to pay for a certain good, assuming certain market conditions were satisfied. Economic theory was then formulated to explain how value could be determined by the demand and supply for goods (for a useful introduction, see Morris, 2012; Santerre & Neun, 2000). Allocation of goods was determined simply by how much one was prepared to pay (i.e. price paid) for that item – leading to French economist Jules Dupuit (Ekelund, 1999) to surmise in his 1844 paper that 'the value of a good is the amount someone is prepared to pay for it' – or how much one is willing to pay (WTP) for it.

In the context of health, the buyer is not necessarily the same as the consumer. The buyer of the health product is likely to be a government institution or an entity responsible for healthcare provision. The consumer is the patient. In other words, allocation of healthcare goods is based on the price that governments (taxpayers) are prepared to pay. This is not necessarily true in all countries however, and it will depend on the structure of the healthcare system of each country.

Valuing health, or for that fact, any product, by how much people are prepared to pay does not take into account the impact on the wider society – or the welfare of everyone. For example, richer people are less likely to suffer from prices going up than the poor. This was not considered equitable, therefore, to address this, a further development in economics: (extra) welfare economics took place, which need not concern us here (see bibliography for more details). What is important for our purposes is to appreciate that the economic evaluation techniques encountered in this book are tools for decision-making to determine which treatments or health technologies offer the greater relative value in terms of a price (or cost) people (i.e. society) are prepared to pay, termed the cost-effectiveness threshold.

1.6.1.2 Allocative Efficiency

Allocative efficiency is where health resources are deployed across an economy in the most efficient manner to match patient needs and preferences. Allocative efficiency is where decision-makers use the evidence (results) from economic evaluation to determine the best set of allocations of treatments that gives an optimum for a given medicines budget. For example, if only £100,000 were available for providing two cancer treatment options, drug A and drug B, the question might be how best to spend the £100,000 on these two treatments. If the price of drug A is £2,000 per year and B is £5,000 per year, one could treat 50 patients with treatment A or 20 patients with treatment B. The other option is to have some patients take treatment A (so long as it works) and some take treatment B. The exact mixture of treatments A and B that will make up the £100,000 is for the decision-maker to determine. The comparative value that A and B offer will influence this decision.

Following the above example further, with £100 million to spend, treatment A could be effective in patients with a particular genetic disposition (biomarker). An optimal allocation might be to treat some patients who have the presence of the biomarker (e.g. EGFR +ve) with the new treatment and treat those that are EGFR-ve with the current treatment.

One technique for such comparative economic evaluation is called cost–utility analysis (CUA), which seeks to address the question of (optimal) allocative efficiency within the health sector. In the assessment of the cost-effectiveness of cancer drugs, CUA is the one that is most pertinent. By using such methods, it is hoped patients will have access to 'value for money' treatments through an efficient allocation of various medicines subject to a 'budget constraint.'

1.6.1.3 Technical Efficiency

Technical efficiency is when the minimum amount of resource (e.g. lowest dose, or shortest duration of dosing) is used to elicit a given level of response, i.e. when one produces a certain level of output with the least amount of input – for example, the lowest dose that achieves a 20% reduction in lipid levels. Economic efficiency occurs when the production cost of a given output is as low as possible: for example, the least costly way of resolving a peptic ulcer. Cost-effectiveness analysis (CEA) is one such tool used to address the issue of economic efficiency.

In health economics, we distinguish between efficacy, e.g. whether a drug or intervention actually works in a technical sense, which is mainly assessed through randomized clinical trials (RCT) when feasible. Effectiveness is whether the same intervention actually works in everyday operating conditions, e.g. after market authorization or a license is given. Generally, (clinical) effectiveness will be lower than, or at best equal to trial effectiveness due to the inherent limitations of clinical trials.

Reimbursement

In the context of pharmaceuticals, once a drug has been approved for licensing by the relevant regulatory body, such as the Food and Drug Administration (FDA), European Medicines Agency (EMA), or some other national agency, the pharmaceutical company will seek a price for its newly licensed drug. Reimbursement, in simple terms, means the price the pharmaceutical company would like to obtain from the decision-maker (payer) for the new drug it has produced. For example, the pharmaceutical company might want £120 per tablet, but the payer might want to pay only £95 per tablet, based on the assessment of evidence of 'value' presented by the company. The price could be on a per tablet basis or for a supply of 28 days – such as £50 per tablet, or for 28 days £1,400. The price of, say, £50 is what the payer has agreed to pay for each tablet. The price set is usually agreed between the payer (e.g. the Department of Health in the UK) and the pharmaceutical company. For example, the price per tablet of lenolidamide (in 2011) was agreed at £249.60 for a single 25 mg tablet. This price is recorded in publications such as the British National Formulary (BNF, 2017).

In some countries, a dual-price system exists, whereby a market price is set at a certain level and then, at a second stage, a reimbursement price is set at a fraction of the market price. The difference between the two is the price charged to patients; it constitutes the so-called patient's 'out-of-pocket expense.' The market price is typically calculated to cover the research and development costs of the pharmaceutical company as a minimum, and to make a profit to sustain future R&D activities. From the payer perspective, the lower the price, the better. However, the price should not be set so low that innovation is discouraged. A premium price is usually a price higher than the current market price for similar existing products (for example when there is a similar reference price set for all drugs within a therapeutic group). A premium price may be awarded if the drug demonstrates improved 'value for money' through economic evaluation techniques.

It is for this reason that, when a health economic evaluation is undertaken, the payer perspective is considered carefully. That is, who is the economic evaluation for? Is it from the perspective of a health insurance company (in the US and some other countries, there is no equivalent of the NHS) or for the local or national government (as in Spain where local provinces can influence decisions)? In short, who will be reimbursed?

In the UK, the Pharmaceutical Price Regulation Scheme (PPRS) is a voluntary agreement between the payer (the government) and industry with the objective that (effective) medicines are available on reasonable terms to the NHS, and this in turn maintains a strong, efficient, and profitable pharmaceutical industry. The workings of these groups are complex, but details can be found in the official publications, such as those of the UK Department of Health and Healthcare. Similar schemes exist for other countries. In France, for example, the Health Products Pricing Committee (Comité Economique des Produits de Santé) and drug manufacturer sign a number of agreements allowing a variety of flexible means to monitor prices and drug use while ensuring that public resources are properly allocated.

1.6.1.4 Opportunity Cost

A very important concept in health economics, and economics in general, is the notion of opportunity cost. Opportunity costs are defined as "the value of the next best alternative" (Polley, 2015; Folland et al., 1997). This applies especially for health resources without market prices, such as informal care. A shadow price is then derived from alternative marketed resources (for example the cost of hiring a home-visiting nurse) to approximate the social value of the non-marketed resource. However, market prices are only considered as adequate under ideal market conditions in perfect competition. This may not apply to many resources in the healthcare sector. (For a recent discussion on the application of opportunity costs to hospital bed days see Sandmann et al., 2017.)

For some activities, like childcare, alternative market prices exist that yield an upper price limit for these services; for others (e.g. the market price for studying) one could use an opportunity cost approach by valuing the activity performed by the cost of forgone leisure time (this implicitly assumes that everyone prefers leisure to work, or 'work as punishment'). In this case, a 'proxy price' needs to be established using contingent valuation methods, such as willingness-to-pay or willingness-to-accept elicitation for non-market, or some other stated preference method (Ryan, 2008; McIntosh et al., 2010). Opportunity costs also arise in fixed-budget constraints.

Economic evaluation is often set against the background of an opportunity cost when comparing treatments. In the context of medicines, for example, assuming a fixed budget of £100 million, the payer may have the difficult decision of allocating all £100 million to pay for drug A for 10,000 patients, which might improve survival by 1 year (cost of £10,000 per year per patient). The opportunity cost might be spending the £100 million on treatment B for 20,000 patients, which might improve survival on average by 6 months (£5,000 per year per patient). In practice, a combination of treatments A and B may give an optimal allocation of available funds.

1.6.1.5 Discounting

Most people prefer to receive benefits sooner and pay costs later, rather than sooner. For example, people prefer to enjoy smoking now and give less importance to their future health. As someone becomes older, his or her time preference may change.

In health economic evaluation, future costs and benefits are discounted so that their value can be judged in present terms. This is achieved by applying an annaul constant discount rate, e.g. 3.5% in the UK (based on the Treasury Department's so-called 'Green Book'). The consequence of the discount rate is that less weight is given to later costs than to the present costs. We use the discounted values of future costs and benefits in cost-effectiveness calculations.

Some cancer trials run for a long time and costs of any health resource used at the beginning of a 7-year trial starting in 2015 may be different to costs at the end of the trial, finishing in 2022. If the trial stops following up patients after 4 years, costs might be determined at 2019 prices. However, for the remaining 3 years (2020, 2021, and 2022), in each year, the future costs would be discounted.

For example, the future costs of treatment for a single patient who experiences disease progression in 2015 (and withdraws from the trial) in each of years 2020, 2021, and 2022 are expected to be: £3,000, £5,000, and £7,000 (total £15,000 over 3 years) – because the patient may have other subsequent treatment or care. After discounting at 3% per year, the future costs are valued as:

Year 2020 $£3{,}000 \times 1/(1+0.03)^1 = £2{,}912.62$ 1 year after withdrawal
Year 2021 $£5{,}000 \times 1/(1+0.03)^2 = £4{,}712.98$ 2 years after withdrawal
Year 2022 $£7{,}000 \times 1/(1+0.03)^3 = £6{,}405.99$ 3 years after withdrawal

The total future costs of £15,000 for this patient after discounting are £14,031.59. In this example, only costs are discounted. In practice, health benefits are also discounted. The debate about whether or not we should discount costs only and not benefits or discount them at different rates, is discussed elsewhere (e.g. see Drummond, 2002) and not considered further. The current practice, however, is to discount both future health benefits and costs. Note that if a trial is 7 years long (1-year recruitment plus a further 6 years follow-up) then discounting is important. However, if in a 7-year trial where recruitment is over 6 years with a 1-year follow-up (e.g. a very rare tumor), then a key concern is the application of a consistent price year. Discounting is applied on expected future costs and effects beyond the first year of follow-up.

1.6.1.6 The Incremental Cost-Effectiveness Ratio

The incremental cost-effectiveness ratio (ICER) is the basis of most economic evaluations. It is a numerical quantity that expresses the relative (mean) differences in costs between two or more treatments compared to the relative effects. It is often written as a simple equation:

$$\text{ICER} = \frac{\text{Mean Costs A} - \text{Mean Costs B}}{\text{Mean Effect A} - \text{Mean Effect B}} \tag{1.1}$$

The numerator is called the mean incremental cost. The denominator is called the mean incremental effect. The higher the value of the ICER, the less cost-effective a treatment is (A vs. B). As can be seen from the denominator, when two treatments are similar regarding their effectiveness, the ICER is likely to be large. Hence cancer treatments that are cost-effective are expected to show mean differences in effectiveness to be somewhat larger than zero. The ICER is judged against a willingness-to-pay (WTP) threshold, a term introduced earlier. The WTP is a value that is also referred to as the cost-effectiveness threshold expressed by the term λ, or the shadow price. The value of λ represents the cost in terms of health forgone elsewhere when resources are reallocated within the healthcare system. In the UK, λ is set at £20,000 to £30,000. If the ICER is $<\lambda$, then it is considered evidence the new treatment is cost-effective. More recently, lower values of λ (e.g. £15,000) have been used for promising treatments (Claxton et al., 2015).

As noted, when the denominator is very small, or zero, the ICER is very large or undefined. When the ICER is negative, its interpretation is ambiguous. A more useful approach might be to convert the formula in (1.1) into a difference expressed in money value whatever the size of the denominator (whether it is small or large). This could be used when drugs might be 'similar' (e.g. biosimilars):

$$\text{Expressing the ICER as} = \frac{\text{Mean Difference Costs}_{A-B}}{\text{Mean Difference Effects}_{A-B}} < \lambda \tag{1.2}$$

This can be rewritten as an incremental net monetary benefit (INMB):

$$\text{INMB} = \text{mean Difference Costs}_{A-B} - \lambda * \text{Mean Difference Effects}_{A-B} \tag{1.3}$$

If the INMB is >0, it means that the new treatment supports a hypothesis of cost-effectiveness. Rewriting the ICER this way gets around the problem of very small ICERs when treatments are similar, as is the case with a class of cancer drugs called biosimilars. Ideally, we would like a high chance or probability that the INMB is positive (>0). This means the net benefit from a new treatment (after taking into account differences in costs and how much one wishes to pay for a new treatment) should have a high chance (e.g. 80%), that it is >0.

1.6.1.7 The Cost-Effectiveness Plane

In economic evaluation, the main results are usually reported in one of two ways:

(i) The incremental cost-effectiveness ratio (ICER) and
(ii) The incremental net monetary benefit (INMB).

There is a relationship between the two that we identified above. In the previous section, the ICER was informally introduced as relative costs to benefits. We now formally present the ICER in the context of the cost-effectiveness plane, which is how the results of an economic evaluation are often reported and interpreted.

The ICER is defined as:

$$\frac{\text{Mean Costs (A)} - \text{Mean Costs (S)}}{\text{Mean Effect (A)} - \text{Mean Effect (S)}} \tag{1.4}$$

$$= \mu_A - \mu_S / \varepsilon_A - \varepsilon_S = \lambda\mu_{A-S} / \Delta\varepsilon_{A-S} = \Delta_c / \Delta_e$$

where $\Delta_c = \Delta\mu_{A-S}$ and $\Delta_e = \Delta\varepsilon_{A-S}$, the mean difference in costs and mean difference in effects between treatments A and S, respectively.

Parameter	Interpretation
μ_A	Mean costs of treatment A
μ_S	Mean costs of treatment S
ε_A	Mean effect of treatment A
ε_S	Mean effect of treatment S
$\Delta\mu_{A-S} = \Delta_c$	Mean difference in costs between A and S
$\Delta\varepsilon_{A-S} = \Delta_e$	Mean difference in effects between A and S

The numerator in (1.4) expressed as $\Delta\mu_{A-S}$, is called the *incremental cost* and the denominator, $\Delta\varepsilon_{A-S}$, is termed *incremental effectiveness*; A and S are two treatments (A is typically the new drug and S is the standard). It is this ratio quantity (Δ_c / Δ_e) and the uncertainty around it that lies at the heart of economic evaluation in clinical trials. This ratio is displayed on the cost-effectiveness plane shown in Figure 1.4.

In Figure 1.4, the X-axis represents incremental effectiveness, or the mean difference in effects between the treatments A versus S (Δ_e). For example, positive values of $\Delta_e(\Delta_e > 0)$ exist where the new drug is more effective. Effective does not necessarily mean efficacy in equation (1.4). It could be a measure of efficacy (e.g. survival time) combined with quality of life to get a QALY (or life-years gained/saved – see Chapter 3). Negative values ($\Delta_e < 0$) indicate the new treatment has worse effectiveness.

The Y-axis in Figure 1.4 is the mean difference in costs (Δ_c), measured in some unit of currency (£s in this case). For example, if the new drug (treatment A) costs £2,000 more than the standard (treatment S), the value of Δ_c is +£2,000. If Δ_c is < 0 then the negative value means that treatment A costs less than S, on average.

In quadrants 2 and 4 in, the decision as to which treatment is more or less cost-effective is relatively easy. If the value of the ICER from equation (1.4) lies in quadrant 2, the new treatment is cheaper and more effective. This is the ideal scenario where pharmaceutical companies would like to have their new drugs positioned. On the other hand, a very much less desirable scenario is where the new treatment is worse, but also costlier (quadrant 4). Values of the ICER can, however, be altered by changing parameters, such as the price of the new treatment. Reducing the price (or increasing efficacy, if possible) might be a strategy adopted so that the ICER can move into a different quadrant in order to show a more favorable ICER – possibly at a reduced profit. A new treatment that has an ICER falling into quadrant 4 is unlikely to be considered as having a high chance of demonstrating value. Even if the price was changed, the fact that the new treatment has poorer efficacy still needs to be addressed.

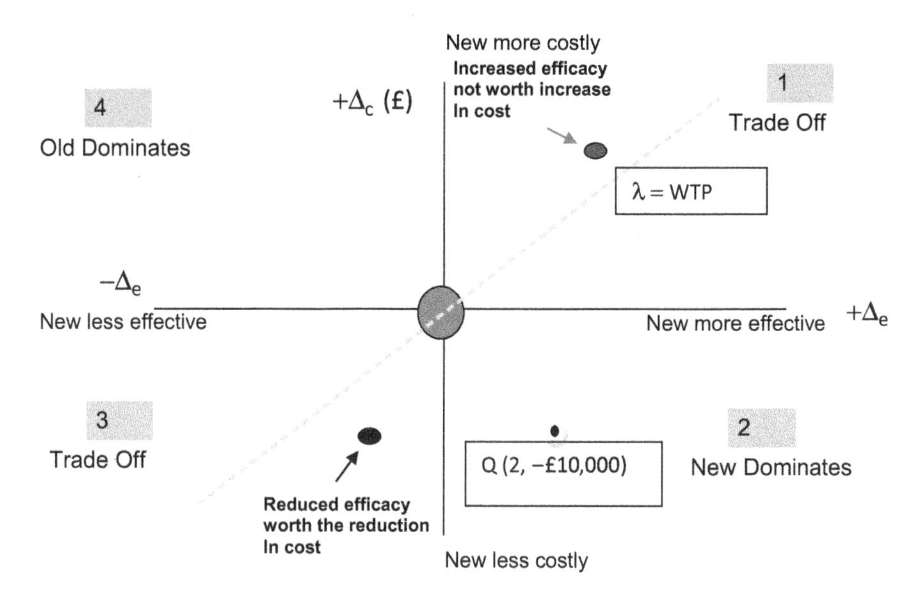

FIGURE 1.4
The cost-effectiveness plane.

Example 1.3

Referring to Figure 1.4, we note that in quadrant 2, the point Q (2, –£10,000) shows that a new drug is more effective (an improved effect of 2) and cheaper by £10,000, on average. Hence the ICER is –£10,000/2 = –£5,000 per unit of effect (e.g. the unit could be QALY). The new treatment is said to dominate the standard treatment. Most decision problems relating to the value of the ICER are concerned with quadrants 1 and 3, and in particular quadrant 1 where justification of value is often sought.

The line that passes through the origin in Figure 1.4, denoted λ, is called the willingness-to-pay or cost-effectiveness threshold. This is the threshold ratio or amount in £ (or other currency) that a payer would be prepared to pay for a new drug. Any ICER values calculated from data that are to the right of this line (e.g. in quadrant 1) show that the new treatment is cost-effective. In this example (Figure 1.4), the incremental effect value (Δ_e) is +2 and the incremental cost value (Δ_c) is –£10,000, resulting in an ICER = –£5,000, shown as the point Q(+2, £–10,000) in quadrant 2. Had the new treatment showed poorer efficacy compared to the standard (e.g. a value of –2.8), the ICER would be –£10,000/–2.8 = £3,571. The ICER is now positive and has shifted from quadrant 2 to quadrant 3 (Figure 1.4).

Example 1.4: Changing the Cost-Effectiveness Threshold

Figure 1.5 shows two slopes λ (dashed line) and λ^* (solid line) – the cost-effectiveness (CE) thresholds. The value of the CE threshold has changed from λ = £30,000 (dashed line) to λ^* = £12,000 (solid line). Initially, the new

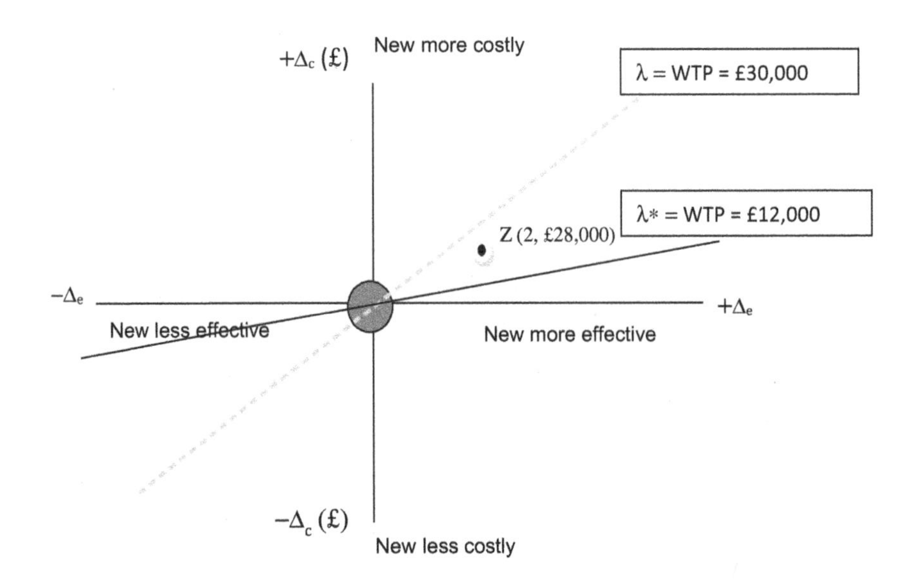

FIGURE 1.5
The cost-effectiveness plane: changing WTP/CE threshold.

treatment (not the same as in Example 1.1) showed a treatment benefit of 2 units, but it was more expensive (£28,000) – the point Z (2, £28,000) in Figure 1.5. The point Z initially lies below the line λ = £30,000, but as the value of λ = £30,000 changes to λ^* = £12,000, the point Z is above the new CE threshold. The observed slope, the ICER, is £28,000/2 = £14,000, which lies to the left and above the new CE threshold. At this new threshold, treatment A is no longer considered cost-effective (because the point Z is above the line).

In general, in quadrant 1, if $\Delta_c/\Delta_e < \lambda$, and so long as $\Delta_e > 0$, the new treatment is cost-effective; values of $\Delta_e > 0$ suggest a benefit with the new treatment. In quadrant 3, Δ_c/Δ_e is always ≥ 0 (for $\Delta_e \neq 0$), so the ratio is $<\lambda$, and the new treatment is considered cost-effective.

In the CE plane, the value of the CE ratio (the ICER) needs to be compared to various values of λ, and the number of points above or below the line is difficult to visualize for changing values of λ.

1.6.1.8 Quality-Adjusted Life-Years (QALY)

A QALY is used as a generic measure of the utility of a (new) intervention on the disease, which involves both the quality and the quantity (length of life) lived. This is a key measure for assessing the cost-effectiveness of healthcare interventions. One QALY is interpreted as equivalent to one year of 'full health.' If a patient's HRQoL over the course of a year is less than in 'full health,' the QALY will be less than 1. QALYs are often accumulated at a rate of less than (or equal to) 1 per year. The EQ-5D, a generic HRQoL instrument completed by patients (or carers), is often used to construct QALYs.

The EQ-5D is an important HRQoL measure and merits a separate discussion (see Chapter 3).

In the economic evaluation of cancer, the QALY is a composite measure of HRQoL and survival time. If the OS is the survival time of a patient measured from randomization (or the start of treatment) until death, or until the last date the patient was assessed, the QALY combines the survival experience with the HRQoL. The HRQoL is often measured on a scale of 0 to 1, where 0 represents a health state equivalent to death and 1 as 'full health.' In some cases, a health state worse than death is also possible and a value less than 0 is used. As a simplistic example, if the HRQoL for a patient who lives for 6 months is 0.60, on average, then the QALY is $0.60 \times 6 = 3.6$ months. This is like saying that 6 months of living in a less than full health state (i.e. an HRQoL of 0.60), is equivalent to living 3.6 months in 'full health' or $3.6/12 = 0.30$ years. In practice, the HRQoL is measured at multiple time points, and an area under the curve (AUC) (time HRQoL curve) is constructed to derive the QALY. This will be described further in later chapters.

1.7 Health Economic Evaluation and Cancer Drug Development in Practice

Figure 1.6 displays the traditional drug development process and the approaches to reimbursement and providing patient access. The square box with broken lines in Figure 1.6 shows how the role of economic evaluation has reshaped this process. In the past, less effort would be planned for demonstrating the value of a new treatment. The traditional route was to perform Phase I to Phase III trials, obtain a market authorization license and then agree with each country separately a price for the new treatment. Evidence of

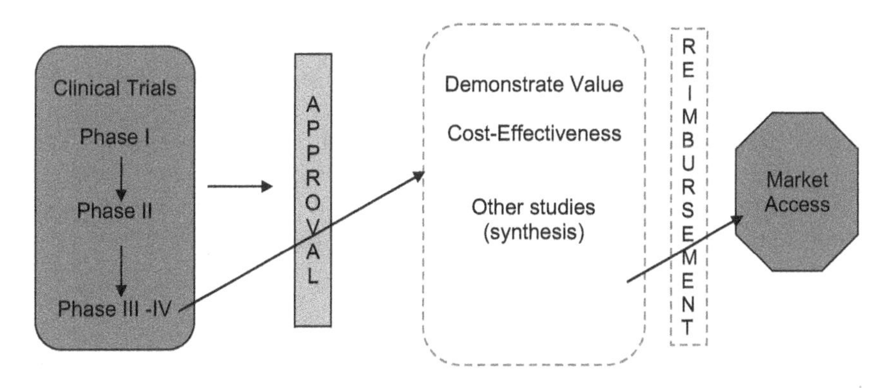

FIGURE 1.6
Drug development and reimbursement.

'value' would not have been formally requested. Only efficacy concerns were considered important at the time of pricing (not relative efficacy or costs). Therefore, one approach to providing patient access to new drugs would be to agree at the local (country) level, a price at which they would buy the new drug – often agreed relatively shortly after the drug was approved. The evidence for informing a pricing decision is often based primarily using the Phase III clinical trial data submitted for market authorization.

In Germany, for example, the concept of 'free pricing' allowed innovator companies to exert greater control over their prices and set them with considerable flexibility. However, the AMNOG law in 2011 (Neuordnung des Arzneimittelmarktes, see Bundesministerium für Gesundheit website) effectively restricted free pricing for a one-year period only, with the pharmaceutical company being required to assess value for money of the new treatment within the first year. German payers no longer found it acceptable to pay for expensive drugs that were seen to offer little value for money. In particular, oncology drugs are likely to feel the impact of the Institut für Qualität und Wirtschaftlichkeit im Gesundheitswesen (Institute for Quality and Efficiency, also known as IQWIG) decisions more sharply because some of these drugs are particularly expensive and have been reviewed judiciously from the perspective of demonstrating value. Previously, approaches to providing patient (market) access to treatments were not influenced by the concept of 'value for money.' There was a lesser need both to formalize the health economic argument and to package the data in a way that demonstrated the uncertainties of value for money.

In the US, drug manufacturers may be free to negotiate prices with payers and insurance companies; however, recently some organizations have raised concerns about 'financial toxicity' associated with cancer care in the US. In June 2015, the American Society of Clinical Oncology unveiled its 'conceptual framework' to assess the value of new cancer treatment options, noting that cancer care is one of the fastest-growing components of US healthcare costs and the growth in healthcare spending, and stating that costs have not been "accompanied by commensurate improvements in health outcomes" (Lowell et al., 2015). This framework assigns a 'net health benefit' to oncology therapies that take into account efficacy, toxicity, and cost. Indeed, in addition to ASCO, the National Comprehensive Cancer Network (NCCN), a not-for-profit alliance of 26 leading cancer centers, also recently decided to include cost as a parameter in its guidelines. In addition to these professional organizations, the Institute for Clinical and Economic Review (ICERev), a non-profit organization, started publishing their own 'value-based' prices for newly approved prescription drugs entering the market.

1.7.1 The Modern Paradigm

The modern drug development paradigm requires formal evidence of the cost–benefit/value relationship. A multidisciplinary team (MDT) is set up that considers as early as possible what is needed from the clinical trials data to form a 'value' argument. Although the analysis of data for economic evaluation occurs after the Phase III trial results are finalized, the design and planning for both efficacy and showing value must be considered well before then. The MDT bridges the working relationship between individuals from clinical research, biostatistics health economics, and other disciplines, to formalize the evidence from clinical trials to obtain access for patients by demonstrating value.

The implication of Figure 1.6 is that if the innovator drug cannot demonstrate value for money to the payer, the price desired may not be achieved. This does not mean that a drug is not efficacious, but the decision-making process should utilize all available information to minimize uncertainty.

Example 1.5: What Might Happen When Economic Evaluation is not Considered in the Study Design Planning Process

A drug to treat myelodysplastic syndrome (MDS) was developed by a manufacturer to reduce the need for blood transfusion in patients with a specific subtype of the disease. Despite this benefit, the manufacturer was unable to secure reimbursement for its drug. The reason for this was because NICE determined that the price requested by the manufacturer did not offer sufficient value compared with patients who receive a blood transfusion. Also, the health resource utilization related to blood transfusion, e.g. hospital admissions for transfusion, day unit or clinic chair times, long-term side effects of blood transfusion (e.g. iron overload and its side effects), etc., were not collected during the trial. This routinely collected information may have added useful information to the economic evaluation of the drug by showing not only a reduction in need for blood transfusion but also a reduction in the health resources utilization cost associated with blood transfusion.

In this example, the clinical research and manufacturing teams were focused on producing a clinically excellent drug that reduced the need for blood transfusion. However, the value argument was overlooked. Had the company considered the reimbursement argument earlier the story might have been different.

The relationship between the drug development program over time, market authorization (getting a license), access for patients (as measured by sales volume), and the importance of reimbursement is shown in Figure 1.7. After license approval, there is a period between approval and a decision for reimbursement. For most drugs, sales are usually somewhat flat during the period between market authorization and reimbursement. This is because reimbursement authorities are either undecided as to whether the new treatment offers value, or a decision is pending. However, when a decision has been made by a reimbursement agency that the new treatment does offer value for money, the sales are likely to increase (the difference between K and W is shown in Figure 1.7) because the new treatment has more value and would be recommended for use. The premium price agreed would also influence profits. The loss in revenue can be substantial if preparations have not been made adequately for reimbursement.

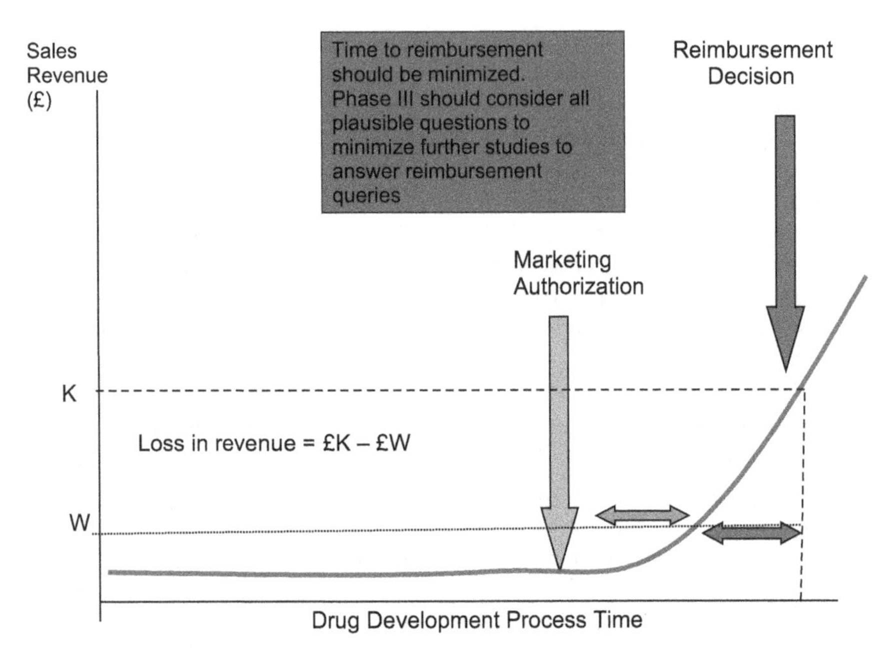

FIGURE 1.7
Relationship between drug licensing, patient access, and reimbursement. W: Sales at some amount £W are flat until £K is achieved (after reimbursement). Consequently, the loss of revenue is £K – £W.

1.8 Efficacy versus Effectiveness

The concept of efficacy is well understood in the context of an RCT. The RCT with its restricted inclusion criteria and very controlled monitoring of efficacy and safety outcomes gives the RCT framework a 'gold standard' status regarding internal validity. The possibility of selection bias is considered to be well accounted for (Pockock, 1983). However, the RCT provides less external validity because any inferences are restricted to the population under investigation and lack generalizability (Sculpher, 2006). In most cancer trials, efficacy is of paramount importance. Even if a new cancer treatment is not cost-effective in the sense that a health system may not wish to pay for it, this does not mean that the treatment does not work. The treatment may still be bought privately, or health insurers may offer to pay for it.

Effectiveness, on the other hand, is where a new treatment is tested in less restrictive (real-world) conditions. One objective of a clinical trial where cost-effectiveness is a key component should be to measure some aspect of the clinical effects of the new treatment in a real-world setting (if feasible). Measuring efficacy in patients with comorbidities, longer-term follow-up, alternative dosing regimens, and poorer patient compliance, may not have been considered in the Phase III RCT. The target population of patients may be broadly similar to those in the clinical trial, but additional questions need to be addressed, such as "How well does the drug work in real practice?"; "How well does the new treatment perform over a longer duration?"

If carefully designed, the RCT offers a good opportunity to collect such data. For example, a clinical trial follow-up period might be suggested as 12 months; however, a follow-up of 24 months might offer an opportunity to collect data in order to gain a sense of how the new treatment is working in a real-world setting when double-blind, and some of the other restrictive conditions, are relaxed. Also, a measure of compliance over a longer period would provide valuable information on the use of the new treatment in practice – especially maintenance therapy, which, in cancer trials, can be particularly expensive causing the ICER to be very large.

In RCTs, compliance is often closely monitored and highly protocol-driven compliance rates may be artificial. True compliance may be as low as 60%, well below some commonly stated compliance rates of 80% (often suggested for per protocol analyses). Although the impact of a per protocol population (a population of patients who are deemed to have complied with the protocol as far as possible) is made on the efficacy endpoints, the importance of the protocol violators on costs are often not considered (Ordaz, 2013; Briggs, 2001; Noble, 2012).

The intention-to-treat (ITT) population, which usually includes all patients randomized (as a minimum), is not always useful for assessing effectiveness. If a patient is randomized but does not receive any randomized treatment, should this patient be evaluable for treatment-related costs? For efficacy evaluation, the ITT principle is that analyses should be conducted based on the randomized treatment (even if patients took the alternative treatment or did not take any treatment). For cost-effectiveness analyses, costs (and effects) incurred from a randomized patient, who did not take the medication (e.g. costs associated with side effects of other drugs), may not reflect the true cost-effectiveness of an intervention. Hence, a modified ITT (mITT) could be defined whereby patients included for analysis must be randomized *and* have received at least one dose or exposure to the randomized intervention. In cancer trials, it can happen that the period between randomization and treatment is long (e.g. several tests, biomarker status, radiotherapy planning, illness). During this 'waiting' period a patient could deteriorate or progress. How such issues of dropout and missing responses are handled can result in biased estimates of treatment effects. This should be no less a concern regarding estimates of cost-effectiveness.

1.9 Real-World Data

A more recent development related to effectiveness that has come about recently is 'real-world data' (RWD). RWD often refers to data collected in real health practice and not just later phase clinical trials with relaxed inclusion/

TABLE 1.4

Relationship between Types of Study and Design Features

	Clinical Trial (Phases I–III)	Clinical Trial (Phase IV)	Real-World Data
Objective	Efficacy	Effectiveness	Longer-term effectiveness/ value
Design	RCT	Observational studies RCTs Retrospective	Observational and RCT Retrospective Electronic health records National/local cancer registries
Population	Protocol defined	Broader population not in the main protocol	Patients in routine clinical practice
Measures	Survival Tumor response HRQoL	Survival Tumor response HRQoL Patient-reported Health resource use	Patient-based outcomes Resource use Impact on health economy
Time frame	Short term or long term	Long term	Long term
Based on	Ideal clinical practice (restricted population)	Normal clinical practice (wider population)	Routine healthcare, hospital setting

exclusion criteria. Data are often collected in electronic medical records once patients leave the clinical trial. For example, a cancer patient completes 12 months of follow-up in a RCT and then is monitored outside a clinical trial through routine visits (e.g. for scans). These data are often held in scattered local hospital records or possibly located centrally through a national registry – such as the National Cancer Registry (NCR). The NCR may collect rich data on systemic anti-cancer therapies (SACT), and there may be an opportunity to link this data with other routine data (general practice data, hospital visits). These can be crucial for evaluating longer-term (real-world) effectiveness of new cancer treatment – especially when a cancer treatment has been given an accelerated approval using data based on a single Phase II trial. There will still be uncertainty around longer-term effects and RWD may help to reduce this.

Table 1.4 shows the relationship between study objectives and key features for particular types of studies. The 'gold standard' to address confirmatory efficacy is the RCT with primary efficacy and safety outcomes; the time frame can be long term or short term – although longer trials (e.g. cancer, cardiovascular, mortality endpoint) can become expensive to run. A study with a primary objective of effectiveness (including economic evaluation) may use a combination of evidence from RCTs or observational studies: outcomes such as resource use (costs), quality of life (QoL), and compliance are examples of the type of data collected in such studies to assess efficiency. In practice, there may be a hybrid type of approach that optimizes the potential to do as much as possible in a single trial.

1.10 Economic versus Clinical Hypotheses

Table 1.5 shows the relationship between the potential clinical advantage envisaged in a clinical trial and how this can translate into a potential economic hypothesis to demonstrate value. It is unlikely that an economic hypothesis can be postulated unless some form of clinical advantage is plausible. In some clinical trials, no clinical advantage is possible – such as 'equivalence' trials where treatment benefits are considered to be 'similar' to, or not worse than, a standard treatment. Bioequivalence trials are also equivalence trials, and even though there might be a change in the mode of administration (e.g. where absolute bioavailability is required for intravenous vs. oral dosing), this type of trial, usually with very few subjects, is unsuitable for any economic evaluation because healthy volunteers are used, and clinical benefit is not assessed.

(a) Hypotheses of Superiority

A superiority trial is when a new treatment is clinically better than the usual treatment or current standard of care. The average treatment difference, Δ_{A-S}, where A is the new treatment and S is the standard treatment. The symbol Δ_{A-S} represents a numerical value for the difference between treatment A versus treatment S; this could be a mean difference, the difference in proportions, or a hazard ratio. For a hazard ratio, used for time-to-event outcomes (commonly for survival times), the lower (or upper 95% confidence

TABLE 1.5

Relationship between Clinical Objective and Plausible Economic Hypotheses

Clinical Advantage	Possible Economic Hypotheses
Superior efficacy	Saves life years Averts disease Improved QoL/QALY gain
Better side-effect profile	Improved QoL
Change in half-life	More convenient administration Improved compliance Improved QoL/QALY gain
Improved delivery	Better compliance Improved QoL/QALY gain

limit) excludes the value of 1. When this happens, a new treatment is said to be 'superior' to the comparator. For example, a 95% confidence interval (CI) for a hazard ratio (HR) of 0.7 (30% less risk of death on treatment A compared to S) of 0.41 to 0.95 is statistically significant because the value of 1 is not in the interval (0.41, 0.95).

The value of Δ_{A-S} (e.g. 0.70) should be large enough to postulate a cost-effectiveness hypothesis. The value argument may depend on observed differences in mean costs between treatment A and B relative to the mean difference in costs. For example, an HR of 0.95 reported from a large trial (n = 2,000 patients) might be statistically significant with a 95% CI of (0.89, 0.99). The value of $\Delta_{A-S} = 0.95$ suggests only 5% of patients more likely to survive with the new treatment, on average. Whether this difference is large enough to demonstrate cost-effectiveness is a separate question. This is an example of a large trial with a small treatment benefit that is statistically significant but that may not necessarily yield a clinical benefit that is cost-effective. On the other hand, even if Δ_{A-S} was large, but the costs associated with this benefit were also high, then a cost-effectiveness argument may still not exist, because the difference in costs may be too high relative to clinical benefits. Table 1.6 gives a summary of how clinical hypotheses can be translated into cost-effectiveness statements.

TABLE 1.6

Summary of Hypotheses for the Primary Endpoint of a Trial

Hypothesis	Hypothesis in Clinical Terms	Average Difference (new vs. standard) at the End of Trial	Example of Possible Cost-Effectiveness Argument
Superiority	New treatment is better than standard	Improved with new ($\Delta_{N-S} > 0$)	Improved efficacy and possibly better safety
Non-inferiority	New treatment is not worse than standard	Improved with new ($\Delta_{N-S} > 0$)	On average, efficacy a little better with new, safety better with new: consequently new is more cost-effective
Non-inferiority	New treatment is not worse than standard	New is worse ($\Delta_{N-S} < 0$)	New is worse on average, but not clinically worse; safety profile is much better with new: cost-effectiveness driven by better safety profile
Equivalence	New treatment is not worse or better than standard	New is neither better or worse	A variation of the above is possible

Note: N, new; S, standard.

Example 1.6

In the above example, a difference between treatments in terms of survival reported an HR = 0.95. If drug A is $10,000 more expensive than S (difference in costs of $10,000), the HR might translate into an average survival difference of 1 week, or about 0.02 years (1 year divided by 52 weeks). The cost for each life-year gained here is $10,000/0.02 = $500,000. That is, the relative cost of treating patients with a new cancer drug A compared to the standard of care, S, costs $500,000 per year (for only a 1-week improvement in mortality). A payer may decide that $500,000 is better spent elsewhere (for example, treating 100 dementia sufferers at the cost of $500 per patient).

(b) Hypotheses of Equivalence: Biosimilars

Several cancer drugs, e.g. Herceptin, are termed 'biologics,' which are considered to be very expensive. Biologics are prepared through complex manufacturing processes (cells, DNA, proteins, tissue), which makes them difficult to copy. Many chemical medicines are manufactured using a predictable chemical process from which we can get an exact copy – these are called generics. At the time of writing, a number of these drugs will come off patent and competition is underway to prepare generic versions of these, more correctly termed 'biosimilars.' In this sense, biosimilars are not the same as generics. To develop a biosimilar, a clinical trial is often needed with the objective to demonstrate 'similar' or 'equivalent' efficacy and safety. The biosimilar market is worth more than $11 billion. The European Medicines Agency estimates savings to the health economy >1.5 billion (year 2009 estimate) annually through the use of biosimilars.

If two treatments are equivalent regarding efficacy, then it would appear that price and costs are the only driving force behind determining cost-effectiveness. Given that some biosimilars are also considered to be expensive, cost-effectiveness is a particular challenge when the clinical and statistical hypothesis of interest is likely to be one of equivalence. The budget impact on the health economy is likely to be important when considering a cost-effectiveness argument between a choice of biosimilars.

Example 1.7

Consider the use of a biosimilar for Trastuzumab for breast cancer in a Croatian population (Cesarec, 2017). The approach to demonstrating cost-effectiveness was not made regarding improvements in efficacy, but on the basis that the price of the biosimilar (test product) was 15% below the reference (branded product). This led to the conclusion that the Croatian health economy could save between €0.26 to €0.69 million euros. In contrast, Brito et al. (2016) compared the drug Nivestim, with a biosimilar for chemotherapy-induced neutropenia. They reported the potential for greater cost-effectiveness in a secondary endpoint (febrile neutropenia) using a cost-effectiveness model.

One approach here could be to use the method described in section 1.5 using equation (1.3) to derive the INMB since the denominator of equation (1.1) (the ICER) will be small in this scenario.

(c) The Hypothesis of Non-Inferior Equivalence

In this situation, the objective is to demonstrate that the new cancer treatment is, on average, not worse than the current standard. In cancer trials, such hypotheses would be rare, since patients are unlikely to enroll in trials where there is an acceptance that a new treatment would result in worse clinical outcomes. In this situation, as far as the new treatment is concerned, a clinical advantage is unlikely or does not exist, and therefore cost-effectiveness is unlikely – unless perhaps other secondary endpoints come into play, or enhanced safety is observed (e.g. lower dose, leading to slightly lower efficacy, but better safety). If there is a value argument, it is likely to be based on 'equivalent' treatment benefit and lower costs, or improved safety.

Example 1.8

In this example, for treatment of infection, a twice-a-day regimen is currently standard. A new once-a-day modified release formulation is developed, which is a more convenient form of administration. The value argument might be based on showing that 'once-a-day versus twice-a-day' is likely to lead to better compliance and that it is cheaper. The manufacturer would seek a premium price as a result of this added value. The treatment effects might be similar or perhaps even worse (although unlikely) with the once-a-day regimen. Since the costs associated with the new (once-a-day) regimen are likely to be lower, the formulation with the lowest cost is likely to be more efficient (efficacy assumed similar). An example of this situation might be a twice-a-day form of clarithromycin (an anti-infective drug) versus a modified (once-a-day) formulation.

1.11 Summary

In this chapter, we have discussed the importance of cancer from an epidemiological and economic perspective. We have shown that expenditure on cancer care is a challenge for almost any health economy. We also introduced some important health economic concepts that we will refer to again in this book. We have also shown that the old paradigm of obtaining a license from the FDA, EMA, or other agency is unlikely to be sufficient and the value of the new treatment needs to be demonstrated. Finally, we have shown the relationship between clinical, statistical, and economic hypotheses and how these need to be aligned so that the tools of economic evaluation can be used appropriately. In the next chapter, we identify the key outcomes in cancer trials, how they are derived, and their relevance and use in economic evaluation.

1.12 Exercises for Chapter 1

1. A biosimilar drug is unlikely to demonstrate cost-effectiveness. Do you agree?
2. What is a risk factor? Explain how a risk factor might influence the cost-effective argument in each of breast, lung, and prostate cancers; compare and contrast your findings. Are there any risk factors in common?
3. The primary endpoint from a clinical trial is the only outcome that is important for determining the value of cancer treatments. Discuss.
4. Biosimilar drugs are drugs that are aimed to show similar effectiveness and yet remain expensive. Therefore, it is not possible to demonstrate an economic advantage for these types of drugs. Do you agree?
5. How would you decide on whether a new cancer treatment was cost-effective in the following situations (assume two treatments being compared against each other)?
   a. The primary endpoint was very positive (i.e. a good outcome for the new treatment) and all secondary outcomes were also better for the new treatment.
   b. The primary endpoint was very positive (i.e. a good outcome) and all secondary outcomes were worse for the new treatment.
   c. The primary endpoint was negative and all secondary outcomes were worse for the new treatment.
   d. The primary endpoint was no different between treatments but all secondary outcomes were superior for the new treatment.
6. Is there a limitation in the way current economic evaluations of cancer drugs are performed based on your answers to the above?

2

Important Outcomes for Economic Evaluation in Cancer Studies

2.1 Introduction

Cancer is a global health problem. There is an increased focus on oncology research to discover and develop safer, more efficacious treatment options. Well-designed clinical trials play an essential role in research and development activities. A fundamental component of clinical trials research is identification of a measurable outcome to delineate clinical benefit of new cancer treatments and further estimate the value they offer for patients and the healthcare system.

Different types of clinical trial endpoints serve different purposes over the phases of drug development. In early phase trials, the focus is to evaluate safety and identify the maximum tolerated dose (MTD) or the minimum effective dose (MED). In Phase I cancer trials, evidence of anti-tumor activity is also investigated, followed by further trials that investigate preliminary evidence of efficacy for designing later confirmatory trials.

Endpoints for confirmatory trials for drug registration (when a new drug becomes available for general patient use by being issued with a license) often define clinical benefit in terms of prolongation of overall survival (OS), progression-free survival (PFS), or an improvement in symptoms (FDA Guidance to Industry, 2018). In this chapter, we discuss the importance of cancer endpoints and their relevance for economic evaluation. Such endpoints can be grouped into two broad categories: (i) patient-centered endpoints and (ii) tumor-centered endpoints. We start with a discussion of common, surrogate, and emerging novel endpoints used in oncology trials.

2.2 Important Common, Surrogate, and Novel Cancer Endpoints

The two general categories of common cancer outcomes in clinical trials can be grouped into are: patient-centered endpoints and tumor-centered endpoints (Fiteni et al., 2014). These are identified below and summarized in Table 2.1.

Patient-centered endpoints

(i) Overall survival (OS)
(ii) Health-related quality of life (HRQoL)

Tumor-Centered Endpoints (Surrogate Endpoints/Intermediate Endpoints)

(iii) Progression-free survival (PFS)
(iv) Disease-free survival (DFS)
(v) Time to progression (TTP)
(vi) Time-to-treatment failure (TTF)
(vii) Event-free survival (EFS)
(viii) Time to next treatment (TTNT)
(ix) Objective response rate (ORR)
(x) Duration of response (DoR)
(xi) Tumor measurements

Tumor-centered outcomes may not always reflect the ultimate goal of the therapy; that is, to increase life expectancy. In the case of an incurable disease, the objective may be to improve the HRQoL during survival as much as possible (increase the QALY).

2.2.1 Overall Survival

OS is measured from the date of either randomization, registration (if not an RCT), or start of first dose until the date of death (due to any cause). For patients still alive by the time the trial has finished (or follow-up could not be completed because the patient withdrew or was lost to follow-up), the survival time is said to be 'right censored.' Hence, a patient's survival time may be censored at the date the patient was last known to be alive. This also means the survival time for a patient that is censored is the minimal survival time. Had the patient been followed up, survival time might have been longer.

Survival data are often presented using Kaplan-Meier (KM) curves for one or more groups. Figure 2.1 shows an example of a KM plot with several types of endpoints, OS, PFS, and post-progression survival (PPS). The Y-axis

TABLE 2.1

Commonly Used Patient-Centered and Tumor-Centered Endpoints in Oncology Clinical Trials

Endpoint	Definition	Comments/ Issues and Relevance to Economic Evaluation
(i) Overall survival (OS)	Time from randomization* until death from any cause (or date of censoring)	• Primary measure for estimating QALYs • Long-term survival often unknown, which is critical for longer-term evaluation of cost-effectiveness • Also considered gold standard by regulators for the purpose of drug registration and approval • Easily and precisely measured • Affected by crossover and subsequent therapies • May require large trial population or longer follow-up in case of less aggressive cancer types • Includes deaths unrelated to cancer
(ii) Health-related quality-of-life (HRQoL)	HRQoL end-points measure physical and psychological status, participation in social activities, and other indicators of well-being, such as the ability to work	• Generic HRQoL used (may not be sensitive) for cost-effectiveness • Rarely used as a primary endpoint • Tend to supplement other patient-centered or tumor-centered endpoints by describing patient treatment experience
(iii) Progression-free survival (PFS)[†]	Time from randomization* until disease progression or death	• Less important for cost-effectiveness although is needed to compute the post-progression survival period • May be a marker of treatment duration and/or duration of benefit from treatment (related to cost) • Progression defined by several types of independent criteria such as RECIST[a] • Smaller sample sizes and shorter follow-up time compared with OS • Not affected by crossover or subsequent therapies • Less influenced than OS by competing causes of death • Not influenced by treatments administered after progression • No international consensus standard for the definition of PFS and DFS • Requires frequent radiologic or other assessments
(iv) Disease-free survival (DFS)	Time from randomization until tumor recurrence or any-cause death after treatments given with curative intent	• Requires balanced timing of assessment among treatment arms • Less important for cost-effectiveness evaluation

(Continued)

TABLE 2.1 (CONTINUED)

Commonly Used Patient-Centered and Tumor-Centered Endpoints in Oncology Clinical Trials

Endpoint	Definition	Comments/ Issues and Relevance to Economic Evaluation
(vi) Time-to-treatment failure (TTF)	Time from randomization* to discontinuation of treatment for any reason, including disease progression, treatment toxicity, and death	• Useful in settings in which toxicity is potentially as serious as disease progression (e.g. allogeneic stem cell transplant) • Does not adequately distinguish efficacy from other variables, such as toxicity, therefore not used in the cost-effectiveness assessment
(vii) Event-free survival (EFS)	Time from randomization* to disease progression, death, or discontinuation of treatment for any reason (e.g. toxicity, patient preference, or initiation of a new treatment without documented progression)	• Initiation of next therapy is subjective. Generally, not encouraged by regulatory agencies because it combines efficacy, toxicity, and patient withdrawal, therefore not used in the cost-effectiveness assessment
(viii) Time-to-next treatment (TTNT)	Time from end of primary treatment to institution of next therapy	• For indolent or incurable diseases, TTNT may provide a meaningful endpoint for patients. Rarely used as primary endpoint as TTNT is subject to variability depending on subsequent treatment options available for patient and physician
(ix) Objective response rate (ORR)	Proportion of patients with reduction in tumor burden of a predefined amount	• Measures direct effect of drug in objective fashion • Earlier assessment compared with survival endpoints • RECIST[a] or other relevant criteria applied
(x) Duration of response (DoR)	Time from documentation of tumor response to disease progression	• Response to treatment may not result in better survival, therefore not a comprehensive measure of drug activity • Commonly used in Phase I or Phase 2 trials • Extrapolation of response rate and duration of response to survival is required, however, due to single arm design of most of these trials, indirect comparison with either historical control and/or best supportive care is performed
(xi) Tumor measurements	Often by RECIST or similar criteria	• Used for solid tumors (RECIST[a] criteria) • Not used for confirmatory trials; often used in Phase I or II trials • Useful for identifying anti-tumor activity

[a] Eisenhauer et al., 2009. RECIST: Response Evaluation Criteria in Solid Tumors. This is a criterion which determines how much a tumour has shrunk. This criterion is used for solid tumours and not blood/haematological tumours. The criteria are shown in Appendix I based on RECIST version 1.1.

* In nonrandomized trials, time from study enrollment or treatment initiation is used.

† TTP and PFS are similar, with the exception that TTP does not include patients that die from other causes (e.g. cardiovascular events)

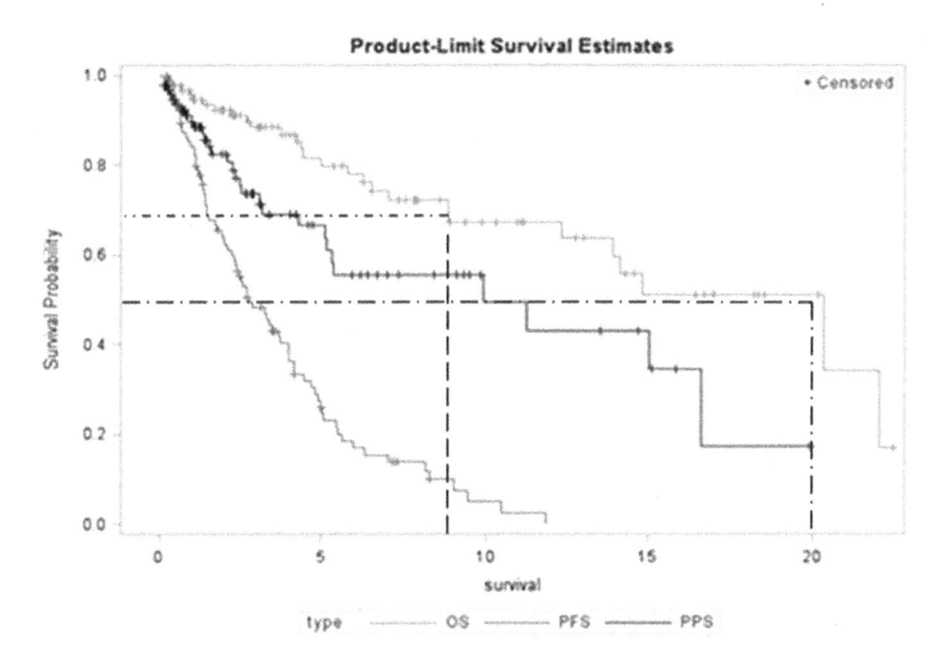

FIGURE 2.1
Example of time-to-event curves.

shows the proportion of patients alive at a time point. In Figure 2.1, about 70% of patients are still alive at around 9 months. One important statistic used to measure clinical benefit is the median survival time. The median OS in Figure 2.1 is about 20 months (draw a horizontal line starting at 0.5 on the Y-axis, until it meets the OS curve). This means that by 20 months, half (50%) of the patients are still alive and 50% have died. The median PFS (brown line) is about 4 months.

Comparing median survival times between treatments is a common way of showing clinical benefit in cancer trials and is useful when such effects are unambiguous. An alternative measure of treatment benefit might be to compare the proportion of patients alive at a fixed time point. In Figure 2.1, at 9 months, around 70% of patients are still alive. This value could be compared with patients in a control treatment group. However, for comparison of the survival rates over the entire KM curve (i.e. comparing the curves) an alternative, more complicated, statistic called the hazard ratio (HR) is often reported. An HR of 1 implies there is no difference between treatments in terms of the event of interest. When the HR is either <1 or >1, then the survival (event) rates for one treatment, on average, are either higher or lower compared to the other. One difficulty involved in interpreting such effects occurs when the KM curves cross (Figure 2.2). This is called a nonproportional hazard and essentially means that treatment differences are not constant across time and may depend on other factors.

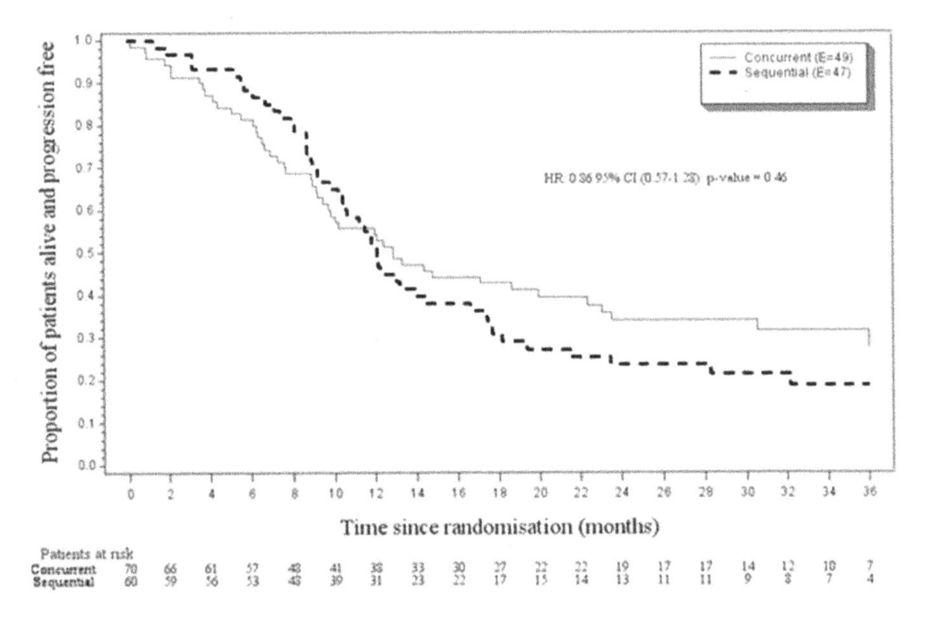

FIGURE 2.2
Survival curves for comparing concurrent versus sequential chemoradiotherapy.

Source: Maguire et al., 2014.

In Figure 2.2, treatment consisting of either concurrent or sequential chemoradiotherapy (chemo-RT) shows that prior to 12 months the sequential treatment group showed higher survival. After 12 months, however, due to the intensity of treatment, survival became worse than concurrent chemo-RT (see Maguire et al., 2014). This is an example where the area under the KM curve(s) can be used to estimate the mean OS for economic evaluation – the so-called restricted mean.

The approach to measuring treatment benefit described here can also be used for most time-to-event endpoints such as PFS, DFS, TTP, TTF, EFS, and TTNT. An important point to mention here is that whereas clinicians use the median OS as a measure of clinical benefit, for cost-effectiveness the mean OS is used. This can be calculated as the area under the KM curve in Figure 2.1. It is sometimes referred to as the restricted mean because the final time point at which all patients die might be unknown by the end of the trial, and hence the area is calculated for a restricted set of survival times. We will discuss further statistical issues for analyzing survival data for cost-effectiveness analyzes purposes in later chapters.

One final point to mention on the use of OS is that the required sample size can be large. Sample sizes in cancer trials (for time-to-event endpoints) depend on the number of events. The events here are deaths (due to any cause). Clearly if we had a trial with 1,000 patients per group and only 5 deaths after 1 year, the statistic of interest would not be of much use if patients died mostly after 2 years. In this case there would be substantial censoring after 1 year making interpretation of the KM curve less useful, and estimates of the median (and mean) OS may not be calculable. The lack of events also has implications for estimating survival patterns over a much longer time horizon. Using OS as an endpoint may therefore require waiting for a long time to achieve the required number of events, resulting in little or no information on longer-term effectiveness (because if death events take a long time anyway, further longer-term effects will take even longer to evaluate). The consequence of this might be that decisions on providing access may be delayed due to uncertainty around the longer-term cost-effectiveness of the intervention. This is neither beneficial to patients nor to industry. In this case special statistical methods can be used to estimate (extrapolate) long-term survival using complex models (parametric survival models). Moreover, such estimates of long-term survival can be confounded by the effects of additional or subsequent treatments taken after disease progression.

2.2.1.1 OS and Economic Evaluation

There are several factors relevant to economic evaluation when using OS in cancer trials:

(i) Whether the OS benefit is achievable

OS is often the main endpoint that is of interest for drug licensing and for payers. Since cancer often results in early death (shortening lifetime), the value of a new treatment must be demonstrated in terms of extending OS. OS is readily accepted by patients and oncologists as evidence for improving patient benefit. In addition, payers of drugs, whether through health insurance or through local or national health systems, value OS as an endpoint of importance for assessing whether to pay for any given cancer drug. About one-third of approved cancer drugs come to market on the basis of reporting improvements in OS through randomized controlled trials (Kim & Prasad, 2016). However, OS is not so straightforward a measure when it comes to assessing cost-effectiveness, even if some form of clinical benefit has been demonstrated.

One limitation of OS is the low likelihood of showing large improvements in OS, especially in elderly patients where some cancers are diagnosed at a much later age (and stage). Fojo et al. (2014) reported median improvements in overall survival from confirmatory trials to be just 2.1 months (Kumar, Fojo, & Mailankody, 2016); colleagues examined 47 consecutive approvals for cancer drugs and found that only 9% showed an absolute increase in OS by 2.5 months (91% showed increases of less than 2.5 months). Even if an OS difference was shown to be statistically significant, this 'significance' does not imply it is a clinically meaningful benefit and moreover it may not have high economic value, especially if the price for a drug is high. In the UK, value thresholds are commonly set at £20,000–£30,000 per QALY (McCabe, 2008; NICE Guidelines, 2013). In some cases, reaching this hurdle is unlikely, as shown in Example 2.1.

Example 2.1: QALYs Reported in Some Published Cost-Effectiveness Analyses for Lung Cancer Using OS

In Chapter 1, Table 1.3 showed that among the 47 ICERs identified from lung cancer trials, about 70% did not yield QALYs below the NICE required thresholds of £20,000–£30,000 per QALY. The implication of such thresholds (say £24,000) is that the new treatment should not cost more than £2,000 per patient per month (or £2,500 per month for a £30,000 cost-effectiveness threshold). This reinforces the challenge to researchers and clinical trialists when designing cancer trials for both efficacy and cost-effectiveness.

(ii) Clinical Trial and Real-World Setting

Clinical trials for registration (trials that demonstrate evidence for efficacy for licensing of a drug) are often performed in highly selected populations, unrepresentative of the general target population. Differences in the magnitude of treatment benefit between experimental (protocol) conditions and real-world settings can be explained in part by the type of (highly selected) patients that present and the nonrandom choice of trial centers and physicians. Economic evaluation of cancer drugs is of greatest interest when used in a real-world or routine clinical practice context and often over a lifetime horizon.

Data on survival from a real-world setting often means in tracking patients well beyond trial follow-up. Such tracking might involve using national (public) cancer registries and possible private data. A recent development has been the use of private enterprises involved in working with public sector institutions to help extract outcomes collected retrospectively from routine hospital and/or clinical practice databases. One difficulty with data collected outside clinical trials, such as cancer registries, is that there may be little or no information on what other treatments were taken that might have impacted the survival, nor what toxicity was experienced. Patient-reported outcomes too, an essential data component for economic evaluation, may not be available. It is better to plan for such real-world collection rather than 'get lucky' from what may or may not be in scattered data registries. It is important to note that regulatory agencies for marketing authorization may not consider registry data as a basis for proof of efficacy, although this might be acceptable for reimbursement agencies.

An important consideration is the recent General Data Protection Regulation (GDPR) (EU) 2016/679 directive within the European Union, which intends to primarily give control back to citizens and residents over their personal data. This includes the use of real-world clinical data. How this law will impact access to outcomes needed for longer-term survival effects is not immediately clear. Often though, by anonymizing the data, sufficient privacy protection for patients is possible.

(iii) Incomplete Follow-Up Data

Complete information on OS may not be available until the last patient in the trial dies. This might only happen for some cases where the life expectation is not too long (see Wang & Li, 2012). As pointed out earlier, this may lead to (right) censoring of patients who have not died at the time of analysis or end-of-study follow-up, resulting in less statistical power to detect differences between groups. This runs the risk of inconclusive results. For economic evaluation, estimates of OS are required over the lifetime of patients, taking into account those still alive at the end of the trial. Hence censoring impacts both costs and effects in an economic evaluation. Methods are available to adjust for censored costs (e.g. see those described in Khan, 2015; Menon et al., 2017). The method of Lin (Lin et al., 1997) is one such method. This method provides an estimate of the mean cost by taking into account patients who are followed up to a particular time point and then are lost to follow-up (censored). The estimate of mean costs uses Kaplan-Meier methods (Chapter 4) to generate weights that are multiplied by the mean costs for specified intervals. A worked example is provided in Chapter 5 (Example 5.7).

(iv) Confounding from Subsequent Anti-Cancer Therapies

Estimates of long-term survival can be confounded by the effects of additional treatments taken after disease progression. In patients with advanced or metastatic disease (not amenable to curative surgery), successions of different lines of treatment are employed. For example, initially a first-line treatment will be given and after some time patients may progress (see Figure 2.3); this will be replaced at some point by different treatments. Figure 2.3 shows how some of the important outcomes relate to the various lines of therapy. The second line (or choice) of therapy for example, starts when the first line of therapy fails, often determined by when disease progression occurs. It is the use of these subsequent lines of therapies that may confound the estimates of OS.

In most, if not all cases, the subsequent treatment options will be less standardized (patients may receive different doses or regimens that impact OS in different ways). For economic evaluation, this creates challenges in handling the heterogeneity (variability) of these differing regimens in the way they influence OS. This issue also extends to estimates of costs from taking other anti-cancer treatments – specifically the costs associated with side effects and the administration of later lines of therapies. When PFS is a primary endpoint, the need for estimating longer-term OS becomes important for

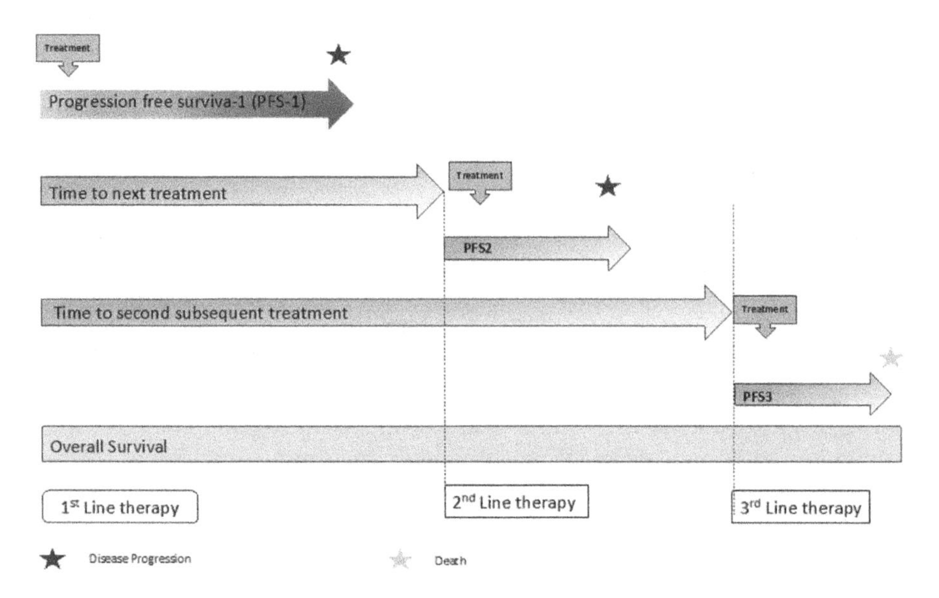

FIGURE 2.3
Relationship of different surrogate endpoints and overall survival.

Source: Adapted and modified from Matuolonis et al., 2014.

estimating the ICER. Hence, although PFS might be acceptable for licensing, OS is still needed to determine the value of a new cancer drug. OS, costs, and QALY estimates can be biased if the impact of subsequent treatments is not considered. This leads to the issue of adjusting effects for 'crossover.'

(v) Crossover or Switching from the Control Drug to the Experimental Drug

Slightly different to taking additional anti-cancer treatments after progressive disease (PD) is the issue of patients being allowed to cross over to an experimental treatment once the primary endpoint (e.g. after the target number of events has been reached or disease progression has occurred) or follow-up is complete. This may happen for ethical reasons to avoid delaying potentially effective treatments for trial patients. If patients who crossed over to the experimental treatment are excluded from the analyses, selection bias may exist because those patients who switched from the control arm to the experimental treatment may not be representative of patients in the entire control arm. It has been noted that over half the health technology assessments (HTAs) have been affected by some form of treatment switching (Latimer, 2015).

Although crossover may confound and bias the treatment benefit, it may be argued that since statistical analysis follows the 'intent to treat' (ITT) principle (analyze patients according to what they were randomized to and not what they actually took), crossover is what is likely to happen in routine practice and may be a more realistic assessment of treatment benefit, despite the potential biased estimate of treatment benefit. Moreover, several statistical methods used in some cost-effectiveness analyses that attempt to adjust for treatment switching have been rejected by decision-makers (Latimer, 2015).

The impact of switching on the ICER and QALY can be significant because the OS benefit can be either over- or underestimated. As an example, the NICE HTA TA269 (NICE, 2012) reveals how switching had a large impact on the cost-effectiveness results in a melanoma trial. In this submission (vemurafenib), adjusting for switching in 34% of control group patients, reduced the ICER from £75,500 per QALY to £51,800 per QALY. The adjusted analyses were considered acceptable resulting in vemurafenib's recommendation for reimbursement, despite the ICER being (marginally) above £50,000 per QALY (used for end-of-life settings).

An example to the contrary involves an HTA of everolimus from the RECORD-1 confirmatory trial in patients with advanced renal cell cancer (RCC). The decision-makers felt that the estimates provided by the manufacturer's economic model were overly optimistic and instead suggested a smaller overall mortality benefit based on alternative statistical estimates – *adjusting for crossover.* The decision-makers noted:

> any estimate of OS obtained using statistical modeling would be subject to some uncertainty because a number of assumptions would have to be made.

Everolimus for advanced RCC was not considered to offer value because the magnitude of its effect was highly uncertain, as were estimates of cost-effectiveness, with several analyses showing cost-benefit ratios that exceeded NICE's standard recommended thresholds (£20,000–£30,000 per QALY).

In a further example, in TA381 (NICE, 2013) for the treatment of BRCA +ve (a biomarker), platinum-sensitive, relapsed ovarian cancer, the hazard ratio for PFS was 0.18 (95% CI 0.10–0.31, $p < 0.0001$) for olaparib versus placebo. The OS was not significantly better ($p = 0.19$). There was some crossover after disease progression and, after crossover-adjusted analysis, the treatment difference was statistically different ($p = 0.039$). However, although the analysis adjusted for licensed treatments, it did not correct for unlicensed treatment with an experimental drug (olaparib) beyond disease progression (patients on the control arm switched to olaparib).

Additional work undertaken by the review group suggested that the incremental cost-effectiveness ratio (ICER) for olaparib versus routine surveillance in BRCA mutated platinum-sensitive, relapsed ovarian cancer patients who received >2 lines of chemotherapy, was likely to be greater than £92,214 per QALY gained. The manufacturer's economic model produced a higher estimate of effectiveness (1.43 QALYs) without adjustment for treatment crossover compared to that generated by NICE experts, found to be 0.52 QALYs after adjusting for crossover (and hence the ICER exceeding £92,214/QALY).

Although OS has limitations, it is nevertheless a strong objective endpoint that has clear meaning and value to both patients and clinicians. Where a disease is known to shorten the lifetime of patients, an improvement in OS is still the most important outcome when it can be measured.

2.2.2 Surrogate Endpoints

There is no agreed definition of surrogate endpoints. According to the National Institute of Health (NIH) Biomarkers Definitions Working Group (NIH, 2001), a clinical endpoint is a characteristic or variable that reflects how a patient feels, functions, or survives, and a surrogate endpoint is defined as a biomarker or intermediate endpoint intended to substitute and predict for a patient-relevant final endpoint (Ciani et al., 2016).

In the absence of OS, surrogate or intermediate endpoints are used in the majority of clinical trials as indirect measures of clinical benefit for several reasons:

(i) One reason is because surrogate endpoints can generally be achieved in a shorter time frame than OS. For example, progressive disease is a prelude to death. An event of 'disease progression' will occur earlier than death.

PFS and objective response rate (ORR) are the most commonly used tumor-centered surrogate or intermediate endpoints in cancer trials. PFS is defined as the time from randomization or patient enrolment (if not an RCT) until first disease progression or death. Disease progression is determined by either clinical signs and symptoms (which can be subjective) or objective criteria such as those of the Response Evaluation Criteria in Solid Tumors (RECIST) – (Eisenhauer et al., 2009). Other similar criteria exist for nonsolid tumors.

The purpose of such criteria is to remove the possibility of bias when judging patients to have disease progression. Typically, RECIST requires measuring the tumor dimensions and calculating an approximate area. The target or primary tumor of interest is measured at baseline (before treatment starts) and post-baseline (after treatment is given). The difference between the two measures is expressed as a percentage and the amount of reduction is classified as either complete response (CR), partial response (PR), or stable disease (SD).

If the tumor size increases or evidence of new lesions is observed in any other part of the body (metastases), this is called progressive disease (PD). PD is judged against the minimal (the nadir) of previous measures, whereas response is always assessed when comparing post-treatment tumor measures with baseline measures. The exact timing of the progression is often unknown. Discrete assessment points (e.g. every 3 months) for clinical or radiological assessment are used in practice and therefore the PD is interval censored. The actual time of PD is therefore also design dependent – dependent on the schedule of assessments and the growth rate of a cancer. Given the open label design of many oncology clinical trials, PFS may be subject to assessment bias. Discrepancies between investigator and independent adjudication of response need to be minimized.

(ii) Fewer Patients and Trials of Shorter Duration

An advantage of surrogate endpoints is that successful treatments can be identified much earlier compared to OS and therefore reach patients and providers more quickly. Such intermediate endpoints are most frequently used when it would be impractical to follow patients for a long time (until death), as in for example indolent, less aggressive cancer types or patients in the early stages of disease. This may also help to reduce the cost of the trial and be commercially beneficial for the manufacturer (less costly trials). Depending on factors such as effect size, duration of effects, and the comparative benefits of other available treatments, surrogate endpoints can lead to accelerated approval by regulatory authorities. An example of approved drugs using surrogate outcomes is venetoclax for treating chronic lymphocytic leukemia.

In reporting the results of venetoclax, it was noted that:

> The committee was concerned that the single-arm design of the trials made it difficult to assess the efficacy of venetoclax (that is, there was no comparator arm of patients having best supportive care)
>
> The committee was aware that in M14-032, neither the median progression-free survival nor median overall survival had been reached, and that because there was uncertainty associated with the efficacy of venetoclax, the European Medicines Agency had granted the marketing authorization for venetoclax conditional on the company submitting more mature data from M14-032, which is due to report in March 2018...

Hence, approval was based on a single-arm trial conditional on more mature data being available. However, for cost-effectiveness, extrapolation was used to predict future survival patterns. Consequently, even if marketing authorization is based on a combination of surrogate and other outcomes, cost-effectiveness will still be evaluated over a lifetime horizon.

(iii) Translation into Final Outcomes

For economic evaluation, surrogate endpoints may need to be translated into final patient-relevant outcomes (OS and HRQoL). The European Network of Health Technology assessment (EUnetHTA, 2019) considers surrogate endpoints to be important and admissible for cost-effectiveness assessment, provided these have been validated. The NICE Methods Guide (NICE, 2013) acknowledges that when the use of a 'final' clinical endpoint is not possible 'surrogate' data on other outcomes can be used to infer the effect of treatment on mortality and HRQoL. This would support the surrogate-to-final endpoint outcome relationship so long as this relationship can be quantified and justified. Note that if a surrogate and final outcome do not generate consistent results (e.g. hazard ratios for OS and PFS in different directions or of vastly differing magnitudes), the uncertainty of treatment benefit is much higher in terms of both market authorization and cost-effectiveness.

The usefulness of a surrogate endpoint for estimating QALYs will be greatest when there is strong evidence that it accurately predicts HRQoL and/or survival. However, it must be noted that in all cases, the association between the surrogate endpoint, HRQoL and the final outcome (OS) may not be strong and needs to be explored, quantified, and justified. Table 2.2 shows the OS and the PFS for a number of clinical trials in glioblastoma:

The plot of OS versus PFS in Figure 2.4 shows the relationship is good (correlation of around 0.78) but not perfect. Hence, one cannot be entirely certain that the surrogate PFS outcome will lead to clinical benefit in OS in the case of glioblastoma.

(iv) Not Affected by Treatment Crossover

PFS is central to understanding the effect of an intervention on tumor burden and is not affected by treatment crossover and subsequent treatments. It therefore potentially offers a direct ('cleaner') assessment of the effect of the experimental anti-cancer treatment. For these reasons, regulatory authorities around the world, including the US FDA and the EMA (European Medicines Agency) (EMA, 2012) consider PFS to be an accepted regulatory endpoint to support cancer drug approval (FDA, 2007), although not always in isolation.

(i) Relationship between OS and Response

Figure 2.4 shows the relationship between OS and PFS. A patient-access (reimbursement) strategy might be to treat patients for their cancer so long as they are responding (either complete or partial response). This could be attractive to reimbursement authorities because if PFS is long and the costs of treating until PD are also large, only patients who respond could be considered for treatment. For example, if the treatment duration is 6 cycles (1 cycle = 3 weeks), then treating beyond 6 cycles (18 weeks) might be expensive if the vast majority of patients have a tumor response by say 8 weeks. In other words, for patients who are responders or have stable disease (SD) by 8 weeks, their treatment would continue until progression. For those who do not respond by say 12 weeks, future response is unlikely. This approach may reduce the ICER.

Where objective response rates (ORR) or other intermediate endpoints are secondary endpoints in clinical trials, these have been used by NICE to set

TABLE 2.2

OS and the PFS for a Number of Clinical Trials in Glioblastoma

Author*	Year	Phase	Population	Design	N	Treatments	OS (months) (median)	PFS (months) (median)
Brandes	2016	II	Recurrent	2:1 RCT	91	Bevcmb vs.fotemustine	7.3 vs. 8.7	3.4 vs. 3.5
Herrlinger	2016	II	Newly diagnosed	2:1 RCT	182	TMZ vs. Bev+Irinotecan	17.5 vs. 16.6	6.0 vs. 9.8
Taphoon	2015	III	Newly diagnosed	RCT 1:1	921	BEV+RT/TmZ vs. pl+RT/TMZ	16.8 vs. 16.7	9.0 vs. 6.1
Gilbert	2014	III	Newly diagnosed	RCT 1:1	637	Bev vs.. pl vs. (TMZ/RT)	15.7 vs. 16.1	10.7 vs. 7.3
Gilbert	2013	II	Newly diagnosed	RCT 1:1	833	TMZ vs. Dense TMZ	16.6 vs. 15	5.5 vs. 6.7
Batchelor	2013	III	Recurrent	RCT 2:2:1	325	Cediranib 30mg Cediranib 20mg vs. Lomustine+placebo	8.0 vs. 9.8 9.4 vs. 9.8	3.1 vs. 2.7 4.25 vs. 2.7
Omuro	2013	II	Recurrent	Simon 2 stage	47	TMZ 50mg	7.0	2.0
Norden	2013	II	Recurrent	Single arm	58	TMZ 75-100mg	11.7	1.9
Vredenburgh	2010	II	Newly diagnosed	Single arm	75	TMZ -> Bev+irinotecan	19.6	13.6
Brada	2010	II	Recurrent	RCT 1:1	447	PCV vs. TMZ	6.7 vs. 7.2	3.6 vs. 4.7
Friedman	2009	II	Recurrent	RCT 1:1	167	BV vs. BV+Irinotecan	9.2 vs. 8.7	4.2 vs. 5.8
Fabrini	2009	II	Recurrent	Single arm	50	Fotemustine	24.5	9.1
Kong	2010	II	Recurrent	Single arm	38	TMZ metronomic 40mg ->50mg	10.0	4.3

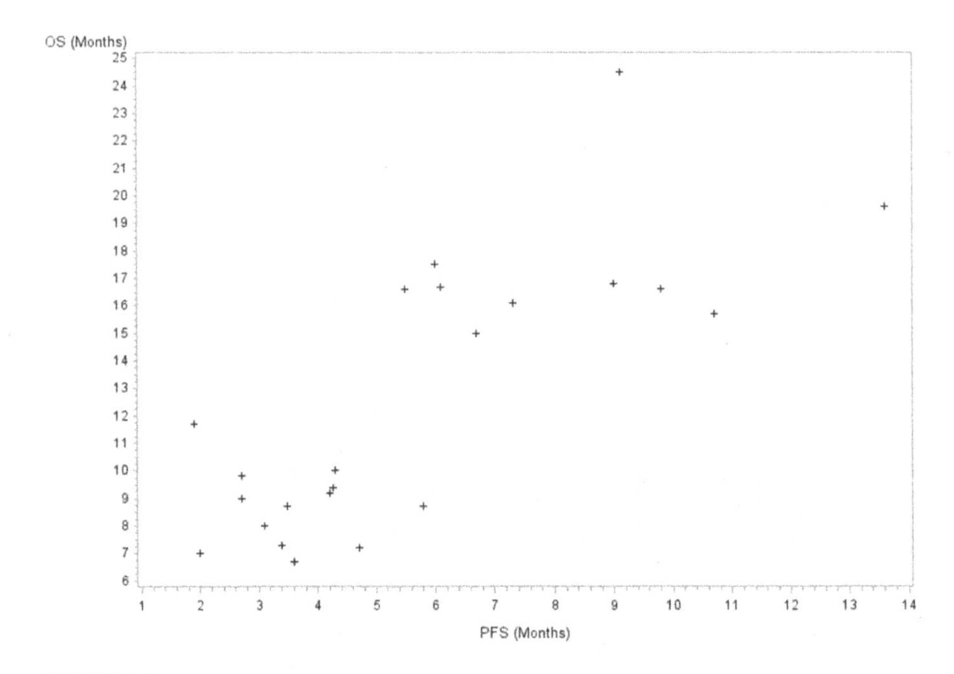

FIGURE 2.4
Relationship between ORR and survival in glioblastoma trials in Table 2.2.

up performance-based patient-access schemes based on response to therapy (see, for example, HTA, TA129, 2007).

(ii) Relationship between PFS and OS

Over the past decade, between 27% and 50% of HTA submissions to several European and other reimbursement agencies (e.g. NICE, the Pharmaceutical Benefits Advisory Committee (PBAC) in Australia, and the Common Drug Review (CDR) in Canada) were based on surrogate endpoints, such as PFS (Clement et al., 2009). However, several issues around PFS require further consideration.

Despite its wide use in cancer trials, PFS is not a statistically validated surrogate for OS in all settings (e.g. follicular lymphoma, ovarian cancer) due to a variety of different challenges. For example, a change in tumor burden with defined disease progression might be insufficient to affect the time to death in all cancer types. A recent analysis by Kim and Prasad (2016) showed that in a sample of 65 studies the correlation between surrogate markers such as PFS and OS was 'weak' in 48% of these trials (31 of 65 studies). Although, as shown in glioblastoma trials, the correlation between OS and PFS can be higher (Figure 2.4), in general the absence of a strong relationship between OS and PFS is reported widely across several tumor areas.

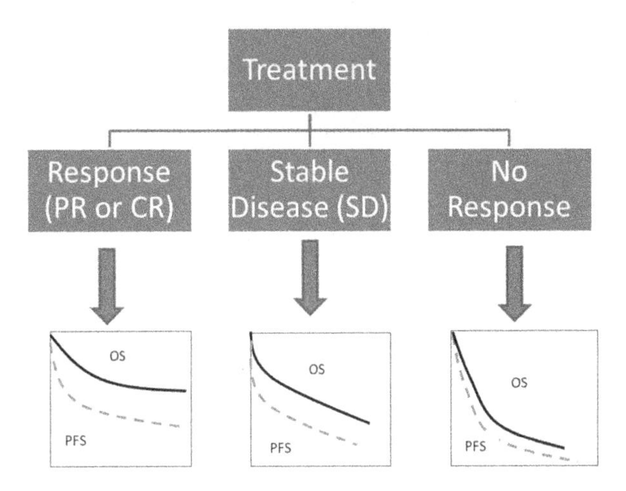

FIGURE 2.5
Relationship between PFS and OS in glioblastoma trials.

Some statistical modeling indicates there is a strong concordance between PFS and OS (Clement et al., 2009), but only when the median survival after PD is short, i.e. <12 months. The relationship between post-progression survival (PPS) and OS is however much poorer when PPS is longer. This may be explained by the fact that survival after PD is more variable because of the number of available treatments after disease progression (see Figure 2.5). Another possible reason for the poor correlation between PFS and OS may be a lack of consistent definition of PD across studies and, indeed, different tumor types (e.g. changes in RECIST criteria, blood cancers use different definitions for disease progression). In addition, in recent years with the advent of immunotherapy, an increase in the size of the tumor on radiological scans that are classed as PD may actually be due to the mobilization of patients' immune systems by such immunotherapy drugs.

(iii) Prolonged Treatment until PD

Prolonged exposure (e.g. maintenance treatment or multiple sequential lines of therapy) might lead to a different evolution of tumors, thus offsetting the advantage from the treatment shown initially through delaying disease progression (PFS1). This was noted by recent EMA anti-cancer guidelines that highlighted the need for prolonged follow-up until the second progression (PFS2). PFS2 is the time between randomization and evidence of second progression. However, treating beyond first progression is likely to make the cost of treatment expensive and will reduce its value (higher ICER). One would expect that by the time the second progression occurs, the HRQoL is likely to be worse compared to the first progression with a much diminished QALY.

Treatment until disease progression or maintenance treatment is a strategy that can be employed across all tumor types. It might be used in mainly indolent or incurable cancers. The argument for using this approach is for long-term disease control by continued exposure to the drug. However, there are important issues with this approach and several unanswered questions remain.

First, this approach does not accurately isolate and quantify the clinical benefit of maintenance therapy as compared with the standard approach of fixed-duration induction followed by the second-line treatment at progression (see Figure 2.5). To address this, RCTs need to utilize an OS (or HRQoL) endpoint; or, in settings where this is not feasible, utilize endpoints that incorporate the effects of subsequent lines of therapy (e.g. time from randomization to second progression or death). Toxicity and symptom information over both the study treatment (maintenance) and the second-line treatment should also be collected and reported. However, trials continue to be designed with PFS as the primary endpoint in most cases. To reduce the economic burden, a possibility is to cap the duration of continued treatment to a fixed period to reduce cost (see, for example, pembrozulimab (NICE, 2018d), nivolumab (NICE, 2017a), and atezolizumab for NSCLC (NICE, 2018).

(iv) Assessment of PFS

Frequent radiological or other additional assessments may not reflect clinical practice and may actually lead to increased health resource utilization. For this reason, PFS and other surrogate endpoints can be prone to error and bias because they are contingent on consistent timing of tumor assessment in both control and intervention groups. That is, PFS is a design dependent outcome. If one chooses to scan more frequently, a different median PFS could be obtained. It could also artificially increase the total cost of treatment (more or less frequent scans influence costs).

(v) Missing Data between PPS and Death

After PD, the potential for collecting post-progression data is limited by clinical protocol requirements. For example, if the 'end of a trial' for a patient is defined as when progression occurs, no further collection can be justified. This will have obvious implications for collecting costs and consequences over a lifetime horizon. Importantly, if no data are available post-progression, extrapolation between progression and death is even more uncertain. Usually data on some patients after PD is required to entertain a plausible model for extrapolation. Extrapolation methods are increasingly being used to predict survival beyond the trial observation period to estimate the expected future health benefits and costs.

(vi) Combined Risk

Another concern relating to PFS during economic evaluation is that PFS may not be suitable for capturing the combined risk–benefit profile. A short observation period may mask the true incidence of serious or detrimental side effects with limited knowledge about longer-term toxic effects of novel treatments, which could make the new treatment less cost-effective (e.g. if the trial stops after first evidence of PD). Delaying disease progression might decrease a patient's emotional distress but, on the other hand, it needs to be balanced against understanding fully (longer-term) drug toxicity and patient preference.

2.3 HTAs with Surrogate Endpoints

Some examples and case studies with surrogate endpoints are now discussed.

Example 2.2: Chronic Myeloid Leukemia

In chronic myeloid leukemia (CML) a number of different tyrosine kinase inhibitors (TKIs) are approved based on surrogate endpoints of complete cytogenetic response (CCyR) and major molecular response (MMR). In 2012 NICE assessed three of these TKIs, dasatinib, nilotinib (Ciani et al., 2013), and standard dose imatinib as first-line treatment of CML. A systemic review and meta-analysis were undertaken to quantify the association between CCyR and MMR at 12 months and OS. This was acceptable to some agencies and a favorable cost-effectiveness conclusion was reached (Ciani et al., 2016).

Example 2.3: Increasing Use of Surrogate Outcomes

The trend over the past two decades suggests that tumor-centered endpoints are increasingly being used as a basis for oncology drug licensing and approvals. The number of FDA approvals based on trials with time-to-event (tumor-centered endpoints) as a primary endpoint has increased while the number of approvals for cancer drugs using OS as their primary endpoint has decreased. Del Paggio et al.'s review (2017) of 277 RCTs involving breast, non-small-cell lung cancer, colorectal cancer, and pancreas cancer showed 35% of trials used OS as the primary endpoint, while 62% had a tumor-centered primary endpoint. The remaining 3% of trials used HRQoL, toxicity, or another type of endpoint.

Figure 2.6 shows the number of trials for each type of primary endpoint used over the two decades 1990–1999 and 2000–2011. The chart shows a clear increase in the number of trials that used tumor-centered

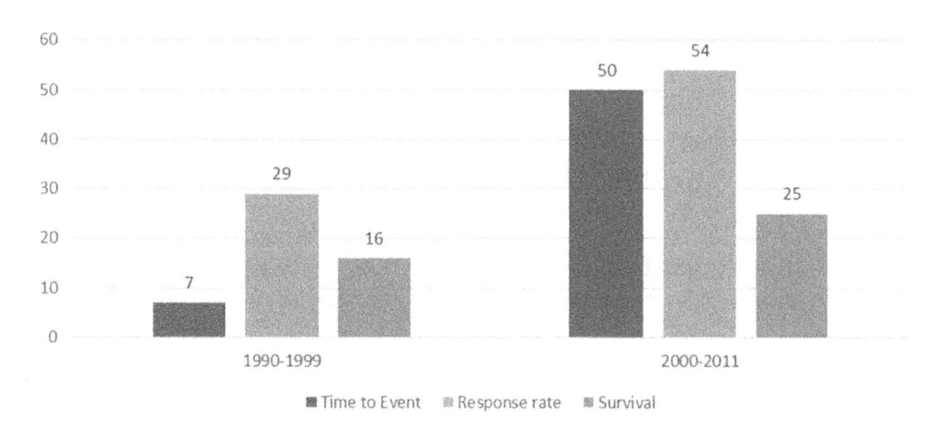

FIGURE 2.6
Changes in the use of primary endpoints for FDA drug approvals since 1990 split by decades.

Source: Adapted from Martell et al., 2013.

endpoints for successful FDA approval (Martell et al., 2013). For example, between 1990 and 1999 there were 36 approvals and, by 2011, this increased to 104. This increase does not take into account recent approvals (e.g. 2014 onward) where 16 out of 17 oncology drugs were approved based on a surrogate endpoint (of these 17, 6 were based on PFS, 1 DFS, 8 ORR, and 1 using a complete remission with partial hematologic recovery rate outcome).

Figure 2.6 shows the changes in the use of primary endpoints since 1990 split by decades (Martell et al., 2013).

Example 2.4: Types of Endpoints used for Approvals (License) based on Common and Novel Cancer Endpoints

Table 2.3 shows endpoints used as the primary basis of drug approval (for licensing). What is noticeable is that whereas cost-effectiveness of cancer treatments is evaluated over a lifetime horizon (using OS as a primary outcome), several of the endpoints above demonstrate that clinical benefit can be determined using outcomes other than OS.

Considerable uncertainty exists if extrapolation of survival is required. In some cancers, survival may be very long and therefore trial follow-up will be curtailed for practical and logistical reasons. Consequently, the proportion of the extrapolated survival as a fraction of the total survival (i.e. extrapolated time divided by the total survival time) might be very large. This means that cost-effectiveness is based on modeled survival patterns and not actual or overall survival for the most part. In some tumor types, this is less of a problem because survival time is so short that most of the survival time is observed during trial follow-up (in contrast to being predicted) (e.g. Lee et al., 2011).

TABLE 2.3

Examples of Drug Approvals Based on Different Endpoints

Endpoint	Drug Name/Year	Indication/Tumor Type
OS	Pemetrexed/2004	Non-small-cell lung cancer
PFS	Sorafenib/2007	Advanced hepatocellular carcinoma
DFS	Anastrazole/2010	Adjuvant postmenopausal estrogen receptor positive breast cancer
TTP	Gemcitabine/2004	Advanced breast cancer
ORR	Atezolizumab/2016	Urothelial carcinoma/2016
DoR	Fludarabine/2007	Chronic lymphocytic leukemia,
pCR	Pertuzumab/2015	HER2 positive locally advanced, inflammatory or early stage breast cancer

2.4 Emerging Tumor-Centered Endpoints

In addition to the traditional tumor-centered endpoints listed above, a number of novel endpoints have become available for cancer patients. These include:

(a) Immune-related response criteria (irRC)
(b) Minimal residual disease (MRD)
(c) Pathological complete response (pCR)

These outcomes are related to how the body's own immune system is used to fight cancer. In some types of cancer such as acute or chronic leukemia and early breast cancer, such novel endpoints based on disease burden have been used selectively.

(a) Immune-Related Response Criteria (irRC)

Immune-related response criteria are appropriate for investigational medicinal products that require frequent repeated assessments and measurements of tumor burden). One important consideration for the development of the irRC is based on the observation that in some cancer patients, based on a scan, the tumor may give the appearance of disease progression whereas the tumor is in fact responding to treatment. Complete response (CR), partial response (PR), and stable disease (SD) may only occur after an initial increase in tumor burden. If conventional RECIST criteria were used, patients would have been classified as having "progressive disease" (Wolchok et al., 2009). For this reason, some have termed the appearance of initial progression as 'pseudo-progression'. That is, even if tumor size is increasing, for certain drugs (e.g. checkpoint inhibitors) the immune system may take some time to 'kick in,' which will eventually lead to a decline of tumor burden in many patients. Hodi et al. (Hodi et al., 2014) report that about 12% of patients (51 of 411 patients) with melanoma treated with pembrolizumab would have been classified as having PD by RECIST but as SD or responding using iRECIST. There appears to be a small percentage of patients who achieve responses using irCR but not RECIST (Chiou & Burotto, 2015).

Although, widely used in cancer immunotherapy trials, at present, regulatory authorities have not approved any drug based solely on irRC, and currently its role is limited to an exploratory assessment tool only. For cost-effectiveness analysis, it may not fall directly into the calculus of the ICER, but it could be considered as an endpoint with the potential to offer further value.

(b) Minimal Residual Disease (MRD)

MRD identifies traces of cancer cells that may otherwise elude other testing techniques before clinical symptoms and signs of cancer become apparent. Sophisticated technology now enables the detection of the persistence of blood cancers at lower thresholds than conventional methods, a level of disease burden known as MRD (e.g. 1 leukemia cell in 1 million compared to 1 cell in 100). This endpoint applies to blood cancers, e.g. acute or chronic leukemias and requires sophisticated technologies to detect traces of leukemia cells. This is measured as a continuous outcome similar to laboratory-type measures, and one objective is to measure effectively a reduction in cancer cells below a pre-specified threshold (e.g. 1 leukemia cell in a population of 1 million normal cells). Although MRD is increasingly used in clinical practice, it is not currently accepted by regulatory agencies for registration of new drugs, and its relevance for an economic evaluation at this time may be limited.

(c) Pathological Complete Response (pCR)

Pathological complete response is limited to neoadjuvant (treatment given before surgery) trials. pCR is a biological reflection of therapy's ability to eradicate micro-metastatic disease. Neoadjuvant therapy has permitted the assessment of tumor response on this basis. Pathological complete response can be assessed quickly (unlike progression or death, which can take longer) and has been used as a surrogate for accelerated approval in patients with operable breast cancer. The FDA accepted definition of pCR is "the absence of residual invasive cancer on hematoxylin and eosin evaluation of the complete resected specimen and all sampled regional lymph nodes following completion of neoadjuvant systemic therapy" (FDA Guidance for Industry – October 2014, accessed on 13 January 2019). Recent approval of pertuzumab in combination with herceptin in early breast cancer is currently the only example of regulatory approval (for a license) based on pathological complete response (pCR) (NICE, TA424 2016).

However, it may not be suitable for a cost-effectiveness analysis because longer follow-up is required in order to confirm whether pCR is a reliable surrogate for PFS or OS. As an example, in the cost-effectiveness evaluation of pertuzumab (NICE, 2016, TA424) in early breast cancer, NICE acknowledged that although there was some correlation between pCR and survival outcomes (OS) it was, however, very weak (correlation coefficients of 0.03 and 0.24 for event-free survival and overall survival respectively). The expert reviewers noted that the evidence for a beneficial treatment in terms of pCR did not translate into an OS benefit or was not convincing:

> there was considerable uncertainty about whether pathological complete response could be viewed as a surrogate marker of long-term benefit...

2.5 Demonstrating Value from Other Cancer Endpoints

There is no single agreed methodology or definition of 'value' when it comes to economic evaluation of cancer treatments across countries. Different countries and regions around the world use different methods to evaluate value at the time of economic evaluation and/or reimbursement. For example, Belgium, France, Germany, and Italy make reimbursement decisions based on the clinical benefit of a product and take costs into consideration in a subsequent separate pricing process. While Austria, the Netherlands, Spain, Sweden, and the UK combine a clinical assessment with an economic evaluation to make reimbursement recommendations. Where economic evaluations are carried out, the most commonly used integrative measure of the value of healthcare products is the QALY, which captures benefits in terms of reduced HRQoL and improved survival. Values from other endpoints can take shape in various forms such as those listed below:

- Relationship between tumor measurements and toxicity (e.g. demonstrating tumor reduction does not lead to worsening toxicity)
- Relationship between toxicity and PFS, TTP, DoR, and other endpoints, with the objective to show better tolerability while benefit is ongoing

Relationship between tumor endpoints and HRQoL. This is particularly important because, after PD, HRQoL can deteriorate quite rapidly. This will be the subject of the next chapter on using HRQoL in cancer for economic evaluation.

2.6 Summary

In this chapter we presented the different endpoints that are commonly used in cancer trials. We made a distinction between primary endpoints, such as overall survival, and surrogate endpoints. We also discussed the relationship between overall survival and progression-free survival and response types. We introduced the notion for QALYs and presented some examples of their use in HTA. Finally, we discussed some more recent tumor-centered endpoints and their role in demonstrating 'value.'

2.7 Exercises for Chapter 2

1. Discuss the relevance of each type of cancer outcome for an economic evaluation.
2. Is overall survival always relevant for an economic evaluation? When might it not be used and what other outcomes might demonstrate value in a cost-effectiveness of a treatment for lung cancer?
3. What are the concerns around assessing disease progression?
4. Distinguish between irRC and RECIST. How can tumor response be used to demonstrate value?
5. Discuss the challenges for cost-effectiveness of treating a cancer until progression occurs.

3

Health-Related Quality of Life for Cost-Effectiveness

3.1 Health-Related Quality of Life (HRQoL) in Cancer Patients

A universally acknowledged definition of 'quality of life' has not been agreed upon. However, most researchers in healthcare adopt the definition provided by the World Health Organization (WHO): "state of complete physical, mental and social well-being, and not merely the absence of disease and infirmity" (WHO, 2014). Health-related quality of life (HRQoL), however, is affected in a complex way by the person's physical health, psychological state, the level of independence, social relationships, personal beliefs, and their relationship to salient features of their environment.

HRQoL is measured through various methods – often questionnaires, with specific questions about feelings, symptoms, ability, and preferences among others, in relation to their state of health. HRQoL data are often collected at several time points during a study (including clinical trials). In cancer trials, an experimental intervention is often expected to yield at least equivalent or better clinical benefit (efficacy), compared to a usual (standard of care) treatment. However, the new treatment may also offer improved HRQoL in addition to or despite a lack of improved clinical benefit (e.g. the new treatment may be equivalent in terms of efficacy, but with fewer side effects).

3.1.1 Limitations of Anti-Cancer Treatments

Cancer patients are concerned about their HRQoL during and after treatment (Cykert et al., 2000). Anti-cancer treatments have sometimes resulted in some harm without benefit as well as harm with modest benefit (Montazeri et al., 2001), but at the cost of increased toxicity and long-term sequelae. Consequently, HRQoL should be a key outcome measure when assessing the cost-effectiveness of a new cancer intervention (Klein et al., 2009). The implications for HRQoL during palliative therapy, for example, can be particularly acute because symptom palliation may contribute toward improved quality of life, and in some cases impact survival as well (Temel et al., 2010). Since no further treatments e.g. chemotherapy) are likely to be used during the end stages of a patient's life (End of Life, EoL), the HRQoL benefits for patients and their carers from other forms of intervention (e.g. carer support) may yield important HRQoL benefits. Some researchers have suggested that a "treatment can be recommended … even without an improvement in survival if HRQoL is shown to improve" (Goodwin et al., 2003).

The importance of HRQoL in cancer trials is noted by the fact that it can influence the choice of treatment. In about 8% of the RCTs in breast cancer, for example, HRQoL influenced a treatment decision. In prostate cancer studies involving chemotherapy and surgery, 25% and 60% of treatment decisions were influenced by HRQoL, respectively (Blazeby et al., 2006). Due to the increasing number of therapy lines, smaller treatment effect sizes, and increasing costs of drugs, HRQoL plays an important role in treatment, policy, rationing, and decision-making. This is likely to remain an important factor in the short to mid term (Damm, Roeske, & Jacob, 2013).

3.1.2 Why Collect HRQoL Data?

There are several reasons why HRQoL data are collected:

(i) Researchers need to maximize the information about how anti-cancer treatments are working, so that informed decisions for treating patients can be made.

It is essential to know (from both patients' and clinicians' perspectives) not only what the side effects associated with treatments are, but also how these side effects impact the patients' HRQoL. It is now universally accepted that HRQoL should be measured in cancer clinical trials, however, the debate has been ongoing for some time as to what is the most reliable and practical way to obtain, measure, and define clinical benefit from HRQoL data (Slevin et al., 1988).

(ii) The risk–benefit relationship between competing treatments, especially when clinical effects are small, can be guided by HRQoL outcomes (Montazeri et al., 2000).

The value of a new healthcare intervention may also have to be considered through its benefit in terms of HRQoL and not only survival. Although some cancers are curable (e.g. testicular cancer), many of them are still considered to be incurable at this time. Therefore, one of the objectives of cancer patient management should be improving HRQoL, particularly toward the end of life, when few further treatment options are available (Drummond & O'Brien, 1993; Clauser, 2004; Gibbons, 2013).

(iii) Pre-diagnosis (baseline) assessment of HRQoL can help in clinical decision-making because baseline HRQoL may be directly related to a patient's survival time and can also be predictive of survival benefits during chemotherapy (Montazeri et al., 2001). Therefore, baseline HRQoL can be used to determine whether certain patients are more or less likely to benefit from a given treatment. Baseline HRQoL is also useful in controlling the considerable variations to estimate treatment differences for effects and costs (as those patients with better/poorer HRQoL at the start of the trial, may also be the same patients with higher/lower post-baseline costs and effects).

3.1.3 Challenges with HRQoL in Cancer Studies

There are several features about measuring HRQoL in cancer patients that are important. First, HRQoL assessments for the purposes of economic evaluation are often omitted. There are several reasons for this omission. For some countries economic evaluation is not important due to the specific healthcare system. Measures such as QALYs may not be so important (e.g. in the US) for decision-making. The issue becomes more complicated when a study conducted in a region where QALYs are not relevant to decision-makers (who pay for the treatment) is also submitted for licensing to, say, countries where the QALY is important (e.g. some European countries). When this happens, the payer perspective does become important. Countries that require HRQoL for decision-making are likely to criticize or even refuse to pay for cancer drugs, despite the drugs having a license for marketing authorization.

The second reason why HRQoL assessments for cost-effectiveness analyses are omitted is because emphasis is placed on the clinical- or disease-specific aspects of HRQoL. HRQoL measures for economic evaluation are often considered to lack sensitivity. A further reason for not collecting HRQoL for an economic evaluation might simply be because two treatments are considered to be equivalent, and therefore collecting HRQoL for an economic evaluation may not be useful (e.g. as in the case of biosimilar or generic drugs).

One key feature of a disease such as cancer is that patients can deteriorate rapidly thereby leading to an absence of data on both short-term and long-term effectiveness. Economic evaluation is often determined over a lifetime horizon, and without available HRQoL data performing a cost-effectiveness analysis can become challenging. Some studies report at least 50% of the data missing within 3 months of starting treatment (Temel et al., 2010) due to disease progression, death, or loss to follow-up. This may be due to short survival time of patients and/or their rapidly deteriorating health. For example, survival times for patients with NSCLC can be short (e.g. only 32% and 10% alive 1 and 5 years after diagnosis, respectively) (Hollen et al., 1997).

Estimation of HRQoL within a study/trial and beyond protocol-defined follow-up also plays a significant role in the economic evaluation of cancer drugs. Improved methods are needed for estimating long-term HRQoL for the cost-effectiveness of cancer drugs. The short survival time also restricts the opportunity to collect HRQoL data when there is a limited time window. This is often despite inclusion/exclusion criteria in protocols specifying a minimal life expectancy, because patients who progress quickly are likely to die quickly, resulting in missing data. A further challenge is ensuring the appropriate or optimal HRQoL is used. For example, the Functional Assessment of Cancer Therapy (FACT) FACT-L (specific to lung cancer) and Quality of Life Questionnaire (QLQ) QLQ-C30 (general cancer measure) can both be used to measure HRQoL in cancer patients resulting in different descriptions and measures of clinical benefit. HRQoL instruments used for measuring cancer HRQoL are discussed in the next section.

3.2 Measuring Health-Related Quality of Life Outcomes for Common Cancer Types

3.2.1 Condition-Specific Measures of HRQoL

Measuring HRQoL can be broadly classified into the two categories – condition-specific measures (CSM), which measure specific HRQoL symptoms (e.g. a cough, dyspnoea) and generic measures, which measure the broader HRQoL areas (e.g. mobility). Figure 3.1 illustrates the relation between some generic and condition-specific measures of HRQoL.

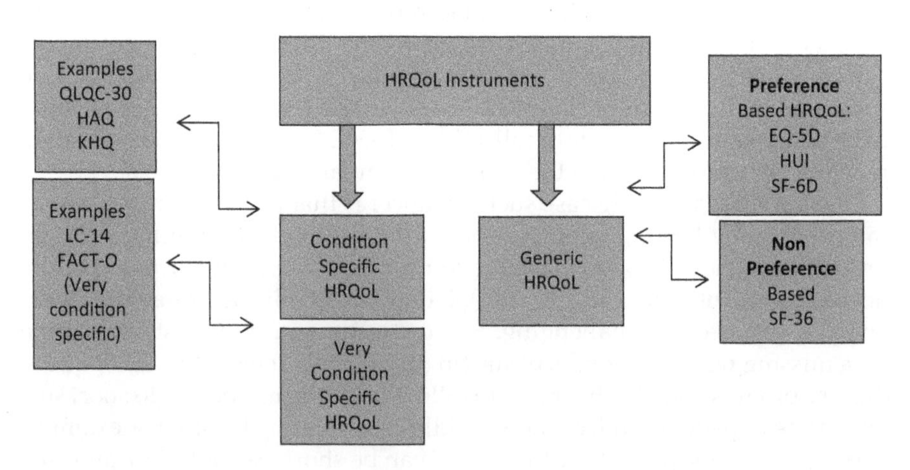

FIGURE 3.1
Relationship between generic and condition-specific HRQoL measures. (Note: LC-14: lung cancer symptom-specific questionnaire; HAQ: health assessment questionnaire; KHQ: King's health questionnaire; HUI: health utilities index; SF-6D: short-form 6D; FACT-O: specific to ovarian cancer.)

In most cancer studies, HRQoL assessments, wherever collected and reported, have been mainly restricted to condition-specific measures. A CSM is an instrument that captures the specific quality-of-life issues in patients who have a given disease. The QLQ-C30 and FACT-G are CSMs, but they are generic for cancer as they are used across several tumors. Very specific CSMs, often called subscales (e.g. European Organization for Research and Treatment of Cancer (EORTC) QLQ-LC13 for lung cancer), attempt to capture information on specific symptoms of the particular cancer and are additional questionnaires to the generic CSM. The wide use of CSMs is due to at least three reasons:

(a) First, CSMs were validated for estimating clinical effects and historically cost-effectiveness was not considered as part of their validation.
(b) Second, CSMs were considered more sensitive than other generic measures for estimating the HRQoL, focusing on specific symptom relief.
(c) Third, economic evaluation was not considered important. As budgets for healthcare became constrained, while demand for health resource use grew, the impetus for rationing healthcare resources became essential. For cost-effectiveness, HRQoL assessments from CSMs are not used unless responses can be converted into a generic preference-based measure. A cancer-specific preference-based CSM (e.g. QLQ-8D (Rowen et al., 2011)) could also be used for economic evaluation, but this is not so common, and, in any case, clinicians may be unlikely to use a short form when the full 30 questions could be used.

As an example, 26 out of 43 (60%) NSCLC studies (including RCTs) that assessed HRQoL included a symptom-specific measure such as the LC-13 (in addition to a generic cancer-specific measure) and only 2 studies (5%) used a generic measure. This suggests that using a generic HRQoL measure was considered inadequate to detect the clinical difference of interest (Gibbons et al., 2013).

3.2.2 Common General Condition-Specific Measures of HRQoL in Cancer

Table 3.1 shows a summary of the main features of some commonly used HRQoL instruments in various cancers. The important thing to note is that none of them are suitable for use in an economic evaluation for deriving QALYs. This is not to say that improved clinical benefits in these measures do not confer additional value. Certainly, if improvements in, for example, physical function are observed, it would not be incorrect to conclude that a treatment did not offer further value in HRQoL just because an alternative generic measure of HRQoL could not demonstrate a QALY difference.

TABLE 3.1

Summary of Cancer-Specific HRQoL Instruments for Common Cancers.

HRQoL Instrument	Cancer Type	Key Features	Outcome	Common Analysis Metric Reported	Useful for QALYs
EORTC-QLQ-C30	Generic across most cancers	15 subscales (5 symptom, 8 function, 1 global and 1 finance) formed from 30 questions Used in Europe	Each scale measured from 0 to 100	Mean difference Time to observe a specified difference Odd ratio	No
FACT-G	Generic across most cancers	4 subscales (physical social/family, emotional and functional well-being) from 27 items. Commonly used in US	22/27 (80%) complete for a total score ranging from 0–108 points.	Mean difference	No
Specific EORTC subscales					
QLQ-LC13	Lung	13 additional symptom specific questions	Each scale measured from 0 to 100	Mean difference	No
QLQ-OV28	Ovarian	28 additional symptom specific questions	Each scale measured from 0 to 100	Mean difference	No
QLQ-MY20	Lymphoma/myeloma	20 additional symptom specific questions	Each scale measured from 0 to 100	Mean difference	No
QLQ-BR23	Breast	23 additional symptom specific questions	Each scale measured from 0 to 100	Mean difference	No
QLQ-PR25	Prostate	25 additional symptom specific questions	Each scale measured from 0 to 100	Mean difference	No
Specific FACT subscales					
FACT-L	Lung	Uses 4 scales of FACT-G plus the lung cancer scale (LCS)	Trial Outcome Index (TOI) – total across 4 scales of FACT-G plus LCS	Mean difference	No

(Continued)

TABLE 3.1 (CONTINUED)

Summary of Cancer-Specific HRQoL Instruments for Common Cancers.

HRQoL Instrument	Cancer Type	Key Features	Outcome	Common Analysis Metric Reported	Useful for QALYs
FACT-O	Ovarian	FACT-G plus the ovarian cancer-specific subscale (OCS)	TOI of FACT-G and OCS	Mean difference	No
FACT-Lymp	Lymphoma	FACT-Lym and fifteen additional disease-specific items FACT-Lymp 15 additional items to the FACT-G (42 in total)	TOI of FACT-G and FACT-Lymp	Mean difference	No
FACT-B	Breast	10 items addressing symptoms and issues specifically relevant to patients with breast cancer on a 4-point scale, from 0 ('not at all') to 4 ('very much')	TOI: PWB+FWB+BCS subscale	Mean difference	No
	Prostate	FACT-P – prostate cancer subscale (PCS) plus including pain scale	TOI: PWB+FWB+EWB+ SWB + PCS + pain scale subscale		
FACT-Ntx	Neurological toxicity	11 items subscale	TOI of PWB+FWB+Ntx	Mean difference	

FACT: Functional Assessment of Cancer Therapy – General; P/F/E/S-WB: Physical/Functional/Emotional/Social/Well-Being

Consider two of the most common HRQoL measures in cancer clinical research: the EORTC QLQ-C30 and the FACT-G: Functional Assessment of Cancer Therapy – General (Hollen et al., 1997; Gibbons et al., 2013; Damm et al., 2013).

(i) The EORTC QLQ-C30 generic cancer instrument

The EORTC QLQ-C30 version 3 is a generic cancer instrument consisting of 30 questions, out of which 28 questions are measured on a 4-point scale ('not at all' (1) to 'very much' (4)) and 2 questions are measured on a 7-point scale. The 30 questions result in: 5 functional domains: Physical Functioning (PF), Role Functioning (RF), Emotional Functioning (EF), Cognitive Functioning (CF), and Social Functioning (SF); 8 symptom domains: Fatigue (FA), Nausea & Vomiting (NV), Pain (PA), Dyspnoea (DY), Sleep Disturbance (SL), Appetite Loss (AP), Constipation (CO), and Diarrhea (DI); and 2 further domains: Financial Impact (FI) and Global Quality of Life (QL).

All raw responses are transformed to a scale of 0 to 100, where a higher value represents better physical function for the function domains (including global and financial scales) and the converse for the symptom domains (a high value implies poorer symptoms).

The QLQ-C30 (Fayers, Aaronson, & Bjordal, 2001) has been well documented, has good psychometric properties, is validated, and is translated into more than 48 different languages with a large number of possible 'health states.' A health state, in economic evaluation terms, means combinations of different responses. For instance, one outcome for a particular patient from the QLQ-C30 could be 11111 … 1 (i.e. 30 responses of a value 1). This combination of 1s represents a 'health state. In this sense, there are $4^{28}+7^{2}$ possible health states. Inferences across all the possible health states are practically impossible. However, summary statistics are often computed for each domain, in terms of the average (mean) scores for which the health states are less relevant. Interested readers may refer to the EORTC's website for guidance on scoring (Fayers et al., 2001).

(ii) FACT-G

The FACT-G consists of 27 items: physical wellbeing (PW, 7 items), social and family well-being (SW, 7 items), emotional well-being (EW, 6 items), and functional well-being (FW, 7 items). Additional subscales can be added as in Table 3.1 to derive the Trial Outcome Index (TOI), a key measure of improvement in HRQoL with this instrument. This instrument also has a large number of possible health states (see Fayers et al., 2001).

The choice between utilizing FACT-G or QLQ-C30 is based on a subjective clinical choice, rather than empirical evidence for the superiority of one over the other. In fact, the empirical evidence presented for their relative superiority can be considered minimal or nonexistent (Gibbons et al., 2013; Calman, 1984).

A related issue is which instrument is more (or less) sensitive to detecting a clinically relevant treatment benefit and what is the clinically and/or economically relevant effect size from these measures (an economically relevant effect in this context refers to a clinical effect size such that the incremental net monetary benefit (INMB) has a high chance of being positive (see Khan, 2015) for sample sizes for cost-effectiveness). This aspect still remains unknown and is not well understood. Maringwa et al. have suggested important effect sizes of varying magnitudes (e.g. a difference of 10 points) (Maringwa et al., 2011). Comparing effect sizes between the varying HRQoL measures has not been widely reported, particularly in NSCLC. In contrast, generic measures of HRQoL have been criticized for the lack of sensitivity to detect HRQoL benefits, something that has implications for later cost-effectiveness (Ades, Lu, & Madan, 2013). A further issue is that a QALY, a key outcome for estimating cost-effectiveness is not usually constructed from CSMs, but from generic measures of HRQoL.

3.3 Measuring HRQoL for Economic Evaluation

Evaluating and measuring HRQoL benefit is an important aspect of economic evaluation. Generic measures of HRQoL capture responses about health in general and not the symptoms that might be associated with toxicity (resulting from chemotherapy, radiotherapy, and surgery). They are useful for comparing effects across a variety of diseases. Some generic measures reflect a patient's preference for certain health states, termed 'preference-based' measures (PBM) because they offer a way in which (subjective or perceived) relative preferences (or values) for specific health states can be expressed by individuals as 'preference weights' or 'utilities.' Utilities are based on subjective judgments by individuals presented with questions such as: "Do you prefer an apple or banana?" and are derived from consumer choice theory in economics. These utilities can subsequently be used to adjust observed clinical effects for later cost-effectiveness analyses or used directly as a measure of effect such as a QALY.

A utility value is often measured on a continuous scale and, depending on which instrument is used, these values have different ranges (lowest and highest values). The health utility index (HUI), for instance, generates utilities on a scale from 0 to 1, where 0 represents 'dead,' which is the worst health state possible and 1 represents 'Full health.' However, not all generic measures of HRQoL generate utilities on a scale between 0 and 1, for example the EQ-5D. Other preference-based generic HRQoL measures include: SF-6D: Short Form 6D; HUI: Health Utilities Index (versions I, II and III); and the more common EuroQol EQ-5D (EQ-5D-3L and 5L) (Carreon et al., 2013; Herdman et al., 2011; Rabin et al., 2001).

Although responses from the cancer specific QLQ-C30 reflects how a given patient might feel with regard to their symptoms, disease, or treatment received, the responses do not necessarily reflect how payers (people who ultimately pay for treatments through taxes) perceive the value of a given patient's health condition, even if the patient is suffering from a disease as severe as breast cancer. It is possible that society (and not necessarily doctors) might regard a specific patient's health (state) as far worse and therefore believe any funds available to treat a patient's illness should be spent elsewhere (e.g. preference for a prostate cancer sufferer over a breast cancer patient). CSMs do not incorporate a relative evaluation of the extent to which a specific symptom or health state affects the overall perception of health. For instance, severe nausea might be considered worse than severe pain for some patients but not for others. The expression of such relative preferences (utilities) is determined through preference-based HRQoL measures. The QLQ-C30 and the FACT are not preference-based measures of HRQoL and, therefore, cannot be directly used as such in an economic evaluation.

The most common preference-based measures used in the UK (and many European countries) for economic evaluation are the EuroQol EQ-5D-3L and the more recent EQ-5D-5L.

3.3.1 EuroQol EQ-5D-3L and 5L

The EQ-5D is a widely used generic measure, which is the shortest and perhaps the least cognitively demanding instrument that appears to be at least as responsive as the other community- (preference-) weighted instruments (Brazier et al., 2007).

EQ-5D-3L consists of a descriptive health state classification system with five questions (mobility, self-care, usual activities, pain/discomfort, and anxiety/depression), measured on three severity levels – 'no problems,' 'some problems,' and 'extreme problems.' Combining one level from each question defines 243 different health states, ranging from full health (value of 1) to worst health or death (value of 0). A health state defined by the descriptive system of EQ-5D can be described by a five-digit number. For instance, 12113 refers to a patient who has no problems with mobility (1), some problems with self-care (2), no problems for usual activities (1) or pain/discomfort (1), and extreme problems with anxiety/depression (3). Full health is indicated by 11111 and the poorest health state by 33333. In practice, the raw responses are converted into a utility scale from –0.594 to 1 (1 is full health and –0.594 represents the worst possible state – even worse than death), depending on the method (called the tariff) of converting the responses into utilities. Some tariffs result in utilities between –0.109 to 1 (Dolan, 1997; Shaw, Johnson, & Coons, 2005). The Dolan UK tariff results in utilities in the –0.594 to 1.0 range.

The term 'health state' requires some elaboration. Given that the EQ-5D-3L consists of a descriptive health state classification system with five domains and 243 different health states ranging from full health (11111) to worst health

(33333). Values such as 11111 or 21333 are not easily analyzed but converting these responses to a utility value will allow analysis. Each of these health states is therefore converted to a single number, called a utility value: a value from –0.594 (worse than death) to 1 (full health). This is true if the conversion from values such as 11111 is based on the 'tariff' provided by Dolan (Dolan, 1997). An alternative tariff of Shaw et al. (Shaw et al., 2005) converts the health states to a range between –0.109 to 1.0 (Lewis et al., 2010; Dunlop et al., 2013). The word 'tariff' refers to the weights applied to health states to generate the final EQ-5D value. Tariffs are country specific (if they exist) and are estimated from general public surveys.

There are various reasons why the EQ-5D is emphasized, at least in some parts of Europe. It is for example recommended for use in economic evaluations in the UK, by NICE (Brazier et al., 2011; Brazier et al., 2016). It is not uncommon that when NICE adopts a decision on the value of a cancer drug, some (but not all) countries follow a similar decision (but not necessarily using QALYs). Hence, the EQ-5D is also used in several countries as a part of economic evaluation and health technology appraisal (HTA). The EQ-5D's properties are well documented (Brazier & Rowen, 2011) and it has been shown to be a reliable and valid HRQoL measure (Hurst et al., 1997; Van Agt et al., 2005).

3.3.2 EuroQol EQ-5D-5L

The EQ-5D-5L is a revision of the EQ-5D-3L. It consists of five questions, identical to EQ-5D-3L (mobility, self-care, usual activities, pain/discomfort, and anxiety/depression), but with an expanded 5-point scale and slightly different descriptors for each of the levels compared to the 3-point scale of the EQ-5D-3L (Carreon et al., 2013). These are: mobility, self-care, and usual activities: 1: 'no problems'; 2: 'slight problems'; 3: 'moderate problems'; 4: 'severe problems'; and 5: 'unable to'; for the pain/discomfort and anxiety/depression scale, these are: 1: 'no'; 2: 'slight'; 3: 'moderate'; 4: 'severe'; and 5: 'extreme.' The scores are on a 5-point scale 1 to 5 (for each of the 5 domains). A perfect health state is '11111' and the worst possible health state would be '55555'. There are 3,125 health states that can be identified using EQ-5D-5L. The corresponding minimum and maximal values are –0.281 for a health state of 55555 and a value of 1 for the 11111 health state.

Predetermined scoring algorithms for EQ-5D have been developed in order to yield community-based health utility estimates (i.e. relative preferences for health states not based on what the patients think but what the general population believes) – specific to a given country. The derived utilities are determined from a predetermined algorithm called a utility function. The utilities from these instruments (such as the EQ-5D, HUI, and other preference-based measures) may subsequently be applied as a weight to clinical measures, such as overall survival or progression-free survival (PFS) time in order to derive a quality-adjusted life-year (QALY).

The primary difference between these two instruments (3L and 5L) is that the latter has responses measured on a 5-point scale, with many more health states (Oppe et al., 2014). EQ-5D-3L is reported to have limited discriminative ability (though it may have higher power to detect differences between groups) compared to EQ-5D-5L (Dolan, 1997; Oppe et al., 2014; Van Hout et al., 2012). Recently EQ-5D-5L tariffs have been developed for the UK and several other countries (Zhao, Li, Liu, Zhang, & Chen, 2017).

3.4 Constructing Utilities

Utility elicitation methods may be classified as direct or indirect methods of health utility elicitation (Figure 3.1) (Sacco et al., 2010). Most direct elicitation methods include some sort of trade-off (standard gamble [SG], time trade-off [TTO]), or a visual analog scale (VAS), but direct utility elicitation is rarely performed in clinical trials. Furthermore, as cost-effectiveness studies are intended to support health policy decisions, utility values from the general population are preferred (Rowen et al., 2015; Batty et al., 2012), and healthcare providers' utilities are considered as valid. Terminally ill patients, children, and dementia patients raise special problems where a proxy person (e.g. a carer) may be used as a substitute for the patient, though as a second-best option.

Direct elicitation, such as time trade-off involves asking people (patients or members of the general public) to trade a given time (e.g. 10 years) in a hypothetical or current health state worse than full health for a lower survival time in full health. The data collected from these choices (trade-offs) are then analyzed to derive a utility score. An example of such elicitation for chemotherapy in breast cancer patients can be found in Simes (Simes & Coates, 2001).

The main indirect methods of utility measurement consist in the use of a generic preference-based instrument (G-PBM), such as the EQ-5D, or a condition-specific preference measure (CS-PBM), such as the QLQ-8D, with their relevant health-profile associated utilities or utility-generating formula (Hao, Wolfram, & Cook, 2016; Lorgelly et al., 2017). Another type of utility generating method is based on mapping utilities indirectly via a generic non-PBM HRQoL questionnaire such as the QLQC30 or the FACT-G via a (published) mapping algorithm that predicts (maps) the components of the HRQoL questionnaire to a PBM utility (Wailoo et al., 2017; Figure 3.2).

The benefit of direct elicitation alongside an RCT is that such valuation of health states within an RCT framework has strong internal validity. In addition, for patients who survive beyond the median survival time, an accurate reflection of the value of health states toward end of life might be possible. However, using direct valuation methods from cancer patients alongside

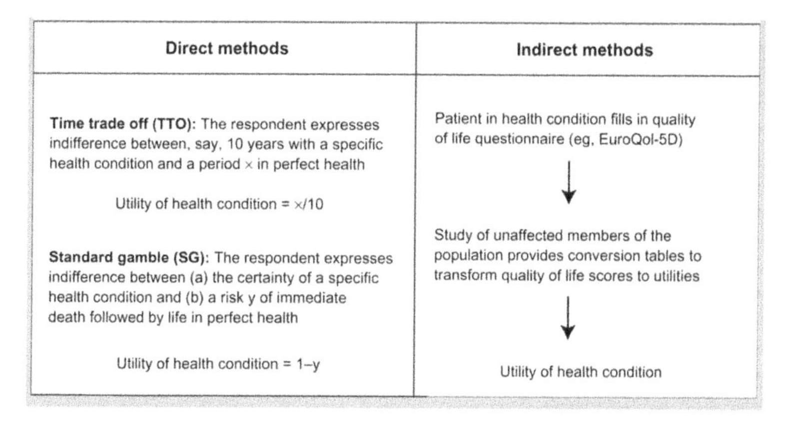

FIGURE 3.2
The EQ-5D utility function in terms of health states.

Source: Sacco et al., 2010.

a clinical trial is difficult in practice because of the poor prognosis, short median survival times, and the complex logistics and ethical considerations involved in clinical trial conduct. It may require extending the duration of the trial perhaps by following up patients until death, which would be impractical in most cases. For example, in order to estimate longer-term HRQoL effects (e.g. valuing health states toward the end of life), some patients would need to be followed up in the trial much longer as part of the same protocol. In practice, after cancer progression, follow-up for many outcomes (other than necessary longer-term safety) is often stopped. Trial governance may also complicate the process of further assessments once a patient's main follow-up has been completed. Moreover, patients in some clinical trials are often extremely ill and there is a serious debate about whether the patients are capable of ascertaining their health status through TTO and SG methods. The complex articulations can be daunting and time-consuming for some cancer patients, especially when they are preoccupied with a variety of other tests such as imaging scans, blood tests, and radiotherapy planning.

In health economics, the concepts of utility and utility functions are central for appreciating why for example health states from EQ-5D assume values between –0.594 and 1.0. A utility function is a mathematical representation of determining utilities for preferences of given health states. Mathematically, for each patient, i, the EQ-5D-3L utility U_i under the assumption of linear additivity is equal to:

$$U_i = 1 - (0.081 * K - \alpha_1 * M_i - \alpha_2 * S_i - \alpha_3 * US_i - \alpha_4 * P_i - \alpha_5 * A_i - \alpha_6)$$

Source: (Dolan, 1997)

where, $\alpha_1 \ldots \alpha_6$ are weights derived from TTO utility elicitation, such that for patient i: $\alpha_1 = 0$ if the mobility score $M_j = 1$, $\alpha_1 = 0.069$ if the mobility score

$M_j = 2$, and $\alpha_1 = 0.314$ if $M_j = 3$ ($j = 1$ to 3, referring to the 3-level response for each question)

Similarly,

$\alpha_2 = 0.104$ if the self-care score $S_i = 2$, and $\alpha_2 = 0.214$ if $S_i = 3$,
$\alpha_3 = 0.036$ if the usual activities $US_i = 2$, and $\alpha_2 = 0.094$ if $US_i = 3$,
$\alpha_4 = 0.386$ if the pain score $P_i = 2$, and $\alpha_2 = 0.123$ if $P_i = 3$,
$\alpha_5 = 0.071$ if the anxiety score $A_i = 2$, and $\alpha_2 = 0.236$ if $A_i = 3$,
$\alpha_6 = 0.269$ if any of the M_i, S_i, US_i, P_i, or A_i is a score of 3, otherwise $\alpha_6 = 0$,

and finally, K is the indicator variable, which takes the value 1 if any health state is dysfunctional (>1), otherwise, it is 0. The utility values are ordered from lowest to highest and a numerical coding can be given to the ordered health states (11111 = 1, 2 = 21112 = 0.878 … 3 = 33333 = −0.549). For example, for a health state of 12123, U_i would be 1 − (0.081 + 0 + 0.104 + 0 + 0.123 + 0.236 + 0.269) = 0.187.

3.5 Quality-Adjusted Life-Years (QALYs)

In economic evaluation, the use of HRQoL is particularly important for cost utility analyses (CUA). CUA is a method of determining the cost-effectiveness of a new health technology by combining HRQoL with clinical outcomes (e.g. survival time) to derive a quality-adjusted life-year (QALY). In Chapter 1, we briefly introduced the QALY in a rather simple way as a combination of the quantity and HRQoL. Utility values determined from the EQ-5D-3L (or 5L) were described in Sections 3.2 and 3.3. A commonly described way of deriving the QALY is by computing the area under the curve (AUC) as shown in Figure 3.3. The difference between the areas under the solid line and the area under the dotted line in Figure 3.3 is the incremental QALY.

In Figure 3.3, the HRQoL responses from the EQ-5D are converted into utilities on a scale from either 0 to 1 or, as in the case of the EQ-5D-3L, from −0.54 to 1.0. Utility measures were collected from baseline (time 0) until 24 months (when the follow-up is final). If continuous measures are available from patients in each of the two treatment groups A and B, then we obtain two curves as shown in Figure 3.3, one for each treatment group describing the behavior of utility over time. In practice only a few HRQoL measurements at fixed discrete time points are available (say every 3 months).

The next step is to calculate the AUC for each utility curve. This area is the QALY. The area can be tricky to calculate sometimes, but it is usually straightforward. For example, if the utility score never changed from

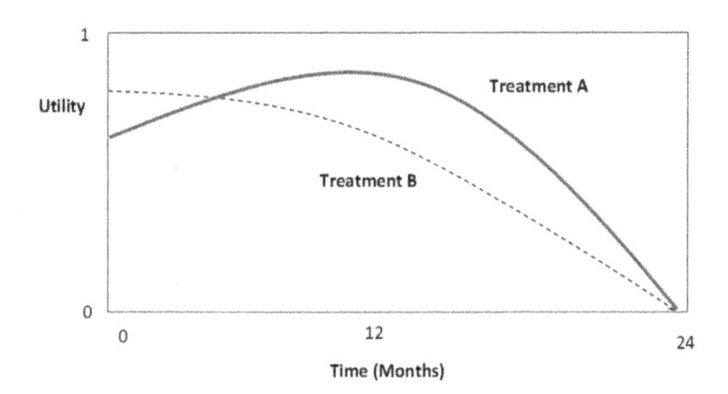

FIGURE 3.3
Theoretical QALY determination between treatment A and B with repeated measurements.

baseline and was always 0.80 every 3 months until 24 months, the area would be the same as the area of a rectangle of 24 × 0.8 = 19.2 months = 1.6 QALY years (i.e. 2 years × 0.80). The difference between the AUC for treatment A and AUC for treatment B is the incremental QALY. When the utility profiles are more complicated, the AUC is computed by dividing the area under the curve into several trapeziums and using the trapezoidal rule to calculate the area of each trapezium and add up all the areas. The area of a trapezium is ½(sum of the parallel sides) × perpendicular height: $½*(a + b)*t$, where a and b are the utilities on the Y-axis and t is the difference between adjacent time points. A more complicated application in a cancer setting is demonstrated in Example 3.1.

3.5.1 QALY Calculation in Cancer Trials

The description above for the calculation of the QALY is reasonably straightforward. There are some complications in that at the end of the follow-up, some assumptions about the (future) unobserved utility need to be made. For example, if the trial is completed after 24 months, and some patients are still alive, what should we assume about the behavior of the utility beyond 24 months? One possibility is to assume it is the same as what was observed at 24 months (last observation carried forward). However, if disease progression occurred at 24 months, we might expect the utility to get worse and therefore the assumption of a constant utility is likely to bias the QALY (upward).

A simple formula that weights the utility by the proportion alive (determined from the Kaplan Meier curve) can be used:

$$QALY_{\text{AUC}} = \Sigma\left[\left(Q_i + Q_{i+1}\right)/2\right]*\left[\left(S_i + S_{i+1}\right)/2\right]*\left[t_{i+1} - t_i\right] \tag{3.1}$$

where Q_i are the mean utilities at time point t and S_i are the survival proportions (e.g. from the Kaplan-Meir curve) at the corresponding time point, t.

The subscript i refers to the time points (e.g. t_0 = baseline, t_1 is the first time point at which utility are observed) and the summation ($\sum$) is over the number of time points. A demonstration of the formula in equation (3.1) follows.

Example 3.1: Deriving the QALY from Survival and Utility Data

Using equation (3.1),

$$\text{QALY}_{\text{AUC}} = \Sigma\left[(Q_i + Q_{i+1})/2\right]*\left[(S_i + S_{i+1})/2\right]*\left[t_{i+1} - t_i\right]$$

we obtain

$$\begin{aligned}\text{QALY}_{\text{AUC}} = &(0.65+0.71)/2*\left[(1.00+0.69)/2\right]*[1-0]\\ &+(0.71+0.72)/2*\left[(0.50+0.69)/2\right]*[3-2]\\ &+(0.69+0.72)/2*\left[(0.32+0.50)/2\right]*[4-3]\\ &+(0.75+0.69)/2*\left[(0.23+0.32)/2\right]*[5-4]+\text{etc.}\end{aligned}$$

Separate to the issue about what to assume about future non-observed utility, is how the QALY is derived when taking into account the pre-progression (progression-free survival) and the post-disease progression periods. A useful feature of the AUC approach is that the AUC is computed by taking into account the corresponding utility during the survival experience. In equation (3.1) the mean utilities are computed for those patients who have and have not progressed. These are then multiplied by the proportion alive. In cancer trials, partitioned survival models (Chapter 7) separate the survival experience into a pre-progression survival (PFS) and a post-progression survival (PPS) period. Hence, OS = PFS + PPS. The mean pre-progression utilities can be used to derive a pre-progression QALY and similarly a post-progression QALY can be derived. This will be discussed in Section 3.7.

3.6 Economic Evaluation in the Absence of Utility Data: Mapping and Utility Studies

Damm (Damm et al., 2013) reports instances where a CSM, in this case the QLQ-C30, was used yet no generic HRQoL was included. Moreover, an economic evaluation of some form was performed using the same data at a later point (e.g. the BR21 trial (Bradbury et al., 2010; Lewis et al., 2010)). In these trials, generic HRQoL data for economic evaluation could have been collected instead of relying on alternative sources (e.g. historically reported). There are several possible reasons why utility data may not be available or collected in a trial, despite cost utility analyses being conducted later:

(i) Several examples in literature report the main results of clinical trials (e.g. Bradbury et al., 2010) where utility data were not collected. One reason is that in some countries the health system does not require cost utility analyses. Therefore, cost-effectiveness was not part of trial design (e.g. submission to the FDA in the US). However, the same clinical data is used for licensing purposes in Europe, where some countries consider QALYs important. Therefore, estimates of patient-level utilities are not available but a CUA is required.

(ii) A second reason might be that EQ-5D are not considered sensitive enough to detect treatment benefit, which may be a reason to avoid them. Clinicians responsible for protocol development may not focus on the 'softer' measures like HRQoL, and even less so on utilities, and therefore do not include these outcomes in the protocols and data collection.

(iii) Direct elicitation studies sometimes involve estimating utilities in separate, smaller specific studies. These can yield biased or imprecise utilities, which affect the QALYs, giving a reason to avoid such an approach (Dunlop et al., 2013). NICE recommends avoiding separate utility studies (Brazier et al., 2011; NICE DSU 2016).

(iv) A further reason is that cost-effectiveness may not be considered important. However, when the cost of cancer drugs is perceived to be high, payers re-evaluate the value of cancer drugs, thus this reason is unlikely to be sustainable. In addition, grant-awarding bodies (for academic trials) request details of the cost-effectiveness of proposed interventions that have potential to become the standard of care.

When utility data are not available, but a cost-utility analysis is required, utilities can be determined by an indirect method called mapping or by using published historical utility data. Mapping or 'cross-walking' can be useful when patient-level utilities are not available in a clinical trial. A statistical model sometimes termed a 'mapping algorithm,' is used to predict (estimate) EQ-5D-3L utilities from a disease-specific measure such as QLQ-C30. If patient level EQ-5D-3L cannot be obtained, then it becomes challenging to conduct an economic evaluation with patient-level data, and reliance is often placed on published aggregate utilities. Mapping is, therefore, another way (and sometimes the only way) to estimate patient-level utilities for a cost-effectiveness analysis. Details of mapping for cancer can be found elsewhere (Crott & Briggs, 2010; Crott, Versteegh, & Uyl-De-Groot, 2013; Khan et al., 2016; Brazier et al., 2010; Doble & Lorgelly, 2016). The alternative approach is to use historical data or published utilities such as those reported in Nafees et al. (2008) (see Section 3.8 for examples).

3.7 Sensitivity and Responsiveness of EQ-5D versus QLQ-C30 HRQoL for Detecting Improvement in Cancer Patients

Some generic instruments may not be adequate to demonstrate HRQoL benefits, compared to condition-specific measures (CSM) (e.g. Lee et al., 2013; De Vine et al., 2011; Malkin et al., 2013; Krahn et al., 2007). This is because a brief and standardized HRQoL instrument across diseases will lack sensitivity due to its nature (Malkin et al., 2013). Concerns about the sensitivity and responsiveness of generic measures such as the EQ-5D-3L (Buchholz, Thielker, Feng, Kupatz, & Kohlmann, 2015; Richardson, Khan, Iezzi, & Maxwell, 2015) have been important enough to lead to the development of the EQ-5D-5L, using a 5-point scale instead (EQ-5D-3L has a 3-point scale). The issue becomes more acute and more relevant where a CSM appears to offer an interpretation for a treatment benefit inconsistent with a generic one (or vice versa).

It is also unclear, not only in cancer studies but also in many trials with HRQoL endpoints (either as primary or secondary endpoints), what a relevant clinical or economic treatment difference is (or the size of the minimum clinical important difference (MCID)). Moreover, which among the common HRQoL measures (in cancer) are more sensitive in detecting HRQoL benefits remains highly uncertain (Buchholz et al., 2015; Richardson et al., 2015). This is relevant whether the HRQoL is primary or secondary because HRQoL effects are often considered to 'add value' to an intervention, especially when the primary outcome result shows modest or borderline benefits.

For instance, with QLQ-C30, there are 15 possible different effect sizes but only 1 for EQ-5D. The precise clinical or economic relevance of such effect sizes still remains unknown or not well understood. Maringwa et al. (2011) suggest important effect sizes of varying magnitudes (Maringwa et al., 2011), although in practice these are rarely stated up-front. A suggested effect size of 10 points (it is unclear whether this is for a particular domain or any domain of the QLQ-C30) is assumed to be an important difference yet it is unclear why this should be the case. Moreover, this suggestion was made many years ago when novel cancer treatments at the time were compared to an older class of drugs. As the standard of care has improved, and because economic evaluation often requires the 'best' standard of care for comparison, treatment benefits are likely to be smaller and this definition, despite its wide used is likely to be redundant (King, 1996; Osoba, 2007; Pickard et al., 2007).

Generic measures are considered to lack the sensitivity to detect HRQoL benefits when compared to CSMs. However, if the treatment benefits are similar between a CSM and a generic measure, then a simpler and shorter preference-based generic measure (e.g. EQ-5D) could be used with a highly condition-specific measure (e.g. such as the lung cancer symptom-specific LC-14 questionnaire, as in Figure 3.1) without losing much information. With preference-based measures, there may be a concern that preference weights from the general population may not reflect the similar relative importance for certain health states that a cancer patient might portray. However, the EQ-5D-3L is considered to lack sensitivity for measuring changes in health states in a cancer setting (Bongers et al., 2011).

In a systematic review of 43 published articles in NSCLC (Damm et al., 2013), for example, 28 of the studies used the QLQ-C30 with the objective of detecting clinical improvements in HRQoL. Among these 28 studies, the vast majority (>80%) did not report improvements with the QLQ-C30, either between treatments or relative to baseline. Moreover, wherever an effect was detected, the sample size was small. Khan et al. (2015) report that condition-specific HRQoL treatment effect sizes in lung cancer trials are rarely large (Khan, Bashir, & Forster, 2015).

Conclusions regarding HRQoL benefits are often provided in terms of 'non-worsening HRQoL' and although a few studies report small improvements, most report no improvements in HRQoL. The conclusions are often presented such that if patients did not deteriorate in their HRQoL, then this is something worthy of comment or a favorable outcome (see Damm et al., 2013). A more complicated situation is when a CSM suggests an HRQoL improvement and a preference-based measure does not. One should recall that utilities for the EQ-5D are based on societal preferences in general populations, whereas CSM measures are determined from cancer patients, which may explain some of the discrepancies.

Small, but important differences in HRQoL should not be ignored (Khan et al., 2015) but investigated further with a view to identifying the implications for an economic evaluation. For example, a small mean difference in EQ-5D (e.g. 0.05 point improvement in physical function) on an odds ratio scale might translate to 20% improvement in HRQoL (this can happen when the data are heavily skewed). It would be misleading to conclude HRQoL improvements do not exist when small mean differences are observed. This approach may help to contextualize borderline QALY differences, particularly where a generic measure lacks sensitivity.

3.8 Measuring Post-Progression (PP) Utility: Some Approaches

Patients with cancer often have progressive disease during or after anti-cancer treatment. The consequence of this on utility estimation can be serious because, as patients deteriorate, the availability of post-progression utility data becomes problematic. In clinical trials, HRQoL is often planned to be collected until disease progression and, in some instances, until death. PP survival can vary depending on factors such as the underlying cancer, severity of the disease, and availability of other treatments. What happens in some clinical trials is that some patients have available HRQoL after disease progression and others do not. A further complication is that even where data are available after progression, the follow-up times may vary from patient to patient.

Earlier, in Section 3.5, we noted mapping as a means to estimate utilities. However, the development of mapping models depends on the availability of both generic measures and CSMs from the same patient sample. Furthermore, many mapping models available in cancer do not specifically offer algorithms for predicting PP utility data. When PD has occurred, both generic measures and CSMs are not collected and the lack of utility data after PD does have a consequence for cost-effectiveness. One approach might therefore be to develop a model to extrapolate utilities after PD (Figure 3.4).

The difference between this approach and mapping is that the estimation of utilities beyond disease progression does not need to depend on a CSM. Mapping involves the use of a CSM to estimate utilities, whereas in this approach, the utilities are extrapolated by modeling available data. In this section, we therefore discuss an empirical examination of patterns of PP utility data and consider the principles of some statistical models for estimating PP utility data and their relevance to QALY estimation for cancer treatments. It is not uncommon to model survival data in a similar way where long-term survival patterns are estimated using complex models.

Why Is Estimation of Utility between Disease Progression and Death Relevant?

There are several reasons why PP utility data are important:

(i) The QALYs computed in economic evaluations of cancer treatments are often computed as a weighted measure of PFS and PPS, using the partitioned survival model approach mentioned in Section 3.4. Therefore, how post-progression utilities are estimated, either directly or in some other way, influences the overall QALY.

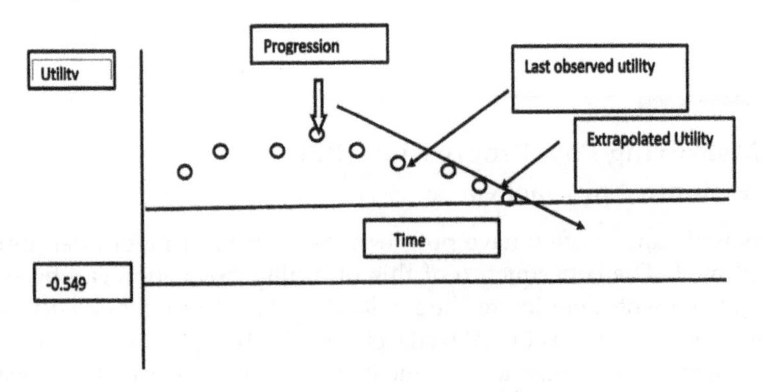

FIGURE 3.4
Post-progression linear decreasing utility function.

(ii) Estimating utility beyond PD is important especially when treatment is planned to be delivered beyond progression (e.g. as in the case of more recent immunotherapy advances like Nivolumab (NICE, 2017; Ulmeanu, Antohe, Anisie, & Antoniu, 2016). This will be important to determine whether it is worthwhile for patients (and payers) to be treated beyond PD.

(iii) For some anti-cancer treatments, late toxicities can occur (e.g. from radiotherapy or surgery), which may have a marked impact on HRQoL for years, or even lifelong, after the treatment has been delivered.

(iv) If no HRQoL data are available after disease progression, then there is likely to be greater uncertainty around the QALY (due to the dependence of utility from external or historical data). In practice, some patients are able to provide HRQoL data after PD as long as it is not too difficult to collect. The EQ-5D is a short and simple HRQoL measure, unlike the QLQ-C30, which facilitates collection of these data. The availability of these data can have significant implications for economic evaluation.

The Behavior of Utility in Cancer Patients between Progression and Death?

One may reasonably expect, as patients' health worsens, HRQoL deteriorates. Therefore, many patterns of post-progression HRQoL are possible:

(a) The utility between progression and death falls linearly at some constant rate from the last observed time (i.e. last time when progression occurred) point it was measured (until death).

(b) The PP utility falls either in a concave or convex fashion (Figure 3.5).

(c) The PP utility oscillates between various health states over time and eventually declines (e.g. due to multiple sequences of treatments).

The assumption that the PP utility falls at a constant rate between progression and death is unlikely to be realistic. A possible situation that might entertain this assumption is in long-term survivors who are no longer at risk for relapse and where the sequelae and the adaptation by the patient to the sequalae has stabilized. However, this is still better than the even stronger assumption that the utility is constant from the last observed utility, like a type of last observation carried forward (see, for example, Dunlop et al. (2012). This may be completely unrealistic in situations where the disease worsens (or improves) over time.

In Figure 3.5, the region below zero reflects the state worse than death. This implies that if a patient has a predicted utility of zero (death) at time t, it is not possible to predict a utility at time t+1 because the patient is assumed

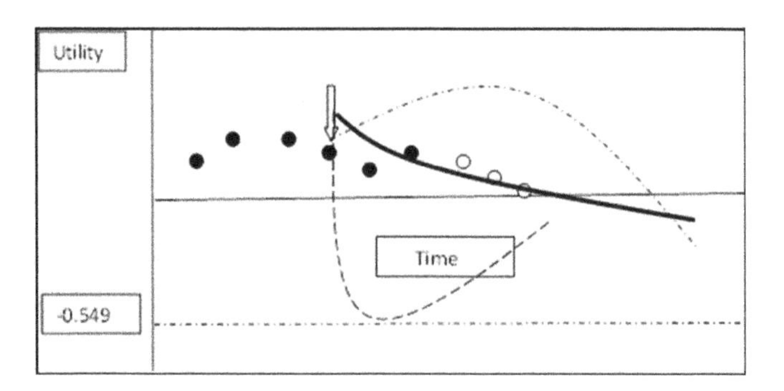

FIGURE 3.5
Post-progression non-linear decreasing utility functions.

to have reached an equivalent of a 'death' state. Using a linear decreasing utility function (or the constant assumption for that matter) does not allow estimates of utilities to weave between states worse than death (utilities < 0) and death (utility = 0). Therefore, either a transformation has to be used to map the utilities on the interval (0 to 1) or a more flexible utility function is needed. A utility value of zero does not mean the patient is not alive (it is representative of a health state equivalent to death).

3.8.1 Plausible Post-Progression Utility Behavior

Figure 3.6 shows the PP behavior from patients collected in an observational study (Khan et al., 2016). The figure appears to show great heterogeneity in

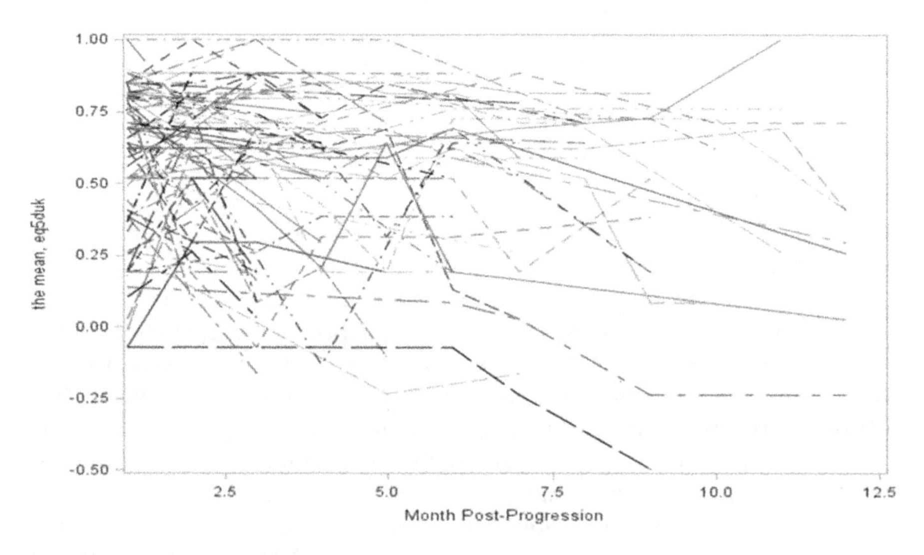

FIGURE 3.6
Post-progression patient profiles.

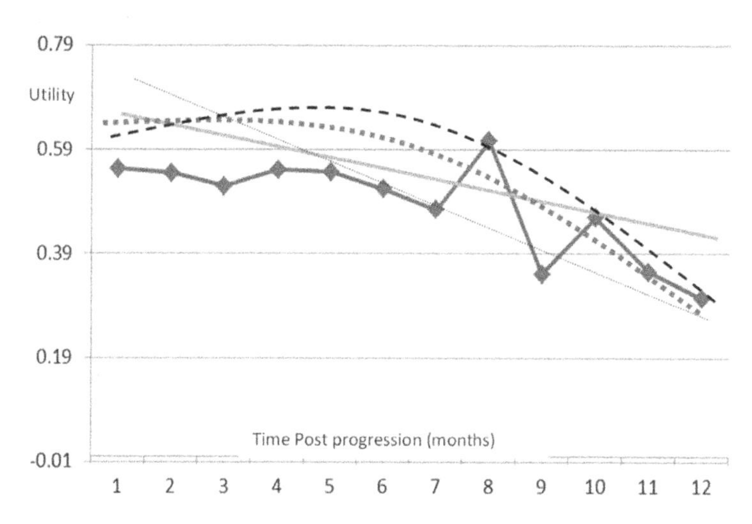

FIGURE 3.7
Mean observed utilities post-progression over time with superimposed possible models (using data from Figure 3.5).

PP utility profiles. Most profiles tend to show a decline in utility after progression, even if there appear to be some spikes.

These profiles can in general be categorized in some key types of behavior (Figure 3.7). Figure 3.8a shows rapidly deteriorating utility after progression, with a 'spike' at around 5 months, followed again by a rapid decline. On the other hand, Figure 3.8c shows an improvement followed by a steadier decline. If a constant value or a linear function is used to estimate PP utility, the estimated utility and QALY are likely to be misleading. Due to the highly variable nature of the PP utility–time profile, a modeling approach using the combined data (for those patients with PP data) who are alive or dead is considered (because fitting a model to each patient's PP utility data profile is likely to be impracticable). Figure 3.7 shows the mean utility plot post-progression with some possible models.

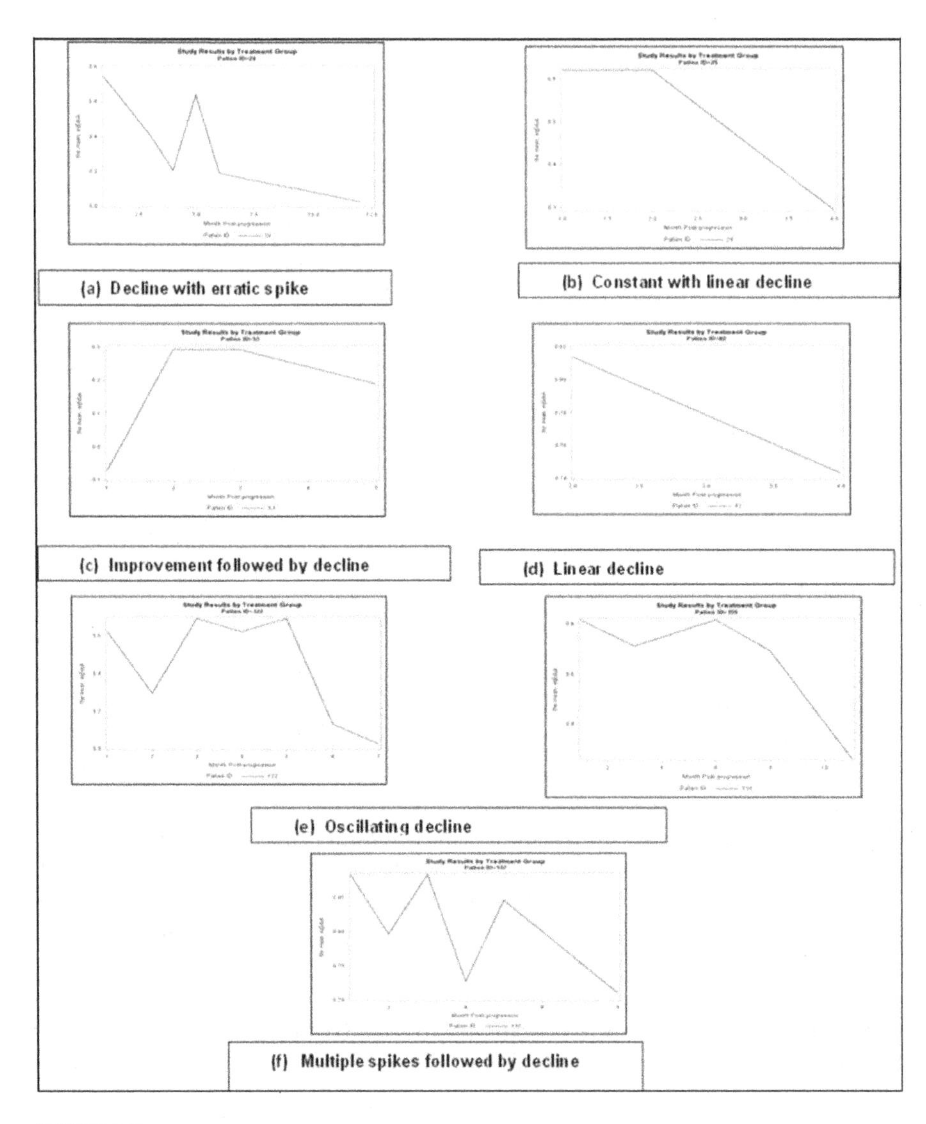

FIGURE 3.8
(a) to (f): Post-progression individual patient profile instances.

Source: Data from Study 3 in Khan et al., 2016.

3.8.2 Non-Linear Models

Several non-linear models are also plausible to model the PP utility: Two graphical representations of models are shown as an example. The Y-axis in each of the graphs in Figure 3.8 shows utilities and the X-axis is a time variable showing the number of months PP:

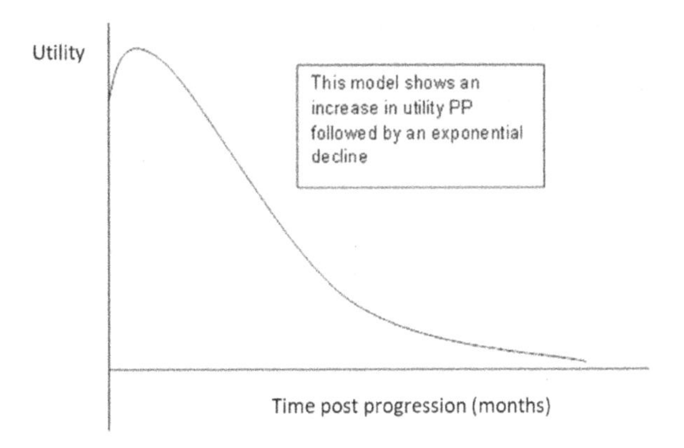

FIGURE 3.9
Bragg and Packer Model (1962) for post-progression utility.

(i) Using the Bragg and Packer (1962) 4-parameter equation (Ratkwosky, 1989)

$$\mathbf{EQ-5D} = \alpha + \beta * \mathbf{exp}\{-\gamma(\mathbf{X}-\delta)^2\}$$

An example of this equation depending upon the parameters α, β, γ and δ shown in Figure 3.9)

(ii) Using a derivation of the Pareto distribution (Ratkwosky, 1989), the equation:

$$\mathbf{EQ-5D} = \mathbf{1 - 1 / X^{\alpha}}$$

where $\alpha < -1$

yields a convex shape that, although it does not allow for an increase, indicates a slower rate of HRQoL/utility deterioration. This function also allows for an estimation of utility at a time that would equal zero (unlike the asymptote in (i) above) – (Figure 3.10).

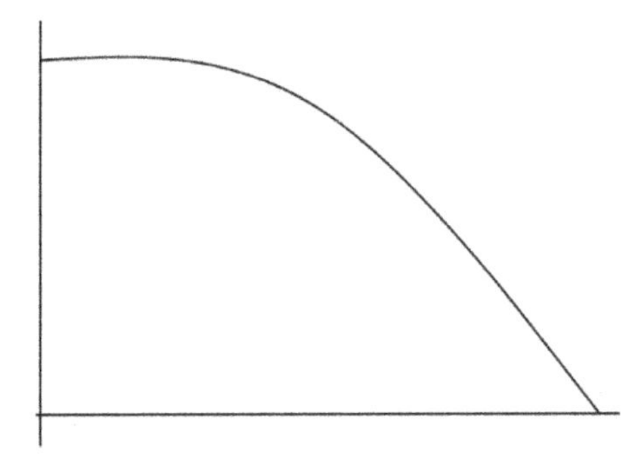

FIGURE 3.10
Pareto-type model for post-progression utility.

Example 3.2: Fitting a Number of Models to PP Utility Data to Estimate the PP QALY

In this example, data is used from Study 3 of Khan et al. (2016) to show how PP utility can be used to estimate the PP QALY. In the economic evaluation of cancer treatments, a partitioned survival model is often used. The total survival experience is partitioned into progression-free survival (PFS) and post-progression survival (PPS):

$$OS = PFS + PPS$$

Consequently, PFS is modeled along with OS and future (extrapolated) survival proportions for each of PFS and OS are generated.

The steps in this approach are:

(i) Extrapolate PP utility.

(ii) Apply the extrapolated utilities to the PP survival data. Compute the AUC (QALY) as the QALY for the PFS plus the QALY for the PPS using: QALY as an area under the curve (AUC) using the formula of equation (3.1):

$$\mathbf{QALY_{AUC}} = \Sigma\left[\left(Q_i + Q_{i+1}\right)/\mathbf{2}\right]^*\left[\left(S_i + S_{i+1}\right)/\mathbf{2}\right]^*\left[t_{i+1} - t_i\right]$$

where, S_i and Q_i are the PP survival and PP utilities respectively

The details are provided in Khan et al. (2019) using data from a lung cancer population. Table 3.2 shows a summary of the PP utility models fitted to extrapolate utilities as far as at least 24 months (the observed follow-up data was 12 months). The five-parameter model had the best fit (smallest value of a model fit statistic called the Akaike's Information Criterion (AIC)).

The results in Tables 3.3 and Table 3.4 show:

(a) The best model to predict longer-term utility data using observed patterns of utility was the five parameter model because the AIC was the smallest (best model fit).

TABLE 3.2

Data for Example 3.2: Construction of the QALY

Month (t)	Utility (mean)	OS (% alive)
0 (baseline)	0.65	100
1	0.71	69
2	0.72	50
3	0.69	32
4	0.75	23
5	0.77	19
6	0.74	4

TABLE 3.3

Models Fitted to Extrapolate PP Utility

Model	Parameter	Estimate	*p*-value	Equation	AIC
Linear	α	0.654	–<0.001	$0.654 - 0.0219 * \text{Time}$	115.7
	β	–0.0219			
Exponential	λ	0.1415	<0.001	$\text{Exp}(-0.1415 * \text{Time})$	198.0
Bragg-Packer	α	–0.08323	0.983	$\alpha + \beta * exp\{-\gamma * (\text{Time} - \delta)^2\}$	106.3
	β	0.693710	0.8617		
	γ	0.005245	0.8990		
	δ	1.697112	0.6575		
Pareto	α	0.4073	<0.001	$1 - [1 - 1/\text{Time}^{0.4073}]$	253.4
Beta	α	0.9595	0.0002	$\alpha\ \text{Time}^{\beta} * (1 - \text{Time})^{\gamma}$	101.2
	β	0.1270	0.1440		
	γ	1.3985	0.0059		
Lorentz	α	–0.4832	0.968	$\alpha + \beta / [1 + \gamma * (\text{Time} - \delta)^2]$	106.2
	β	1.0939	0.927		
	γ	0.00532	0.948		
	δ	1.77192	0.784		
Rational function	α	–0.04831	0.5562	$(\beta + \gamma * \text{Time}) / (1 + \alpha * \text{Time} + \delta * \text{Time}^2)$	106.4
	β	0.5997	<.0001		
	γ	–0.01726	0.8670		
	δ	0.005538	0.7464		
Five parameter	α	–0.01618	0.7419	$(\beta + \gamma * \text{Time} + \varepsilon * \text{Time}^2 / 1 + \alpha * \text{Time} + \delta * \text{Time}^2)$	92.4
	β	0.5985	<.0001		
	γ	0.1000	<.0001		
	δ	0.003861	0.8397		
	ε	–0.00148	0.7431		

(b) Not all parameters were statistically significant, suggesting a model with fewer parameters (and possibly easier interpretation) could be used.

(c) The PP QALY was estimated to be lowest for the Pareto model and the highest for the linear model (which assumes utilities are falling at a constant rate over time).

(d) The model with the greatest uncertainty was also the Pareto because the extrapolated QALY constituted more than 32% of the total QALY. Uncertainty here is determined by how much of the QALY is determined through extrapolation relative to the total QALY.

TABLE 3.4

Extrapolated Mean Utilities Beyond 12 Months for Each Model

Month PP	PPS[a] (%)	Linear	Exponential	Bragg-P	Pareto	Beta	Lorentz	Rational	5-parameter
1	100	0.6323866	0.8680552	0.6087141	1.0000000	0.6035076	0.6077124	0.6082953	0.5783413
2	89	0.6104600	0.7535198	0.6101463	0.6699382	0.6193203	0.6097999	0.6104777	0.5606051
3	80	0.5885334	0.6540968	0.6043310	0.5299948	0.6109764	0.6042279	0.6053164	0.5550958
4	71	0.5666067	0.5677921	0.5914498	0.4488172	0.5919137	0.5912281	0.5924955	0.5720147
5	69	0.5446801	0.4928748	0.5719015	0.3945166	0.5667773	0.5713266	0.5722454	0.5519026
6	63	0.5227535	0.4278426	0.5462812	0.3550638	0.5378116	0.5452932	0.5453433	0.5255827
7	55	0.5008269	0.3713909	0.5153507	0.3248014	0.5063101	0.5140697	0.5130163	0.5140768
8	55	0.4789003	0.3223878	0.4800006	0.3006798	0.4731083	0.4786924	0.4767720	0.5421457
9	55	0.4569736	0.2798504	0.4412078	0.2808945	0.4387921	0.4402168	0.4382009	0.4000281
10	55	0.4350470	0.2429256	0.3999912	0.2643017	0.4038001	0.3996548	0.3987983	0.3997085
11	49	0.4131204	0.2108728	0.3573677	0.2501377	0.3684792	0.3579274	0.3598385	0.3285215
12	43	0.3911938	0.1830493	0.3143117	0.2378708	0.3331174	0.3158357	0.3223101	0.3172918
13*	36	0.3810000	0.1588969	0.2717202	0.2271183	0.2979837	0.2740473	0.2869069	0.2763705
14*	33	0.3600000	0.1379312	0.2303847	0.2175969	0.2632678	0.2330954	0.2540558	0.2368746
15*	32	0.3390000	0.1197319	0.1909714	0.2090917	0.2292018	0.1933870	0.2239648	0.1988992
16*	29	0.3180000	0.1039339	0.1540096	0.2014369	0.1959969	0.1552166	0.1966766	0.1627003
17*	29	0.2970000	0.0902204	0.1198883	0.1945018	0.1638710	0.1187826	0.1721177	0.1284338
18*	25	0.2760000	0.0783163	0.0888597	0.1881820	0.1330590	0.0842040	0.1501403	0.0961758
19*	23	0.2550000	0.0679828	0.0610497	0.1823931	0.1038273	0.0515365	0.1305537	0.0659408
20*	20	0.2340000	0.0590129	0.0364715	0.1770658	0.0764966	0.0207869	0.1131479	0.0376981
21*	18	0.2130000	0.0512264	0.0150440	0.1721430	0.0514822	–0.0080745	0.0977094	0.0113846
22*	15	0.1920000	0.0444674	–0.0033898	0.1675768	0.0293806	–0.0351042	0.0840311	–0.0130844
23*	13	0.1710000	0.0386001	–0.0190427	0.1633268	0.0112157	–0.0603764	0.0719187	–0.0358072
24*	11	0.1500000	0.0335070	–0.0321654	0.1593588	~0	–0.0839771	0.0611935	–0.0568892
PP QALY#		4.648132	3.747115	4.160589	3.732875	4.272484	4.135935	4.304773	4.028435
%Extrapolated@		28.25819	21.88337	18.89631	32.44121	21.13157	18.50418	21.69392	19.02141

[a] *Note:* Using a 3-knot Royston-Parmar model

* Extrapolated utilities using modeling; #using $\sum\left[(Qi+Qi+1)/2\right]*\left[(Si+Si+1)/2\right]*\left[ti+1-ti\right]$

@ percent of PP QALY extrapolated = (Total calculated QALY – QALY without extrapolated)/ Total calculated QALY*100.

3.9 HRQoL Issues in Health Technology Appraisals of Cancer Drugs

In HTAs of cancer drugs, there are several aspects of HRQoL issues that have been identified during the reporting of cost-effectiveness analyses. These are important to appreciate, especially regarding utility data. For example, a summary of the issues from several HTA submissions for lung cancer are presented in Table 3.5. For the moment, we focus on the issues relating to utility (HRQoL) data.

TABLE 3.5

Data Source for Key HTA Submissions

Treatment	Submission[a]	Utilities
Afatinib	920/13 1L (SMC, 2014)	• Lack of details • Data collected from historical sources
	TA310 1L (NICE, 2014b)	Health state utilities derived from LUX-Lung and LUCEOR trials (Chouaid, 2012) in base case and assumed to be the same across treatment arms other sources used in sensitivity analysis (Doyle, 2008; Lewis, 2010; Nafees, 2008) Disutilities sourced from LUX-Lung 1, LUX-Lung 3, and (Nafees, 2008)
Crizotinib	TA296 2L (NICE, 2013d)	Utility collected in PROFILE 1007 using the EQ-5D Calculated EQ-5D in PFS by weighting the value at each time point by the number of patients at each time point A weighted average utility at the end of treatment was extrapolated to post-progression health states No utility decrement was applied to AE occurrences
	865/13 2L (SMC, 2013)	Utility data was derived using EQ-5D from the clinical trials. Values for BSC were assigned using assumptions
	pCODR, 2013 2L (pCODR, 2013b)	Utility data was derived using EQ-5D from the clinical trials
Erlotinib	TA258 1L (NICE, 2012)	Utilities were taken from (Nafees, 2008); a study commissioned for second line NSCLC, with 100 members of the general population, using SG and VAS techniques
	TA162 2L (NICE, 2008)	No detail
	749/11 1L (SMC, 2012)	Primary study derived from a survey that used the standard gamble technique with 100 members of the UK public
	220/05 2L (SMC, 2006)	Primary study from a sample of the UK general population using appropriate methods (not specified)
	07-2013 1L (PBAC, 2013b)	Utilities for patients with stable disease and progressive disease directly from (Nafees, 2008)

(Continued)

TABLE 3.5 (CONTINUED)

Data Source for Key HTA Submissions

Treatment	Submission[a]	Utilities
Gefitinib	TA192 1L (NICE, 2010b)	Most utilities were sourced from (Nafees, 2008) Progression-free and therapy were sourced from an ERG report (2006) Disutility for anemia was sourced externally (2009)
	615/10 1L (SMC, 2010b)	Sourced from literature (not specified)
	07-2013 1L (PBAC, 2013c)	Utilities were adapted from HRQoL data reported in the trial
Pemetrexed	TA181 1L (NICE, 2009)	Utilities were taken from (Nafees 2008); a study commissioned for second line aNSCLC, with 100 members of the general population, using SG and VAS techniques.
	TA309 MTx (NICE, 2014a)	EQ-5D data from a mixed regression model of the PARAMOUNT trial.
	531/09 1L (SMC, 2010a)	Sourced from a utility valuation survey using SG in 100 members of the general population in the UK
	342/07 2nd line (SMC, 2008)	Sourced from a study of 100 members of the general population using SG to value 18 states and adverse events)

Key: AE: Adverse events; EQ-5D: EuroQoL five dimension; ERG: Evidence review group; NICE: National Institute for Health and Care Excellence; NHS: National Health Service; NSCLC: Non-small-cell lung cancer; OS: Overall survival; PBAC: Pharmaceutical Benefits Advisory Committee; pCODR: pan-Canadian Oncology Drug Review; PFS: Progression-free survival; PSSRU: Personal Social Services Research Unit; SG: Standard gamble; SMC: Scottish Medicines Consortium; SPC: Summary of product characteristics; TA: technology appraisal; UK: United Kingdom; VAS: Visual analogue scale.

[a] *Note:* References for the HTAs are provided in the bibliography.

The common features of HTA submissions, including HRQoL issues were:

(i) Utility data were collected from historical sources and limited details were provided on the assumptions. Where assumptions were provided, some of these were problematic (e.g. utilities the same between the two arms of the treatment).

(ii) In some cases, utilities from later lines of treatment were used (imputed) for earlier lines of treatment. In some cases it may also be the case that utilities from earlier lines of treatments are used to impute for later lines of treatments – this might happen when first-line therapy has resulted in progression and utilities collected on the first-line treatment are 'carried forward' while patients take later lines of treatment.

(iii) Utilities were used from separate utility studies (e.g. TTO or SG methods). That is, utilities were not collected in the clinical trial.

(iv) Utilities for patients in the SD and PD health states were determined from an external study (Nafees et al., 2008).

(v) Lack of details about where health state utilities have been sourced from, either directly from the trial or from external studies such as Nafees et al. (2008) or through mapping (Scuffham, Whitty, Mitchell, & Viney, 2008).

3.10 Summary

In this chapter we have discussed the reasons why HRQoL is important. We have also discussed the differences between cancer-specific and generic HRQoL measures. We showed an example of how utilities can be constructed from generic HRQoL measures for economic evaluation, focusing on the EQ-5D. The computation of the QALY was outlined in a general and a cancer-specific context. New methodology was introduced on modeling HRQoL for economic evaluation in cancer by investigating the behavior of post-progression utility – a common issue in many HTAs. We concluded the chapter by reporting the issues around the use of HRQoL measures in cost-effectiveness analyses of cancer drugs.

3.11 Exercises for Chapter 3

1. Generic HRQoL measures should be avoided at all cost. Discuss.
2. Compare and contrast the approaches to estimating HRQoL for economic evaluation.
3. How would you go about designing a study to collect HRQoL data for an economic evaluation in a cancer trial? What challenges would you encounter?
4. Extrapolation of survival data is common and therefore we should be allowed to extrapolate utility data. Discuss.
5. Do you think that treatment effects from CSMs and generic measures are comparable? Can effects from generic measures be understood in the same way as CSMs?

4

Introductory Statistical Methods for Economic Evaluation in Cancer

4.1 Introduction

In this chapter, we will introduce some essential statistical concepts that will allow the reader to appreciate statistical methods used in economic evaluation. Economic evaluation relies heavily on the use of statistical and clinical trial-related methodology to quantify and present cost-effectiveness analyses. When these methods are used in a cancer context, they may be more challenging. Some methods presented are slightly more technical and advanced. However, it is more important to understand the concepts rather than the finer technical details for which statistical software can be used. References in the bibliography can be consulted for interested readers. The statistical methods underlying economic evaluation in cancer broadly consist of appreciating the distribution of data, presenting data using summary measures, understanding survival analyses methods, modeling, and simulation. Some of these will be covered in this chapter. Statistical methods in economic evaluation do not really revolve around complex hypothesis-testing problems and statistical inference. Although many HTAs and cost-effectiveness analyses present *p*-values (the observed treatment difference being due to chance) in some form or another, these are secondary to the important objective of economic evaluation. Statistical methods in economic evaluation are mainly used to quantify the uncertainty in the decision-making process – whether to pay for a new cancer drug (or not). We therefore start with the concepts of uncertainty and variability.

4.2 Uncertainty and Variability

Uncertainty is central to the decision-making process that determines whether a new cancer treatment is cost-effective (or not). Uncertainty is sometimes confused with words like 'variability' 'and 'probability.' It is important to disentangle some of these concepts so that we can be precise in our language.

Indeed, Kaplan (1997) noted that "50% of the problems in the world result from people using the same words with different meanings" and "the other 50% come from people using different words with the same meaning."

4.2.1 Uncertainty

Uncertainty in everyday language suggests we are "not sure" or "we do not know" about some statement. Technically, uncertainty refers to an unknown true value of some measure or quantity. For example, we might believe that the proportion of deaths in the population is 30%. The statement: "the proportion of deaths in the population is 30%" can be true or false. The quantification of this statement is made in terms of probability. That is, we may be certain the statement is true (with a probability of 1) or is highly uncertain, with a probability close to 0, or false if the probability equals 0. Similarly, we might believe some risk factors are related to survival or increased costs. The *choice* of selecting the risk factors (e.g. we choose age and gender, but we could have chosen weight and ECOG) is also subject to uncertainty. Uncertainty can arise from many factors (poor communication, subjective belief, imprecise approximation, etc.) of which one might be statistical variation (variability), which leads us to distinguishing between variability and uncertainty.

4.2.2 Variability

Variability is a feature of observed phenomena, or, for our purposes, data collected from a clinical trial or some other study. Variability occurs where multiple measures are observed. For example, if we measure the HRQoL of 10 'identical' (or similar) cancer patients at 3 months, each value may be different. The dispersion of the values around some central point (e.g. the mean) can be expressed as a numerical quantity – termed the 'variance.' The larger this quantity is, the greater the variability (or dispersion). The question of what the central measure (i.e. the mean) is allows us to make a statement such as "The mean is 5.7." The uncertainty of this statement is quantified through the use of probability. If the variability is large (reflected in say a range of values between 0 to 10), we might be less certain compared to observing values between 5.5 and 5.9 (more certainty about the mean).

In economic evaluation, whether for a cancer intervention or otherwise, we are interested in expressing the uncertainty of a statement such as "The new intervention is cost-effective" in terms of:

(i) The probability (a single value) of this statement being true.
(ii) The range of values (e.g. ICERs) for which the statement is plausible with some level of probability (e.g. ICERs between £18,000 to £22,000 have between 85% to 90% chance of cost-effectiveness at a threshold WTP of £30,000).

The statistical tools used to ultimately determine (i) and (ii) are described in this chapter.

4.2.2.1 Hypothesis Testing

In classical (frequentist) statistics, the hypothesis-testing framework presents two scenarios: the null hypothesis and the alternative hypothesis. For efficacy trials in cancer, with OS as a primary endpoint for two treatments we could have:

H_0 (null hypothesis): no difference in survival between treatments
H_1 (alternative): there is a difference (a target effect size in mind)

After we conduct the trial, we collect the data and are then faced with a decision to choose (declare) one or the other hypothesis to be true/false, based on the data (evidence). The *p*-value (the likelihood of rejecting H_0, when in fact it is true – that is akin to declaring a treatment as being efficacious, when in fact it is not) is used as a way to judge the evidence in favor of one hypothesis over the other (e.g. choose H_0 or H_1).

In a cost-effectiveness framework, we might have the hypothesis presented in terms of incremental net monetary benefit (INMB, introduced in Chapter 1)

H_0 (null hypothesis): INMB = 0 (not cost-effective, for some given WTP)
H_1 (alternative): INMB not = 0 (cost-effective for some given WTP)

Rather than deciding in favor of one or the other hypothesis, a more informative question might be "What is the chance of H_0" being true (or false). In other words, we wish to quantify the uncertainty of a hypothesis rather than simply choose one or the other. There could be several reasons why we may not be comfortable in deciding whether H_0 is true or not (for example, a small sample size, some extreme values, excess variability, and so on). Alternative inference paradigms are possible (Bayesian), which we will briefly discuss later. The statistical measures used to determine uncertainty around cost-effectiveness decisions will take the form of traditional statistical quantities (e.g. mean, median, rates, proportions, variance, probabilities, and confidence intervals) determined from simple to more complicated analyses.

4.3 Distributions: Cost, Utility, and Survival Data

The distributions of outcomes such as survival, health resource use, costs, and utility data are important to appreciate before starting any statistical analyses. Examples of some typical distribution of each are shown in Figure 4.1a–c.

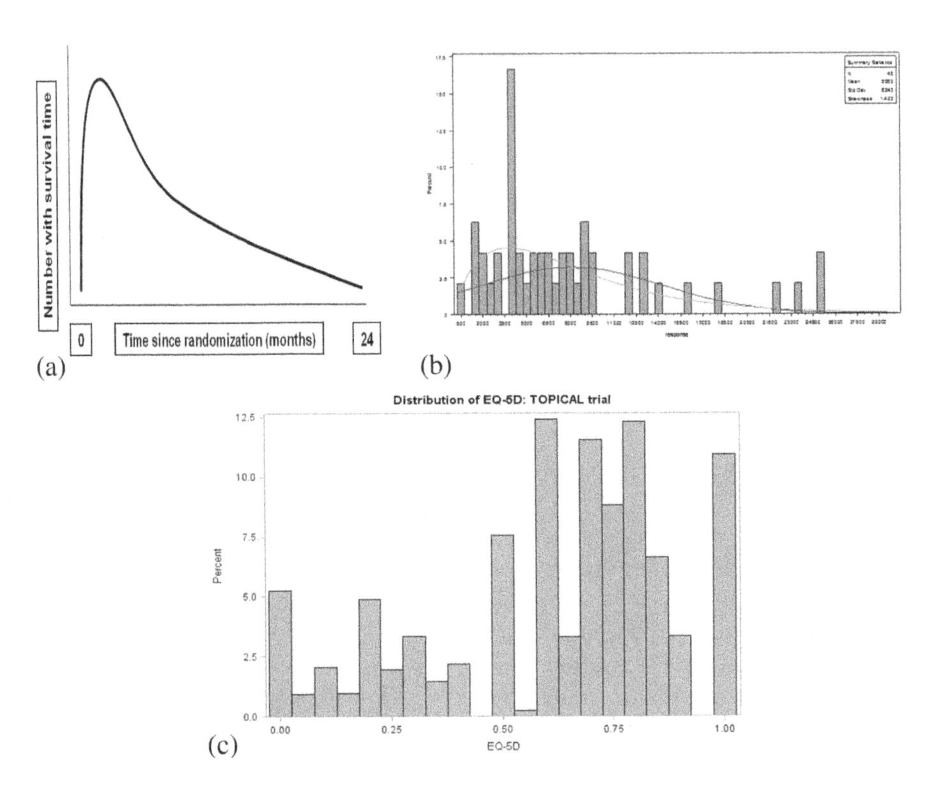

FIGURE 4.1
Distribution of (a) survival times, (b) costs and (c) HRQoL.

Figure 4.1a shows the distribution of survival times typical of OS or PFS. The distribution is skewed, with some patients having longer survival times. These are consistent with a family of exponentially distributed outcomes (see Collet, 2014; Crowther, 2016; Collet, 2017). The extremes of the tail might also indicate patients still alive in the trial at the end of follow-up.

Figure 4.1b shows the distribution of costs and health resource. These are positive (≥ 0) and like survival data also have some extreme values for different reasons (the two could be correlated because those who live longer might also have more extreme costs). Some costs appear often (spike) at some value(s) and are said to be 'over-dispersed.' When data exhibit skewness and over-dispersion, that is, the presence of greater variability in a data set than would be expected, special statistical modeling approaches are needed to estimate the mean cost.

Figure 4.1c shows the distribution of HRQoL data (see also utility data, Chapter 5). The distribution is also over-dispersed particularly at values at 1. That is, there are lots of values near to 1 (ceiling effects) and this can cause problems in presenting mean estimates, unless suitable statistical approaches are used to handle excess variability. Here, over-dispersion may also occur near to the extremes. This makes the distribution look like a 'U' shape and hence the term 'U-shaped distribution.' Special statistical models can be used to analyze these types of data.

It is important to note that regardless of the shape of the distribution, we will need to determine the *mean* value of the data for the purposes of economic evaluation. It might be tempting to use the median or other statistic such as a truncated or trimmed mean (the mean of some data with some extreme values omitted), but that would not be appropriate. At the current time, only the arithmetic mean is considered suitable for an economic evaluation.

4.4 Important Measures Used in Cancer Trials

4.4.1 Time-to-Event Endpoints

The primary outcomes in confirmatory Phase III trials are often time-to-event outcomes such as OS and PFS. The event is often death or disease progression and the time taken to reach the event is the outcome of interest. Since some patients may live for a long time (long after the trial has been completed), there are instances of some very extreme survival times that result in a 'skewed' distribution. For this reason, the median is often used to present the summary statistics. Figure 4.2 shows a Kaplan-Meier (KM) plot of two treatments (A and B) from a cancer trial.

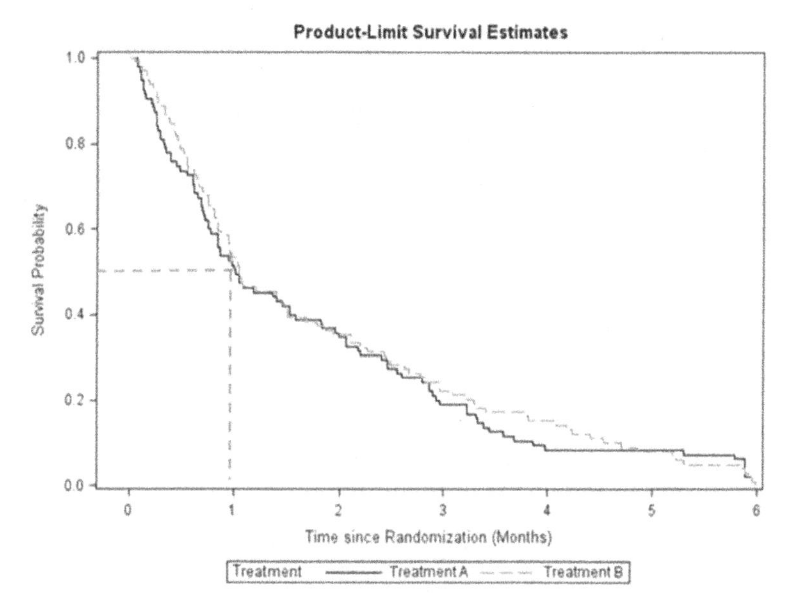

FIGURE 4.2
Kaplan-Meier plot of two treatments (A and B) from a cancer trial.

The y-axis shows the proportion (probability) of patients being alive at given time points. The x-axis is the time since randomization presented in years or months (or days, depending on how often the event occurs.) At time 0 (when the trial started), 100% of the patients are alive. It may happen that some instantaneous deaths could occur after the patient has been randomized or on the day of randomization. Hence, it is not necessary that at time 0 exactly 100% of patients are alive. When reading numbers from survival curves, we should be aware whether the time unit is in days, months, or years. Over time, fewer patients are alive. The maximal follow up is around 6 months (the last time point on the KM curve) in this example.

The median survival is observed by drawing a horizontal line starting from 50% (or 0.50) until it reaches the curves. By drawing a vertical line, we can read off the values. In this example, the median survival times for treatments A and B are each around 1 month. Hence, neither treatment appears to improve median survival time. What is important to know is that the proportions calculated at each time point are determined through calculations involving the number of deaths (events) occurring in the preceding time interval based on those alive (called the risk set). The KM estimates of the (cumulative) proportions alive at each time point are called nonparametric estimates because we do not need to fit a theoretical curve to the overall survival times in order to estimate important measures of treatment benefit.

Figure 4.3 shows a KM curve for PFS. Here, there are more 'steps' in the curve, due to fewer events. The steps get longer over time. These steps are related to the frequency at which 'progression' or 'death' events accumulate. The median is estimated in the same way as for the OS curve. The median for Treatment A is about 3.25 months and for B is about 2.75 months. Hence Treatment A improves survival by 0.5 months (about 2 weeks). The crosses on the lines show the presence of censoring, or patients who have not had an event during the observation time. Over time, as fewer patients live or have not progressed, the curve takes a more discrete shape and is less informative (more uncertain) about the event rates, especially where there are fewer patients and therefore fewer events.

4.4.2 Median Survival

In some KM estimates, the median may not exist (Figure 4.4). The reason for this is because there are insufficient events, or that patients have not been followed up for long enough. It is an important consideration in trial design (Chapter 6) to ensure that patients can have adequate follow-up so that reliable cost and survival data can be determined.

The median is often reported with 95% confidence intervals. A median OS of 5 months with a 95% CI of (3 to 7 months) tells us that the true median lies somewhere between 3 to 7 months with 95% confidence. Note that the median calculated from the survival curve is not the same as the simple raw median when some data are censored (i.e. patients that have not died by the

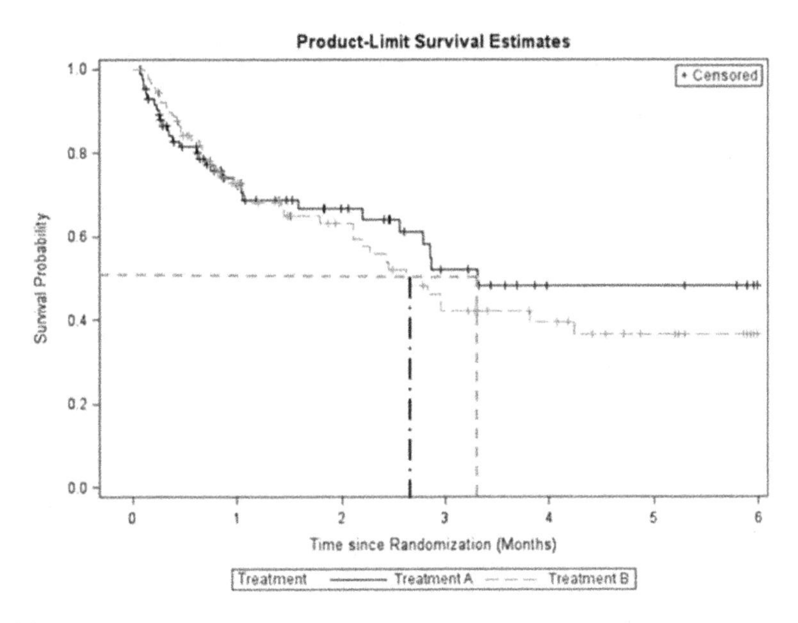

FIGURE 4.3
Survival rates in the presence of censored data (fewer events).

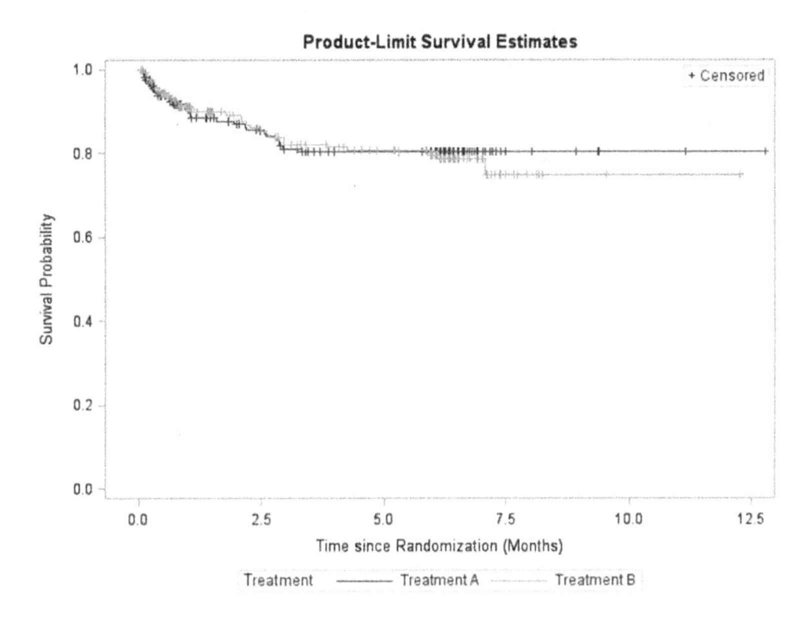

FIGURE 4.4
Kaplan-Meier curve where median does not exist due to too few events.

end of follow-up). If there are no censored data, then the estimate of the raw median and the median from the KM curve are the same.

4.4.3 Hazard Rate and Hazard Ratio

An important concept in analyses of time-to-event data is related to 'hazard rates.' A 'hazard' in everyday language is synonymous with 'risk.' When one says it is hazardous (and often illegal) to drive after drinking alcohol, it suggests there is a risk of an event (e.g. a car crash or death). For patients with cancer, unfortunately, there is a risk of death from their disease. That risk might be immediate or it could happen over time. Sometimes, the potential hazard for death changes. For example, immediately after complicated surgery, the hazard for death is high; then, as the patient recovers, the hazard falls. In other cases, the hazard might be increasing (e.g. as with increasing age or severity of the disease). The hazard might also remain constant (this does not mean patients do not die, but rather the hazard for death during say months 2 to 3 is the same as it is during months 3 to 4). The hazard rates are often depicted using graphs (called hazard functions) as shown, for example, in Figure 4.5. A hazard rate is also referred to a 'failure' rate, where 'failure' might refer to a death event (thought of in simplistic terms as the failure of a treatment to prolong survival or time until disease progression).

An 'incidence' is a measure of the frequency with which a disease occurs in a population over a specified time period and 'incidence rate' or 'incidence' is numerically defined as the number of new cases of a disease within a time period as a proportion of the number of people at risk for the disease. So a failure rate is basically an incidence rate where the incidence is a negative event, namely a failure.

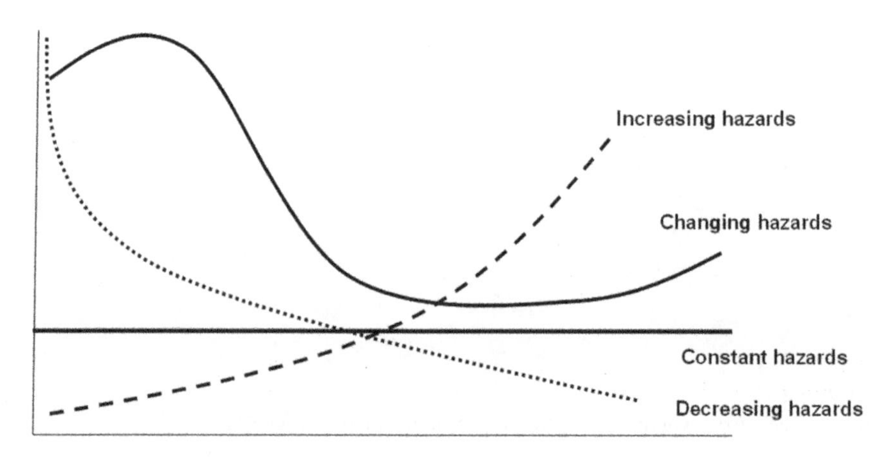

FIGURE 4.5
Examples of hazard functions.

A more technical description of a hazard rate is the chance of an event occurring within a specified time interval, given or conditional on the patient having survived to some time, *t*. If the interval is long (e.g. between 6 months and 2 years), the rate might fall. If the interval is short (e.g. between 2 and 4 weeks), it might increase. The hazard rate, $h(t)$ defined below is not a probability. Its value must be >0 and can be >1. A high value means that chances of death, (death rates) will be high for a given time interval.

$$h(t) = \lim_{\Delta t \to 0} \frac{P(t < T \leq t + \Delta t \mid T > t)}{\Delta t}$$

For example, if the hazard rate of disease progression (for an individual) at 3 months is 0.25, this means that, if the hazard stays at the value of 0.25 (assuming a constant hazard) over the next 2 months, one would expect disease progression 0.25 times. If the event is repeatable (e.g. second disease progression), then the reciprocal of this value (1/0.25) = 4 means that we can expect the next progression for that individual to take place in about 4 months' time, on average. If the hazard was 1.5, then we would expect this individual to have disease progression 1.5 times over the year (assuming the hazard stays constant over that year); and the next progression would be expected to occur in about 8 months' time (1/1.5). This is important because, in some cancers, very few events might be observed. This will involve longer follow-up to get the events, the use of external (real-world data) or extrapolation (Section 4.6.3), or even the abandonment of the trial (due to an inconclusive result).

When one considers hazards, one could imagine that each person has his or her own hazard or risk of an event. For example, as one sits at a computer, the risk of death is small (but not zero). However as one gets into their car to drive, the risk increases, and it will change again when they return home. The true hazard function (the evolution of the hazard over time) will depend on lots of factors and conditions. The combined hazard functions in a group of patients in a cancer trial will include some patients with high (short survival time) and some with relatively lower (longer survival time) hazards, such that across lots of individuals, so that the general trend is captured.

When we have hazard rates for two treatment groups, it is the relative hazard rates that are important. This is termed as the 'hazard rate ratio' or simply the 'hazard ratio.'

4.4.4 Hazard Ratio

In its simplest terms, the hazard (rate) ratio (HR) is the ratio of chances of events occurring in one group compared to the other. A more detailed definition is "the ratio of two hazard rates or of two hazard functions, either at a particular point in time or averaged over a long period" (Day, 2002). The HR determined from two patient groups can be interpreted as a reduction or increase in the risk (the hazard) of an event in a similar way to the relative risk or risk ratio when the time interval for an event is small. In this sense, the HR *describes* the relative risk based on a comparison of events (Spruance, 2004). Time occurrence of the event is not of interest or not available (Saad et al., 2018). The hazard ratio is frequently interpreted as a risk ratio (or relative risk), but these are not technically the same (Stare, 2016).

In a comparison of two treatments for an outcome like death, an HR of 1 suggests no treatment benefit. An HR of 0.8 would be interpreted as the risk of death being 20% lower in the group taking treatment A compared to B. An HR of 1.20 suggests that the risk of death is 20% higher for A versus B. In general, an HR < 1 suggests the experimental intervention is better when compared to a control; and an HR > 1 implies the experimental intervention is worse than the control for the outcome of interest. HRs are important for interpreting clinical efficacy, but they are also important in economic evaluation for simulating survival patterns.

Example 4.1

The following results are reported in NICE TA189 (May, 2010) for the treatment of hepatocellular carcinoma with the drug sorafenib (Figure 4.6).

The HR of sorafenib versus placebo (S vs. P) was 0.69 with a 95% CI of (0.55, 0.88): on average, the risk of mortality was reduced with sorafenib

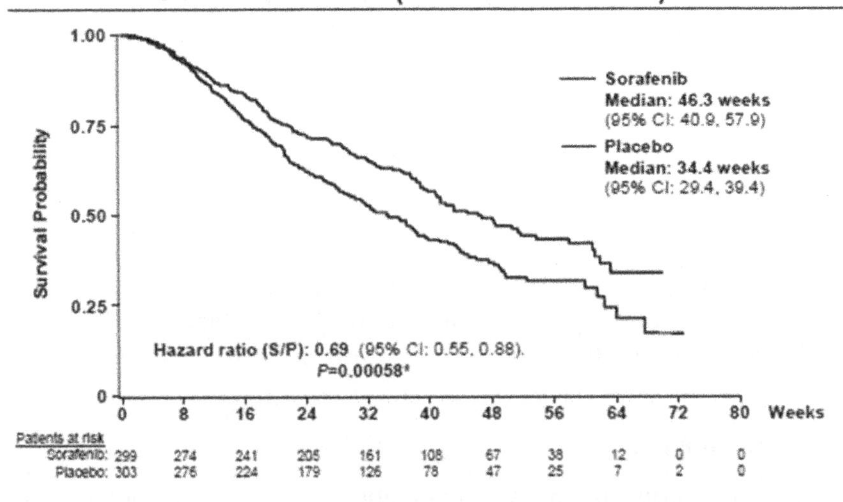

FIGURE 4.6
OS in hepatocellular carcinoma (NICE, TA189).

by about 31% and the true risk reduction lies somewhere between 45% and 12% with 95% confidence. The p-value of 0.00058 shows strong evidence to reject the null hypothesis (of no difference between S and P). An interim analysis was carried out using an adjusted p-value ($p = 0.0077 > 0.00058$) to take into account looking at the data early.

4.4.5 Survival Rates and Proportions

A survival rate is the estimated proportion of patients alive at a given time point. This can be read from the survival curve. As noted, earlier estimates are likely to be more precise than those at the latter part of the curve, where fewer patients are alive. In Figure 4.2, the proportion alive at 2 months was 36%. At later time points (say 5 months), the survival rates are more uncertain. This is likely to be reflected in wider confidence intervals at these and later time points.

A common occurrence is when we might wish to estimate the proportion of patients alive at a given time point (e.g. 12 months) if we are provided with a median. For example, if the median is 6 months, then the proportion alive is 50%. If we assume the KM is approximately an exponentially decaying curve, we can use this information to estimate the survival proportion at 12 months. The survival proportion can be denoted as:

$$S(t) = \exp(-\lambda t),$$

where t is the time to an event of interest. The value of λ is important. It represents the rate of death (event), also called a constant hazard (of death) – i.e. the rate of death is constant over time. Hence, for a median of 6 months, $S(t) = 0.50 = \exp(-\lambda * 6)$ at 6 months, the proportion alive is 50%. We can estimate $\lambda : -\log(0.50)/6 = \lambda$; $\lambda = 0.1155$. The proportion alive at 12 months is estimated as $S(12) = \exp(-0.1155 * 12) = 0.25$ or 25%.

We can convert a hazard rate into a probability and vice versa: The hazard rate λ (or incidence rate of death, assumed constant) can be estimated by the formula:

$$-\text{Log}(1-\pi)/t,$$

where t is the time point of interest, and π = the survival rate at time t. When the hazard function is no longer constant but changes over time, the survival curves may cross as in Figure 4.6a. In this HTA (TA179, 2009) in gastrointestinal stromal tumors, the difference in median survival values was about 8 weeks. Differences in the proportion alive at 5 weeks are larger. In Figure 4.7a, the survival curves cross at the median. Differences at later time points are larger and using the median difference would be misleading.

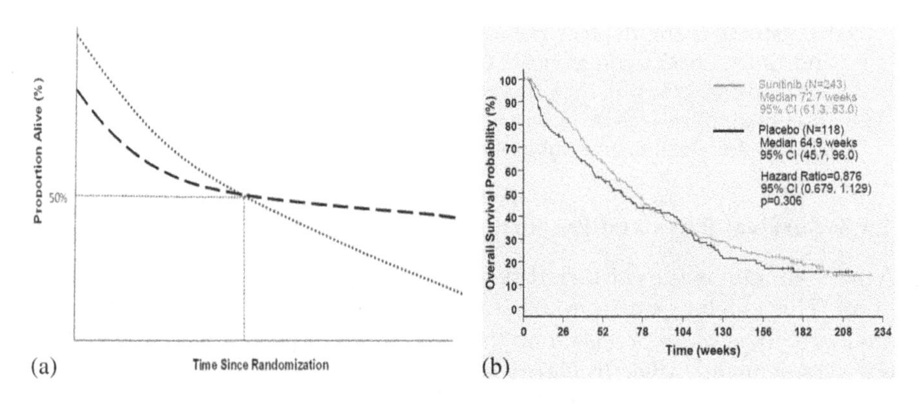

FIGURE 4.7
Nonproportional or changing hazards in general (a) and observed in a comparison of sunitinib versus placebo (b) (NICE, HTA TA179, 2009).

4.4.6 Relationship between Hazard Rate and Survival Rate

In this section the relationship between transition probabilities and survival rates is briefly explored. This is important because in some situations a health economic model (e.g. Markov model, Chapter 7) is used where survival rates are modeled. Determining transition probabilities from survival rates becomes important for this purpose. In some cases, the primary endpoints for cancer trials are survival rates at fixed time points (e.g. two-year survival rates compared between experimental and control treatments). Therefore, the relationship between survival rates changing from one time point to another (or a transition) is related to the death or hazard rate. It is plausible that the hazard for death increase for some patients who progress in their disease and therefore the rates of transition between PD and death are high.

Earlier, we saw how an exponential model had a survival function of the form: $S(t) = e^{-\Phi 06Xt}$. In this expression λ is the hazard rate or the rate of an event (such as death) per unit of time: e.g. 5 deaths per month (unit of time is months). The probability of death can be expressed as a rate, where π is the proportion alive at time t:

$$\pi = e^{-\Phi 06Xt} \text{ and hence } \lambda = -(\log(\pi)/t)$$

For example, if after 2 years 50 patients out of 200 are alive, and assuming the death rate is constant (the same number of deaths each year), the death rate is: $[-\log(1-0.25)][/5 = -\log[0.75]/5 = -0.287/5 = 0.0574$ and the probability of death at year 3 would be: $1 - \exp(-0.0574 * 3) = 0.158$ (15.8%).

To distinguish between a rate and a probability, as an example, 4 patients are followed up of whom 3 die at various times (5, 3, 2, and 1 months).

The rate of death = 3/11 or 3 per 11 person-years or 0.27 persons per year. The probability of death is 3 out of 4 = 0.75.

4.4.7 Transition Probability and Matrix

A transition probability is the probability of moving from a given health state to the next health state in a Markovian process. In other words, the *transition probability* is the chance of moving between health states over (discrete) time. The Markovian process means that the chance of moving into a future health state is determined only by the current health state (and not other, previous, health states). A patient cannot move from a state of 'death' to 'progressive disease,' although the reverse is possible.

The source of the transition probability is also important – where was it taken from, how reliable it is, whether it is a conditional or a joint probability. For example, rates of adverse events are extracted from clinical trial reports. Many adverse events summary tables report percentages using the denominator of the intent-to-treat (ITT) or safety population (i.e. the total sample size). An example of a transition matrix for patients with health states mild, moderate and death after 1 month of treatment with an experimental treatment might be as shown in Table 4.1.

Prior to the computing the transition matrix in Table 4.2, patients would have been randomized to one of two treatments: experimental or control. Patients at the start of their treatment are considered to be in either a mild or moderate state (e.g. based on ECOG or similar inclusion criteria). The proportion of patients who started the trial at baseline in a mild health state and then remained in the same state after treatment was 45%. Very few patients (5%) who started the trial in a moderate state improved into a mild state post-baseline. In fact, 60% of patients who presented with moderate disease did not change states after starting treatment.

In its simplest form, it is assumed that the probability of *moving* from one health state to another (namely the transition probability) is the same for each future time point (i.e. is constant over time) although the probabilities of being in each health state at each time point or cycle will be different. In order to compute how the transition matrix will look like after 1 month, we

TABLE 4.1

Example Transition Matrix on Experimental Treatment after 1 Month Post-Randomization

		Post-Baseline (After Treatment)			
		Mild	**Moderate**	**Death**	**Total**
Baseline	Mild	0.45	0.35	0.20	1
	Moderate	0.05	0.60	0.35	1
	Death	0	0	1	1

TABLE 4.2

Example Survival Times for Determining Restricted Mean

Patient	Survival Time (Months)	Death
1	3	Yes
2	4	No
3	6	Yes
4	7	Yes
5	2	Yes
6	8	Yes
7	3	No
8	9	No

need to know the initial probabilities (or the probabilities at baseline). These are assumed to be $\mathbf{a}_0$=[0.45, 0.35, 0.20] (the fact that these are the same as the first row is coincidental).

After 1 month of treatment, therefore, the transition matrix is $\mathbf{a}_0$ multiplied by the 3 × 3 transition matrix above: $\mathbf{a}_1$ = [0.45 × 0.45 + 0.35 × 0.05 + 0.20 × 0, 0.45 × 0.35 + 0.35 × 0.60 + 0.30 × 0, 0.45 × 0.30 + 0.35 × 0.35 + 0.30 × 1] = [0.22, 0.37, 0.56]

The 1 × 3 matrix $\mathbf{a}_1$= [0.22, 0.37, 0.56] describes the probabilities in each of the health states mild, moderate, and death; 1 month after treatment, this 1 × 3 matrix now becomes the initial matrix needed for further calculations. After 2 months (cycle 2 of the process), this would be: $\mathbf{a}_1$ multiplied by the 3 × 3 transition matrix, and so on. In general, one can compute the proportion of patients for the n + 1th step in any of the above 3 health states by simply multiplying $\mathbf{a}_n$ by the given transition matrix, where $\mathbf{a}_n$ is the 1 × 3 matrix at the current step:

$$\mathbf{a}_1 = \mathbf{a}_0{}^*\mathbf{P}$$

$$\mathbf{a}_2 = \mathbf{a}_1{}^*\mathbf{P}$$

$$\mathbf{a}_3 = \mathbf{a}_2{}^*\mathbf{P}\ldots\ldots\mathbf{a}_n = \mathbf{a}_{n-1}{}^*\mathbf{P}$$

4.4.8 Relation between Transition Probability and Survival Rates

The Kaplan-Meier method estimates probabilities of survival within given discrete intervals. If the survival rate at 2 years = $S(2) = 0.80$, then the survival rate in the previous year before (year 1) can be written as $S(1) = 0.9$. In general, the survival during the previous year u, will be $S(t - u)$, where the current survival rate at time t is $S(t)$.

More technical (can be left out without loss of generality)

If the survival rate is $S(t)$, then the failure (death) rate is $1 - S(t)$. The probability of surviving during an interval of time is $S(t)/S(t-u)$, hence the probability of death (failure) during an interval of time is $1-[S(t)/S(t-u)]$. The transition probability (TR_p) for an event (e.g. death) is defined as $TR_p = 1-[S(t)/S(t-u)]$.

In survival analysis, there is a key relationship between the survivor function, hazard function, and the probability density function (see Collett, 2014 for further details) is defined as:

$$f(t) = h(t)^* S(t) \text{ and further, } S(t) = \exp\{-H(t)\},$$

where $f(t)$ is the probability density function, $S(t)$ is the survival function, and $H(t)$ is the cumulative hazard function. Therefore, the transition probability, TR_p is:

$$\begin{aligned} 1-[S(t)/S(t-u)] &= 1-[\exp\{-H(t)\}/\exp\{-H(t-u)\}] \\ &= 1-[\exp\{H(t-u)-H(t)\}] \end{aligned}$$

Example 4.2

For example, if the survival times follow an exponential distribution, then the probability density function (PDF) is:

$$f(t) = \lambda\exp\{-\lambda t\}$$

Here,

$$h(t) = \lambda, S(t) = \exp\{\lambda t\} \text{ and } H(t) = \lambda t$$

Using,

$$\begin{aligned} TR_p &= 1-[S(t)/S(t-u)] = 1-[\exp\{-H(t)\}/\exp\{-H(t-u)\}] \\ &= 1-[\exp\{H(t-u)-H(t)\}], \end{aligned}$$

then

$$TR_p = 1-\exp\{\lambda(t-u)-\lambda t\} = 1-\exp\{-\lambda u\}$$

The above is the constant transition probability of moving from one time point to another. Typically what is required in cancer trials is the transition probability of moving between health states such as death, progression, and being stable over time.

Example 4.3

For example, if $t = 6$ months and the proportion alive is 30%, the HR = $-\log(1 - 0.30)/6 = 0.0594$. Converting a rate into a constant probability is determined from:

$\pi = 1 - \exp\left(-\lambda^{*}t\right)$ hence, for $\lambda = 0.0594$, at 6 months,

yielding a survival probability of 0.70, which agrees with the above.

We will revisit this in an example when discussing Markov models (Chapter 7). At this junction, we simply need to appreciate that transition probabilities, hazard rates, and survival rates are all related quantities.

4.4.9 Proportional Hazards

Many statistical analyses of survival data rely upon the validity of the proportional hazards (PH) assumption mentioned earlier (strictly speaking, the name PH model can be generalized to allow for non-PH). The PH assumption means that the hazard functions for two different levels of a covariate are proportional for all values of t. For example, if women aged 60, taking treatment A have twice the risk of death compared to women at age 60 who take treatment B, then it is assumed they will also have twice the risk of death (on Treatment A compared to B) aged 70, or for that fact, any other age. Violation of this assumption is often visible when survival curves cross or are not parallel. When that happens, it suggests that the risk of death (or the event of interest) is not constant over time. As another example, in a trial comparing surgical intervention, there is a high risk of death initially after surgery (see earlier Figure 4.5), which later falls as the patient recovers. This is an example of non-constant hazards or changing hazards.

4.4.10 Mean Survival and Restricted Mean

In situations where there exist non PH, as noted from Figure 4.4, the median difference may not be reliable and the HR too might be misleading or at least need some special adjustment using more advanced statistical tests (e.g. adjusted log-rank or Renyi statistics (Li et al., 2015)) that weight the treatment benefit across the survival experience in different ways. An alternative approach suggested is to use the mean survival difference – termed the restricted mean (Royston, 2011).

In economic evaluation, the mean is the choice of statistic despite the median survival time often being cited as a measure of effect size. The mean survival time is computed as the area under the survival curve. Mathematically this is computed as an integral:

$$\hat{\mu} = \int_{0}^{\infty} \hat{S}(t)dt. \text{ With no censoring, } \hat{\mu} = \bar{t}. \tag{4.2}$$

Equation (4.2) is the area under the survival curve between the time 0 to infinity. In practice, the survival times are restricted to some time point t (since no one lives for infinity, at least not in this world). The raw mean and the mean from the KM curve in the absence of censoring are equal.

The method of estimation of the mean is usually carried out using an approximation rather than equation (4.2). Equation (4.2) could only be used if knew the (true) equation of the survival curve (and we could actually use that equation to model survival times). A KM-curve has no equation: it is empirical and determined from observed data. In Section 4.6.2, where parametric survival curves are used, equations like those above may be useful.

When computing the mean survival time from a KM plot, some computer packages issue a warning that if the largest survival time is censored, the mean survival time and its precision (measured by the standard error) may be underestimated. For this reason the mean is sometimes called the restricted mean. The restricted mean cut-off (restricted by either using the maximum overall survival time at which an event occurs, or using the maximum overall survival time regardless of an event, or some other cut-off point) could result in different values of the restricted mean. There are several reasons why the restricted mean might be preferable over a median estimate.

(a) It covers the whole survival curve (up to the restriction point T*).

(b) When used in cost-effectiveness analysis it is coherent with the use of the difference in mean cost in the numerator of the ICER and the definition of the effects.

(c) It is possible for the KM curves to cross at the median (no difference in median survival) or near to where the median difference is small, but the area under the curves (mean survival) might show a larger difference (Dehbi, Royston, & Hackshaw, 2017).

(d) When the follow-up time is short, or a large fraction of observations are censored earlier on, a large part of the (potential) survival curve might be uncertain. The restricted mean may not be appropriate in the presence of heavy censoring (Saad et al., 2018).

As an example, if the survival times were observed as in Table 4.2, the longest survival time is 9 months, where the patient was still alive. A restricted mean could be based on using this value. If however, it was based on the largest survival time with an event (i.e. 8 months), it would give a different restricted mean (a smaller one in this example). In the latter case (8 months) the mean survival time and corresponding standard error would be underestimated because the largest event time was censored.

As survival times are usually right-skewed the mean survival will generally be larger than the median. It is also more sensitive to outliers. An important question is what restriction time point should be used. Several suitable methods to define the restriction time (T*) have been proposed (see for example Miller, 1981; Klein & Gerster (2008); Klein & MoeschBerger (2005). The methods proposed in deriving the restricted mean suggest:

- If the last observation is censored, use this to compute the restricted mean.

TABLE 4.3

Summary of Statistical Measures and Their Relevance for Economic Evaluation

Measure	When/How Used	Relevance to Economic Evaluation
Median	From the Kaplan-Meir or survival curve Describing clinical effects	Limited, expect for contextualizing clinical effect
Mean	Area under the KM curve Useful when non-PH as a clinical measure, but used in the ICER calculus regardless of PH assumption	Used directly in the estimation of effectiveness
Hazard rate	Used for describing the nature of event patterns	Useful for justifying choice of survival model for extrapolation May also be used for deriving transition probability
Hazard ratio	Describes the clinical effect	Not used directly in the ICER, but may be used in modeling survival data and transition probability
Transition probability	Describes the chance of patients moving from one health state to another	Used in Markov modeling
Restricted mean	Area under the KM curve using a specified cut-off survival time Useful when non-PH as a clinical measure, but used in the ICER calculus regardless of PH assumption	Used directly in the estimation of effectiveness
Log rank test	A statistical test to determine if the survival curves are statistically different	Not directly used except to contextualize treatment differences
p-Value	Used as evidence for a decision to reject the (null) hypothesis – often that the experimental and control treatments do not differ in terms of an outcome	Not used for ICER or decision-making
Confidence interval	Describes the plausible range of values for which the true difference (e.g. HR, mean difference) lies with some specified degree of confidence (e.g. 95%).	Not used for ICER or decision-making, but may be used to summarize results
Correlation	Describes the relationship between several variables – e.g. costs and effects	Important to report and understand so that simulation can use the correct correlation matrix for sensitivity analyses
Quantiles	Measures used to describe proportion of patients with the event of interest (usually, 25%, 50%, 75%)	Not used for ICER or decision-making, but may be used to summarize results

- When there are two curves (two treatment groups), define T* as the minimum of the largest overall survival times (with an event) in the different trial arms or groups.
- Use the redistribution to the right (i.e. tail correction) algorithm for censored distributions.

Other suggestions are of a more theoretical nature and have not been widely used in practice like those of Andersen et al. (2004) or Susarla and Van Rizyn (1980)

A summary of important statistical measures and their relevance for economic evaluation are shown in Table 4.3.

4.5 Simulation: Bootstrapping and Monte-Carlo Simulation

An essential part of economic evaluation is using simulation to quantify the uncertainty around cost-effectiveness decisions. The concept of a representative sample revolves around the idea that the data observed in a trial or study is a representative sample from a population. Assume the data supported a conclusion of cost-effectiveness (ICER < £20,000 per QALY). This conclusion is a single realization from numerous possibilities. If the trial were to be conducted repeatedly with a similar (not necessarily identical) set of patients, would it result with the same conclusion? If it were repeated 10,000 times how many of those conclusions would be consistent with our observed finding of cost-effectiveness. If in 80% of these 10,000 simulations we have the same conclusion as the observed data we might feel our decision is more 'credible' or we might feel more 'confident' about it.

Usually, in an economic evaluation, for each patient, there are several types of outcomes used in a cost-effectiveness analysis: costs, utilities, PFS and OS, which are often correlated with each other and with costs). When patient-level data are available, we can simulate individual patient-level data by randomly selecting patients from the observed sample. When only summary data are available and there are no patient-level data, we need to make assumptions in order to generate data from a (probability) distribution. An example of simulation will be demonstrated using two well-known approaches: bootstrapping and Monte-Carlo methods.

Example 4.3: Simulating Using Bootstrapping

Table 4.4 shows ten patients with cost and effectiveness measures, for each of two treatment groups. The example is fictitious to demonstrate the concept.

TABLE 4.4

Observed Data for Bootstrapping

Patient	Treatment	PFS	OS	QALY	Drug Cost	Toxicity Cost
1	A	3	5	0.8	2,000	1,300
2	A	5	7	0.7	2,500	1,000
3	A	6	9	0.8	2,800	800
4	A	2	4	0.6	2,600	700
5	A	7	8	0.5	2,400	550
6	B	4	5	1.2	4,000	230
7	B	6	8	0.9	3,800	220
8	B	7	9	1.1	4,120	420
9	B	4	8	0.8	3,800	330
10	B	3	7	0.9	3,200	190

TABLE 4.5

A Bootstrap Sample of Size 5 from Observed in Table 4.5

Observation	Patient	Treatment	PFS	OS	QALY	Drug Cost (£)	Toxicity Cost (£)
1	1	A	3	5	0.8	2,000	1,300
2	1	A	3	5	0.8	2,000	1,300
3	2	A	5	7	0.7	2,500	1,000
4	4	A	2	4	0.6	2,600	700
5	4	A	2	4	0.6	2,600	700
6	6	B	4	5	1.2	4,000	230
7	8	B	7	9	1.1	4,120	420
8	8	B	7	9	1.1	4,120	420
9	9	B	4	8	0.8	3,800	330
10	10	B	3	7	0.9	3,200	190

A bootstrap sample of ten patients (five in each group) is performed separately for each treatment group. This involves taking a random patient with replacement (as each patient is representative of the population). Hence, in a bootstrap sample of the same original sample size, the entire (row) set of data is sampled for that patient, ensuring that the correlation between costs and effects remains intact.

Table 4.5 shows one bootstrap sample of size ten (five per group). Due to the small sample size here, some patients have not been resampled. In 10,000 bootstrap samples of a larger sample size (e.g. a sample size of n=150 instead of n=10), we would expect a more representative sample (if n=10, it is possible we could resample the same patients 50% of the time). The data from each bootstrap sample is then used to construct the mean (10,000 incremental means costs and QALYs). It is important to note that the bootstrap is conditional on the sample. If the observed sample is biased or of poor quality, the bootstrap sample is also likely to share these characteristics.

4.5.1 Simulating Using Monte-Carlo Sampling

This type of simulation can be used when we need to use summary statistics to simulate the observed mean, or variance, or other parameter of some observed data (patient-level data may not be available). This requires assumptions to be made about the statistical distribution for each outcome. For example, if the data were assumed to be normally distributed with a mean of 3.4 and a standard deviation (STDev) of 1.4, we could simulate a data set (or several data sets) such that when we compute the mean and STDev of the simulated data set, it is close to the observed mean and variance values.

For example in Table 4.4, OS and PFS might be exponentially distributed (see Figure 4.3), costs might be gamma distributed (due to skewed data), and ensuring that the simulation holds, the correlation structure can be very challenging. One difficulty encountered with Monte-Carlo simulation is that sometime a survival (OS) time can be generated that is shorter than the PFS (at the very least) such that OS < PFS; hence care needs to be taken with these methods. Simulation of OS and PFS to generate PPS is commonly employed to generate a distribution of the mean survival times for to derive the QALY. Khan (2015) provides several examples of Monte-Carlo simulations of correlated data from any distribution.

4.6 Analyzing Data from Cancer Trials

The KM method does not involve modeling survival times. Other estimates of survival rates are based on the methods such as the 'life table' approach or the so-called Nelson-Aalen estimates. The KM is a descriptive method for presentation of survival rates and has limited application when it comes to describing the treatment effect over the entire overall survival curve.

4.6.1 Semi-Parametric Methods: The Cox PH Model

The Cox proportional hazards model (Cox PH) is a statistical method for comparing survival times (events) between two or more groups while allowing for other factors or covariates (e.g. age, gender). If we assume that there are two treatment groups and we wish to determine whether treatment is effective, the hazard rate for patients can be written as:

$$h_i(t) = h_0(t)\exp(\beta X_i),$$

where X_i is an indicator variable that takes the value of 1 if the patient takes the experimental treatment and 0 if they take control and $h_0(t)$ is the baseline hazard (which can take any form). The baseline hazard corresponds to the chance of an event (e.g. death) when all the explanatory variables assume a value of 0. The baseline hazard function can be thought of as similar to the intercept in linear regression. When the covariate assumes a value of 0 (e.g. if the control arm was given a value of 0), the baseline rate could be interpreted as the risk per unit time of death for an individual who does not take the new treatment (i.e. takes the control). The Cox model differs from other models because the covariates are used to predict the hazard function, and not a survival time (or failure time). Using the model is reasonably straightforward with a computer program and the interpretation of treatment effects is also straightforward as shown in Example 4.4.

4.6.1.1 Adjusting for Covariates with the Cox Model

The Cox PH model can be used to adjust for covariates when estimating the HR. For example, where survival differences exist between treatments for males and females (e.g. females live longer), an adjusted measures of treatment effect (the HR) can be computed. An HR of 0.70 for treatment A versus treatment B means that patients, on average, are 30% less likely to have the event of interest (e.g. death) on treatment A compared to treatment B. An analysis from a Cox PH model will not give estimates of median or mean survival times. Cox PH models are used because, like KM methods, one does not need to make assumptions (other than the PH assumption) about survival times. Despite the widespread use of the Cox PH model, there are nevertheless limitations. In practice the Cox PH model is used for estimating hazard ratios (or adjusted hazard ratios) and little else (Table 4.6).

Example 4.4: Interpreting Results from a Cox PH Model

Table 4.4 shows that prior to adjusting for treatment, the HR was 0.63 and statistically significant ($p < 0.001$). After adjusting for age, gender, and ECOG, of which only ECOG appeared to be a statistical predictor of survival, the risk of mortality on treatment A was now 27% lower (previously, ignoring ECOG, it was 37% lower).

TABLE 4.6
Example of Interpreting Adjusted Hazard Ratios

Effect	HR	95% CI	*p*-Value
Treatment (A versus B)	0.63	0.34, 0.89	<0.001
Treatment (A versus B)	0.73	0.51, 0.91	<0.001
Age			0.313
Gender			0.105
ECOG			0.002

4.6.1.2 Using Hazard Ratios to Predict Survival Rates

Sometimes it is pertinent to use the HR to compute the percentage increase in survival rates. An interesting example in NICE (TA189, 2010, sorafenib) for hepatocellular carcinoma, is discussed. In the comparison of sorafenib, the manufacturer stated:

> The percentage increase in survival was calculated using the Hazard Ratio, which takes into account the whole K-M survival curve by averaging the treatment effect across the curves. Formula: HR = hazard of sorafenib/ hazard of placebo. Thus the relative improvement of sorafenib = 1/HR, i.e. 1/0.6931 =1.44 (i.e. prolongation in survival by 44%). (Note: Under the assumption of exponential survival distribution, the ratio of hazards is the inverse of that of the medians. Comparing the medians directly is considered the most intuitive, but less reliable since it only takes one point of the K-M curve).

The ERG commented on this:

> The use of hazard ratio (HR) to calculate a % increase in survival time is potentially misleading if the assumption of exponential survival distribution is not supported (see Spruance et al., 2004). HR informs on the likelihood that a random patient from one group will reach an endpoint before a patient selected randomly from the comparator group. When the exponential assumption is not supported HR may inflate (or deflate) the apparent survival benefit.
>
> The ERG extracted individual patient data for the placebo group and tested the exponential assumption. On the basis of this analysis the ERG consider that the assumption is not supported and that a 44% increase in survival benefit probably inflates the apparent benefit. A more reliable indicator in this case is the % increase in median survival, which for overall survival is 34.6%.

In Example 4.1, the HR was 0.69 (Figure 4.6). The relative improvement was computed as 1/HR = 1/0.69 = 1.44 (a 44% improvement in OS). However, before reporting this, it would have been prudent to check that the survival data fitted an exponential model. This means checking the model for both groups. In fact the data did not support an exponential model fit and the conclusion was that the improvement in OS of 44% was an overestimate. The median OS was 46.3 versus 34.4 weeks (a difference of 11.9 weeks). This corresponds to a 35% improvement. When the exponential fit cannot be satisfied, the improvement in OS (across the entire OS curve) can be determined from the median values, or restricted mean, or from a parametric survival model.

Spruance (2004) makes the point that the hazard ratio can be misleading if used to assess the magnitude of treatment benefit. In some cases large treatment effects (small HRs) can be reported along with small median differences (KM curves cross near to the median but diverge significantly over time); in other cases small treatment effects (larger HRs < 1) can result in large median differences. One reason for this is due to the shape of the survival curves combined with non-constant hazards. A more reasonable estimate of the treatment effect size when these situations arise is likely to lie somewhere between these two extremes. The median could be a conservative assessment of OS improvement on the one hand, whereas the HR may be overly optimistic. This leads us now to the issue of parametric survival models.

4.6.2 Parametric Methods: Modeling Survival Data for Extrapolation

The Cox PH model is a useful model for estimating treatment effects in terms of HRs as well as adjusting the effects for covariates. However, a key part of economic evaluation lies in extrapolating survival rates beyond trial follow-up. Prediction of survival rates beyond the last overall survival time point (extrapolation) allows health benefits (and associated costs) to be computed over the entire life time of patients for economic evaluation. Several parametric models are now discussed that may be used for predicting survival rates. Details are also provided in the NICE TSD on survival models (Woods, 2017); Latimer, 2011).

(i) The exponential model

The exponential distribution is a simple parametric model with one parameter λ. It therefore assumes a constant hazard with a survival function;

$$S(t) = \exp(-\lambda * t)$$

This is a PH model and treatment effects are estimated in terms of HRs, interpreted in a similar to the Cox PH model. The model is easy to fit and interpret.

(ii) The Weibull Model

The Cox PH model is often used when the probability distribution of the sampled survival times is unknown, or it might be complicated to fit a model to the data. Since we wish to predict survival rates at specific time points, the survival function using a Weibull model can be used:

$$S(t) = \exp\left(-lt^{\alpha}\right) \quad (4.3)$$

where t is the survival time. Equation (4.3) has two parameters, λ and α, which need to be estimated (here λ is the hazard rate or scale parameter) and 03B1 is the shape parameter. These are used to adjust the shape of the survival curve and provide predictions of survival times at time t, once the shape and scale parameters are estimated. Note that when $\alpha = 1$, this becomes an exponential model.

In practice one might fit this curve to an observed set of survival data, estimate the parameters λ and α, then use equation (4.3) to predict future survival data. The Weibull model is frequently used (sometimes inappropriately) in HTAs. The reasons for its popularity is because it is relatively simple to fit and it is also a PH model (which is helpful for interpreting coefficients as treatment effects as it is similar to the Cox PH model).

The Weibull model has greater flexibility than the exponential model, which assumes a constant hazard. Here the hazard may increase or decrease, but cannot change direction. Where $\alpha = 1$, the Weibull is the same as an exponential. For $\alpha > 1$ the hazard function increases and for $\alpha < 1$ the hazard function decreases monotonically. In order to fit a Weibull distribution, it is important to check the nature of the hazard function statistically and whether it has a sound clinical interpretation. Figure 4.8 also shows how the survival curve takes on different shapes for varying values of α. Example 4.5 shows how an exponential and Weibull function are used.

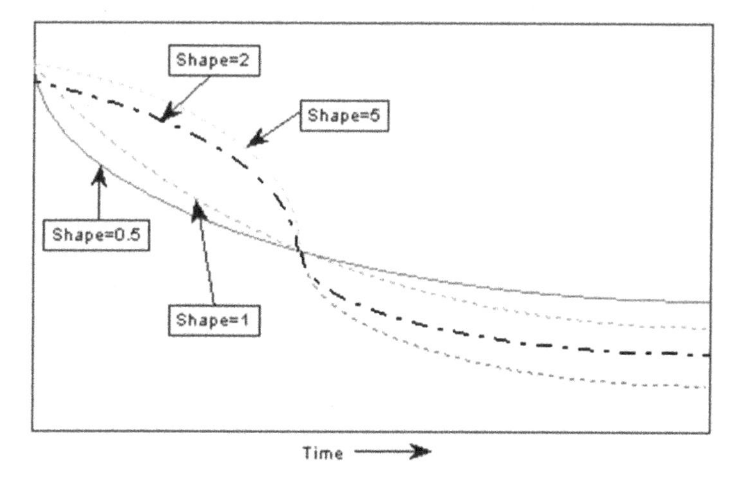

FIGURE 4.8
Changing shape of the survivor function for the Weibull model.

Example 4.5: Fitting an Exponential and Weibull Function to Estimate Survival Rates: Cost-Effectiveness of Lenalidomide

BACKGROUND

The data for this analysis was kindly provided by Reck et al. (2014). Despite lenalidomide and dexamethasone being highly effective, its use in multiple myeloma (MM) is restricted due to a lack of evidence of cost-effectiveness. In this example we performed a cost-effectiveness analysis by using an alternate day dosing strategy where lenalidomide commenced at 25 mg daily; Due to hematological toxicity, instead of giving 15 mg daily, 25 mg was given every two days (alternate days). Subsequent reductions of 5 mg were made due to potentially further toxicity (i.e. 15 mg then 10 mg on alternate days, instead of 10 mg then 5 mg daily). The objective was therefore to compare the cost-effectiveness of lenalidomide and dexamethasone alternate dosing (L+$D_{Alternate}$) versus lenalidomide plus dexamethasone standard (L+$D_{Standard}$) dosing based on the summary of product characteristics.

DESIGN, PATIENTS AND TREATMENT SCHEDULE

The data for this example comes from a real-world setting. It was a retrospective review of patients with relapsed multiple myeloma treated with lenalidomide and dexamethasone in a single UK center (University College London Hospitals Foundation Trust (UCLH)). The main efficacy endpoints were time-to-progression (TTP), progression-free survival (PFS), and overall survival (OS).

Real-world patient-level data were available for a single cohort of L+$D_{Alternate}$ patients (N = 39) who were given an alternate dosing regimen. Summarized data for lenalidomide alone, dexamethasone alone and L+D_{SPC} were taken from published data.

First a Kaplan-Meir curve was generated for TTP for L+$D_{Alternate}$ and then a Weibull parametric function was used to predict survival probabilities beyond 21 months. Figure 4.9 shows the KM curve with a Weibull function for L+$D_{Alternate}$ fitted over the first 55 months. The value of the scale and shape parameters were 0.817 and 0.0276 respectively.

For the comparison of L+$D_{Alternate}$ with dexamethasone, since no patient-level data were available for dexamethasone alone, this data had to be simulated using published statistics. The mean TTP for dexamethasone alone was simulated using published data that compared L+D_{SPC} versus dexamethasone using a reported hazard ratio of 0.427. It was assumed that the TTP followed an exponential model (see Table 4.7).

In Table 4.7, the mean OSs for L+D_{SPC} (4.0 years) and dexamethasone (2.3 years) were determined by simulating survival times from published data. Recall, it is the mean survival times needed for cost-effectiveness analyses. Mean survival times were not reported (only medians were reported) and so had to be simulated. The L+$D_{Alternate}$ group was used for the real-world data for which limited follow-up data were available. Hence, TTP was modeled to compute the mean TTP for the L+$D_{Alternate}$ group. In short, for each group, we required a mean OS, a mean TTP, and a mean PPS, from which we could construct the QALY. The available

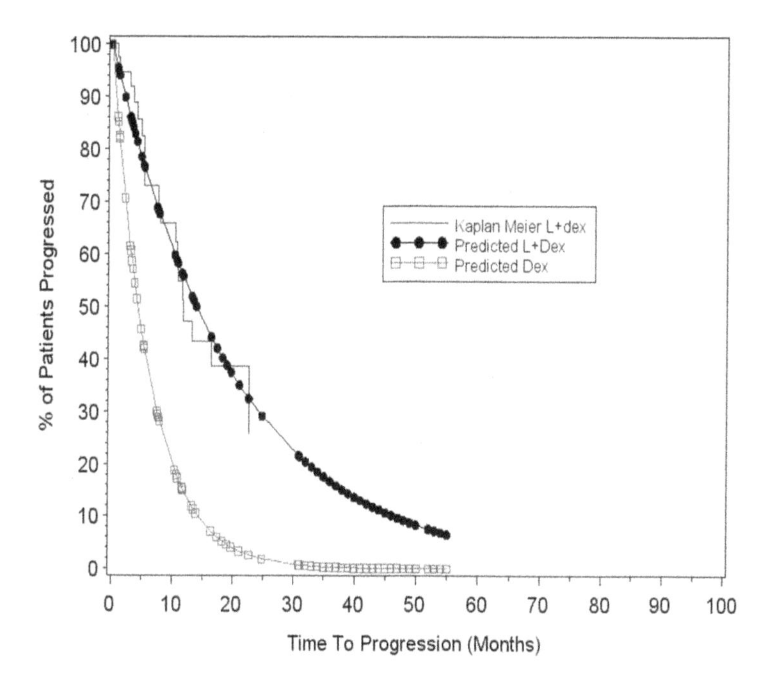

FIGURE 4.9
Estimated shape of the TTP L+dexamethasone and dexamethasone alone survivor function estimated from a Weibull model.

TABLE 4.7

Summary of Estimates Used for Simulation

	Parameter	L+D$_{SPC}$	Dexamethasone alone	L+D$_{Alternate}$
Efficacy	Median OS[1]	2.8 years	1.6 years	2.8 years
	Mean OS[2]	4.0 years	2.3 years	4.0 years
	Median TTP	0.87 years[1]	0.4 years	0.98 years[3]
	Mean TTP	1.7	0.6[5]	1.7 years[4]
	Mean PPS	2.3 years	1.7 years	2.3 years

[1] *Notes:* From ERG report (NICE, TA171, 2008; Stadtmauer, 2006).
[2] Modeled assuming an exponential distribution (mean OS was not reported so had to be simulated).
[3] Observed in the data (also reported in the published studies).
[4] Using a Weibull function for the observed data and assumed to be the same for the standard regimen. The observed TTP was modeled using a Weibull model with a scale parameter of 0.817 and a shape parameter of 0.0276. The log likelihood test for model fit suggested the model fit was appropriate.
[5] Estimated using TTP/log(2) , assuming dexamethasone TTP is exponential (page 88, ERG report, NICE TA171).

data (often medians) were used to construct (simulate) these values as shown in Table 4.7.

From the above we were able to generate the effectiveness inputs for both $L+D_{Alternate}$ and dexamethasone alone. Using the observed OS data for $L+D_{Alternate}$, assuming an exponential model to fit the observed KM curve, we can extrapolate beyond the last time point to the maximum time an 'average' human being could theoretically live – set to 100 years. Consequently, the mean OS for $L+D_{Alternate}$ was 4 years. In order to estimate the mean OS for dexamethasone alone, we used the fact that OS = TTP/log(2) (also used by the evidence review group, NICE TA171, 2008). For the dexamethasone group, therefore, the mean TTP was estimated to be 2.3 years. Similar data for the $L+D_{SPC}$ was already reported (Table 4.7).

A strong and somewhat unverifiable assumption was that mean survival times between the alternative dosing arm versus the dexamethasone arm would yield similar effects to $L+D_{SPC}$ versus dexamethasone. This could have been investigated using a well-controlled RCT; however, it may not be in a manufacturer's interest to conduct such a trial.

(iii) Other Models

The NICE technical support document (TSD) (Latimer, 2011) suggests several other survival function models that can be used, including the Gompertz, generalized gamma, log-normal, log-logistic models. Details of how to fit these models can be found in several references (Collet, 2014; Crowther, 2016; Klein, 2005). A further group of models called piecewise and flexible parametric models are now discussed. For now, we limit our discussion on the statistical aspects of these models.

4.6.3 Advanced Modeling Techniques for Survival Data

4.6.3.1 Flexible Parametric Survival Models

Standard parametric models (e.g. Weibull) can be used to model survival data, but not all will retain the useful assumption of PH or fit the overall survival pattern well. Flexible parametric modeling methodology (Beck & Jackman, 1998; Royston & Parmar, 2002) is based on using 'flexible' polynomial functions that are fitted piecewise. This consists of several functions that are joined together at 'knots' (which act as constraints) so that the overall fitted function is smooth. The idea can be compared with linear spline fitting (basically joining lines), but instead of linear splines (which are polynomial functions in the first degree), 'curves' are joined together to fit the observed data.

The approach to flexible parametric modeling involves joining pairs of data points using higher degrees of polynomial functions (e.g. quadratic for order two and cubic for order three, or fractional polynomials). One useful property of using splines is that the underlying functional form does not need to be specified (Kruger, 2004). Splines can be used in the context of a Cox PH model to smooth the hazard function (Sleeper & Harrington, 1990), however in this section we present the use of splines for fully parametric models.

Although the Weibull model is a useful alternative to the Cox PH model, especially when the assumptions around distributions are reasonable, a more flexible approach (Royston & Lambert, 2011) directly modeling the baseline hazard function $h_0(t)$ as a polynomial function has shown to be a versatile approach to fitting smooth survival functions.

4.6.3.2 Applications in Cancer Surveillance

Cancer registries increasingly collect important prognostic factors of survival useful for oncologists, policymakers, and others in order to make decisions on expected survival rates for subgroups of patients. Calculating patient- and strata-specific survival rates, although possible, is not straightforward using Cox PH modeling. The main reason for using the Cox model is the PH assumption for which the baseline hazard function is eliminated (through special estimation methods called partial likelihoods). For a Cox model, the important aspect is the hazard ratio and not the hazard function. The baseline hazard can be thought of as nuisance parameter, which is eliminated.

For example, calculating the survival probability for an individual (or group of individuals) who are female, aged 50 (on average), with Stage III breast cancer is a particularly useful statistic for policymakers and planners, especially for future costing of cancer treatments. Latimer (2011) and Bagust and Beale (2014) discuss approaches to extrapolating data in survival models, including a selection process as a guide for modeling. Several issues merit consideration.

First, it is recognized that reimbursement decisions depend on having reliable evidence with respect to costs and effects accrued beyond what is often presented, because trial follow-up is curtailed for practical purposes. Second, methods for selecting or checking models/model fit and assumptions (such as PH) should be assessed using appropriate plots and information criterion methods (note model fitting is somewhat determined by the observed data). Third, there is debate as to whether standard parametric functions should be considered as the first choice (e.g. Weibull, log-normal), although it is agreed that the data should determine the most appropriate method through a systematic approach to modeling. In addition, a pre-specified cut-off point should be identified for when the extrapolation should start. Often this is the last observed time point or is dependent on the date of data cut-off, which in itself is dictated by a regulatory constraint that requires a definition in the protocol as to when the 'end of trial' occurs. Lastly, consideration should be given to the physiological process. It is possible to fit a mathematical function to survival data that shows an excellent fit, but the estimates of the parameters may not have sound clinical relevance.

Example 4.6: Modeling Survival Data Using a Flexible Parametric Model in a Lung Cancer Trial

BACKGROUND

The data from Lee (2012) were used to fit a flexible parametric model. Nearly all (98%) of the patients died at the time of analysis (658 deaths). The objective was to fit a parametric survival curve to each treatment

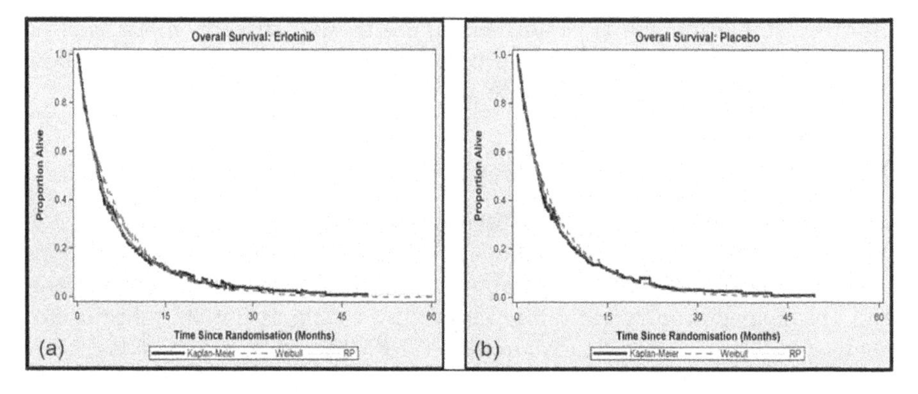

FIGURE 4.10
(a) OS Erlonitib (b) OS Placebo of predicted survival rates from Weibull applied to data from the TOPICAL trial.

group to predict the survival pattern and mean survival time. More details are in Dewar and Khan (2015). Although in this example the practical benefits of extrapolation are negligible, the exercise shows that a flexible parametric model can show a better fit than standard models. The Royston-Parmar (RP) model was fitted using SAS statistical software. In this analysis the OS was used as the time to event variable. The separate curves were joined using 1 'knot' (or '2 separate curves'), hence it was called an RP(1) model.

RESULTS

The empirical survival curve (Figures 4.10(a) and 4.10(b)) is also plotted along with the Weibull model. The Kaplan-Meier (solid line) is approximated well by the RP (dotted line) with three knots. The Weibull (dashed line) is a slightly worse fit (Table 4.8).

In this example, the mean survival times for erlotinib versus placebo were 6.95 versus 6.53, 6.96 versus 6.47, and 7.05 versus 6.62 months for

TABLE 4.8
Estimates of Coefficients and Hazard Ratios from STATA and SAS

	Cox PH	Weibull*	[a]RP(1)
HR(SE)	0.95 (0.08)	0.93 (0.09)	0.95 (0.08)
Lower 95%	0.82	0.78	0.82
Upper 95%	1.11	1.11	1.11
Predicted 6 month survival[b]		40.1 vs. 38.4	34.1 vs. 32.4
AIC	7340	3818	2165

[a] *Notes:* RP(1): Flexible parametric using 1 knot.
[b] Observed 6 month survival rates for erlotinib vs. placebo were 39.1% vs. 36.6%.
* Using PROC LIFEREG in SAS.

the Kaplan-Meier, RP(1), and Weibull models respectively. The Weibull model might therefore overestimate mean survival time and hence QALYs (assuming quality of life is the same between treatment groups).

Example 4.7: Modeling Survival Data Using a Flexible Parametric Model in the Presence of Censoring

In this trial, two treatments A and B were compared in terms of OS. Patients were followed up in the trial for 12 months. Long-term cost-effectiveness was required over a 5-year time horizon by modeling and extrapolating survival time between randomization and death, after examining the overall survival curves (Figure 4.7).

The follow-up period was only 12 months, and there were many patients who were still alive by the end of 12 months. A flexible parametric model using cubic spline (Royston & Parmar, 2002) with a RP(3) (3-knot) model was used. Extrapolation beyond 5 years was considered to be highly speculative and uncertain because most death events occurred between randomization and end of follow-up. The fitted Royston-Parmar model was used to predict the survival rates at each time point (Figure 4.8). The survival rates at each of 3 monthly intervals (3, 6, 9, 12 ... 60 months) were used to determine the expected costs and derive the QALYs (at an aggregate level).

After fitting, a Royston-Parmar 3-knot model (the best model based on lowest AIC) using a 5-year time horizon yielded a mean survival time of about 41.9 versus 33.3 months for A versus B, respectively. From this, the mean overall survival (OS) for A versus B was 4.12 versus 4.07 months based on the observed KM estimates from the within-trial data over 12 months. At 5 years (60 months) post-randomization, 67% of patients were expected to remain alive in group A compared to 45% in group B (Figure 4.8a: KM survival plot). These survival rates are lower than the national average as reported in mortality statistics for the general population with a similar age distribution to this population. These would be 95% at 5 years from a mean age of 63 years, which logically are higher than observed here as these are patients with cancer.

Plots of the log survival (Figure 4.11b and the hazard rate (Figure 4.11c) suggest that A has a trend of decreasing hazards (lower risk of death over time) while B appears to have an increasing hazard (higher risk of death over time). This is mainly due to the spike in hazards after month 6 because of a later death event in group B. Both hazard functions suggest risk of death is decreasing with a similar trend until 4 months, albeit with a more erratic hazard for the group B.

After about 4 months, patients may die at a slightly faster rate (ignoring the spike) in the group B. Due to a lack of further follow-up data, future death patterns may or may not be similar, although the curve trajectory for group B suggests the hazard curve may lie slightly above that of group B. These plots partially support the extrapolated survival curves, suggesting death rates in group A occur more slowly compared with patients in group B, but survival rates over time may converge.

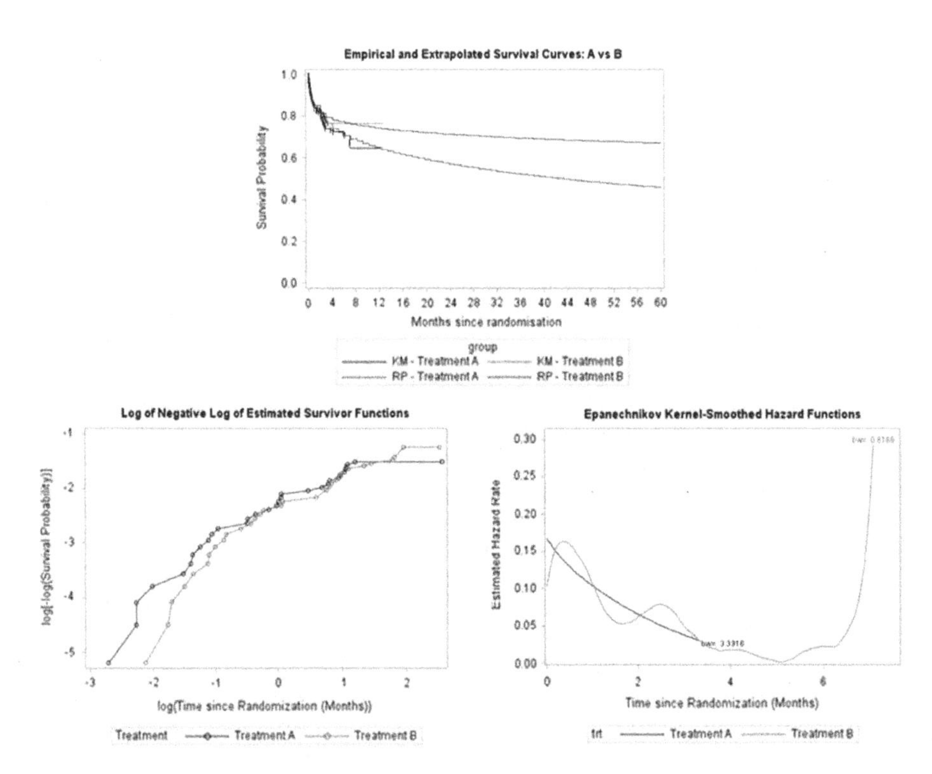

FIGURE 4.11
Observed and extrapolated OS over 5 years using RP (3) log survival (bottom left) and the hazard function (bottom right).

4.7 Issues in Fitting Models

When a parametric model is fitted to survival data, two broad approaches may be taken. One is to fit a single parametric model to the entire data (assuming PH). The second is to fit an individual or piecewise parametric model separately for each treatment group to each treatment arm. If an HR is used (assume two groups) to fit a model for the entire data set, it should ideally be fitted under the PH assumption – that is, the treatment effect is proportional over time and the survival curves fitted to each treatment group have a similar shape. Proportional hazards models such as the exponential, Gompertz, or Weibull could also be used. However, some models (e.g. log-logistic and some accelerated failure time models) will not necessarily produce a single hazard ratio (HR). With such models, the PH assumption does not hold.

Using separate parametric models fitted to each treatment arm requires fewer assumptions (but requires the estimation of more parameters). Fitting parametric models separately to each treatment arm is possible (e.g. a Weibull for one treatment arm and a log-normal for the other) but will require strong justification because different models allow very different shaped hazard distributions. If the PH assumption does not hold, it may be reasonable to fit separate parametric models. Where a PH model is used, justification will be needed. Further details can be found in the NICE TSD report (Latimer, 2011).

In addition to the Weibull, other models such as the Gompertz model can also be used. The approach to determining which model is the most useful fit can be determined by the smallest value of the AIC. In general, where the survival rates are to be estimated, an accelerated failure time (AFT) model form would be most useful. In general, the PH models the hazard rate, whereas the AFT form of the models is used for modeling the survival rates over time. Klein and Moeschberger (2005) present a table of hazard functions and survival functions for each model.

4.8 Handling Crossover, Treatment Switching, and Subsequent Anti-Cancer Therapy

4.8.1 Introduction to Treatment Switching

Sometimes randomized clinical trials in oncology include the possibility for patients in the standard care or comparator arm (i.e. the control arm) to be able to switch to the experimental drug. This is due to ethical concerns that when equipoise is lost, patients should not be forced to remain in a supposedly lower-efficacy treatment. Earlier (in Chapter 1) we introduced the issue of crossover (or treatment switching) in cancer trials, which can make differences between treatment arms appear larger (or smaller) and therefore bias the estimate of the QALY. Jonsson et al. (2014) and Latimer et al. (2014) provide an overview of the issues and implications of crossover for economic evaluation. Crossover allows patients to experience the treatment they did not get because the current treatment a patient has received did not yield the desired effect (efficacy or safety). Crossover often occurs at the point of unblinding (at the patient level) and results in a loss of information. In a (double-blind) trial, at the point of progression (switching over), it would not be known whether an experimental treatment is efficacious or not – that would usually be known after the data analysis is complete or partially complete (through interim analysis).

There are several issues that concern both efficacy and effectiveness relating to crossover. These are likely to be about the methods available for handling crossover, the assumptions for their use, and how to interpret the resulting treatment effects. From the efficacy perspective, we consider that such methods can only be used as a form of sensitivity analysis around the observed treatment effect. For cost-effectiveness, however, the issue may be deeper. Whereas efficacy is essentially about an unbiased treatment effect, effectiveness is often about effects in the real world in which crossover is often unavoidable.

Designing a trial for potential crossover may be impractical or very challenging (i.e. you don't always know if patients will switch over, or who they are, and it is unlikely patients would want to be randomized again to another 'choice' when they have just stopped taking the existing treatment). Moreover, some patients can be treated with experimental treatments (switch over treatment) by moving to a location where the treatment is available. For example, stereotactic whole brain radiation therapy offered to lung cancer patients is only available at some particular hospitals. If some patients decided they wished to receive this despite being randomized to the alternative treatment group, this too would have similar effects as crossing over – biasing treatment effects.

4.8.2 Types of Switching

Figure 4.12a shows the simplest form of switching. Patients in the experimental arm are not allowed to switch to the control arm (arrows moving upward or downward signify direction of switching). Usually switching is allowed when or some time after progression has been detected. However, in practice there may be other reasons for switching, such as the occurrence of a severe adverse event, toxicity, or the treating physician's decision. These are called the (switching) trigger events or reasons (see Green Park Collaborative, 2016). This case is called a unilateral switch as opposed to a bilateral switch where both switches are allowed. Less usual is a bilateral switching process (Figure 4.12b) whereby patients in the experimental group switch to the control as well as vice versa. Switching starts later in the experimental arm. This would be the case if switching was allowed upon progression in the control arm and progression is delayed in the experimental arm.

Other more complex switching patterns (Figure 4.9c) can be observed if switching to other (e.g. second-line treatments) are allowed (including palliative care in metastatic disease). In this case, both patients who received experimental and control treatments, and to different 3rd line drugs H or F. Figure 4.9d shows that both groups switch to treatment A, but some or all control patients might switch to the experimental treatment first. It is important to note that the assumption that patients switching from control to experimental treatment will not be subject to harm or deterioration will be very strong but only hypothetical. Where efficacy is more important than effectiveness, an OS free from confounding factors will be more important.

4.8.3 Implications of Switching

The statistical issues around treatment switching also have similar implications for situations where patients take other concomitant medication, stop

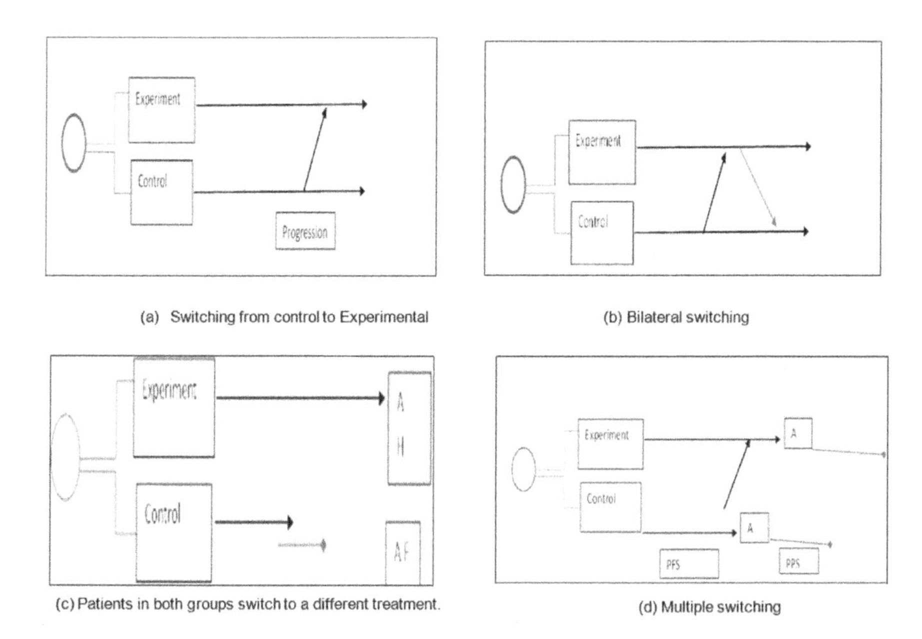

FIGURE 4.12
Graphical demonstration of the types of switching/crossover: (a) Switching from control to experimental; (b) bilateral switching; (c) patients in both groups switch to a different treatment; (d) multiple switching patients on control switch to experimental (A), and then subsequently take another treatment (F). Patients on experimental (A) take a subsequent treatment (H).

taking treatment, take cocktails of treatment, and also take dose adjustments (which are commonly captured through dose modifications in the case report forms). The presence of significant crossover can have serious implications for QALY estimates due to biased efficacy estimates. Hence, this problem is not just a health economic evaluation question, but a more general question on generating unbiased estimates of treatment effect in the presence of crossover in cancer trials. It is also related to a more recent theme called 'estimands,' which is explained in the addendum to the ICH E9 guideline on statistical principles (ICH E9 Addendum, 2017). 'Estimands' attempt to estimate the 'true' value of a new treatment by considering multiple sets of analyses, where each analysis is relevant to a specific stakeholder. Hence, efficacy and effectiveness will have their own corresponding 'estimad' or measure of treatment effect. This ICH E9 addendum seeks to differentiate the types of treatment effects that ensue according to the different ways in which patients are handled for complex issues such as treatment switching or missing data. The addendum may have been needed to clarify the different and sometimes conflicting requirements from reimbursement and licensing agencies for determining efficacy and effectiveness under different scenarios.

In general, a definition of a crossover treatment should be identified and stated up-front. One should also determine whether, for a given reimbursement agency, crossover is likely to be a concern, especially for long-term treatment effects in the presence of crossover. One should identify and distinguish between spontaneous versus treatment-related crossover (e.g. patient decision rather than due to progression). It is always better to design for switching, and where possible, to avoid crossover. It would also be useful to have an idea of the rate of crossover expected based on experience with previous trials. In addition, careful testing of assumptions and beliefs about PPS after switching should be evaluated – this also extends to post-progression HRQoL.

4.8.4 Handling Switching in Statistical Analyses

There are several approaches to handling crossover suggested in the published literature:

(i) ITT analysis
(ii) Per protocol analysis
(iii) Including crossover treatment as a time-varying covariate in a Cox model
(iv) Inverse probability-of-censoring weighting (IPCW)
(v) Rank-preserving structural failure time models (RPSFTMs)
(vi) Two-stage adjustment model
(vii) Other approaches

We will discuss somewhat approaches (iii) and (iv) in more detail since these appear to be the currently recommended approaches (Jonsson et al., 2014; Morden et al., 2011; Ishak, 2014).

No one particular method has been identified as the 'best' approach suitable for all situations. Interested readers may consult the references for specific details. However, each method aims to address particular questions (or estimands). For example, the IPCW estimates the treatment effect as if switching from control treatment to experimental treatment was absent, but the estimate still includes the effects of subsequent therapies. Using RPSFT on the other hand might allow for an estimation of the experimental treatment benefit alone (disentangled from the subsequent treatments), although in practice the estimate of treatment benefit is a combination of experimental treatment and subsequent therapy. More complex statistical techniques have been developed to adjust or correct for the switching problem.

4.8.4.1 Intent-to-Treat (ITT)

In the case of ITT, since patients are analyzed according the group they were randomized to, effects measured after switching are considered as belonging to the treatment group being switched from. For example, a patient is randomized to the control group (C). The group's median OS time (until progression) is 6 months but the PFS time was 4 months. Patients in the experimental arm (E) have a median OS time of 8 months and a median PFS time of 6 months. At 4 months this patient switched treatment to the experimental arm. It would appear this patient lived for 7 months.

Using an ITT analysis, the patient would have an OS of 7 months attributable to the control. If the median OS is 8 months on E, then the patient has an OS of 1 month less than on average in E (Figure 4.13). The fact that the extended survival might be due to post-switch experimental treatment is not factored in. Consequently, the treatment effect is underestimated, as will be the QALY. Conversely, if a switch from E to C happened (because E was too toxic), the ITT analysis may lead to the wrong interpretation. The effects are not necessarily biased (in the statistical sense), because data are treated as belonging to a randomized experiment.

In a usual ITT analysis (where patients are grouped according to their initial randomization therapy), even in the simple case of unilateral control switching, the overall effect is to dilute the difference in OS between the two arms (Δ_E), so that the true drug efficacy is underestimated. In fact, any post-switch subsequent endpoint is affected (e.g. PPS, OS, HRQoL, adverse effects, or dropout). This can be important as in some trials up to 80% of the control arm patients switch to the experimental drug some time after progression. One should bear in mind that in practice, the transitions happen with some delay after evidence of progression and switching is not necessarily instantaneous.

Example 4.8: Impact of Switching on Cost-Effectiveness

In a trial with a mean survival of 12 months for the experimental group E and 6 months for the control group, switchers from C to E gain another

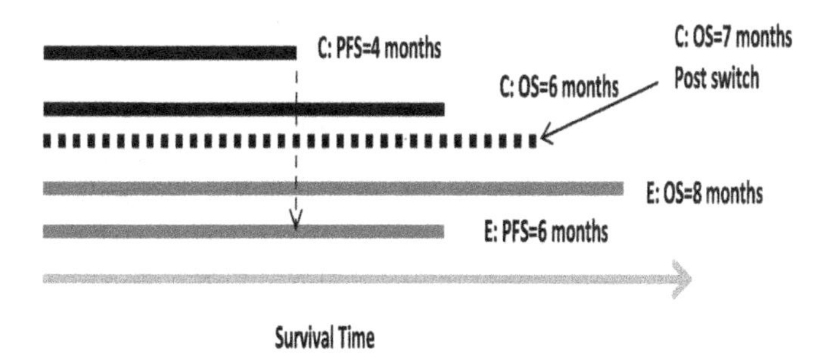

FIGURE 4.13
Relationship between switching and survival; C = censored; E = event.

3 months and 50% of the controls switch at progression (they increase their PPS by 3 months). Had those in C stayed in the control arm, the difference in mean survival would have been 12 – 6 = 6 months. With switching, the mean survival of the controls is now equal to (6 x 0.50) + (9 x 0.50) = 3 + 4.5 = 7.5, or a difference of 12 – 7.5 = 4.5 months in favor of E.

Now imagine also that the average experimental cost for a full treatment is much higher than for the control drug cost, say respectively €5,000 and €1,000. The same switching process also makes the cost higher for C; instead of a cost difference of €4,000 without switching we now face (1,000 x 0.50) + (5,000 x 0.50) = 500 + 2,500 = €3,000 (if all switchers also receive a full treatment with E). These combined effects change the ICER dramatically in favor of the new drug; ICER no switching = (€4,000/6) ≈ €667 per life-month gained (LMG) compared to (€2,000/4.5) = €444 per LMG.

4.8.4.2 Per Protocol Analysis

A per protocol (PP) analysis would censor patients from the date they switched. This analysis can be subject to selection biases: patients who switch may well be those with poorer prognosis. This has two main consequences: first, to diminish the statistical power of the study because their observation is cut short, reducing the number of observable events (deaths) in the control arm. Second, unless switching is random, it will most probably introduce a selection bias as the events (or reasons for it like progression) for switching are likely to be correlated with the final endpoint (death for OS assessment), and therefore distort the initial randomization in treatment groups.

4.8.4.3 IPCW

The IPCW approach (Robins & Finkelstein, 2000) involves calculating the probability of censoring in relation to a set of confounders (e.g. age, performance status, stage, etc.) using a logit model. We assume there are no hidden or unmeasured confounders – an assumption difficult to verify. This is basically an adaptation of the marginal structural model (MSM) first developed for observational studies.

The MSM inverse probability-of-censoring weighting (IPCW) model, frequently used in epidemiology to correct for dropouts, can be used also for correcting for switching. In this approach patients who switch are first censored at their time of switching. Then the bias introduced by the switching is corrected by weighting each patient in the control arm by the inverse of his predicted probability (estimated through logistic regression) of *not being* censored. The predicted probability is estimated based on baseline patient characteristics and further time-varying factors that could influence the switching. Once these probabilities have been calculated they are used as weights. This creates a (weighted) pseudo-population where control patients who did not switch are weighted more heavily. Finally, a survival analysis is performed on this pseudo-population, usually with a standard survival method, such as Cox regression or a parametric model.

The whole method relies on the premise that the probability of switching is correctly estimated from the observed covariates and that, *conditional on these,* switching is independent of the outcome and its timing (the so-called 'no unmeasured confounding' assumption). Consequently, the trial must collect enough information over time on the switching covariates. Trial sample sizes also have to be relatively large as generally the number of potential covariates is large, and in smaller trials the logistic regression will not converge or yield very high weights for some specific patients when the number of non-switchers is low (Jonsson et al., 2014; Latimer et al., 2016).

The method is briefly described below.

For a given data set we identify the date of switching for each patient. If a date is present a switch is considered to have occurred. The logit model is then regressed against a set of covariates:

$$\text{Response} = \text{intercept} + \text{covariates}\ (\text{including time varying covariates})$$

where response is a binary variable with 1 for a censored survival time and 0 if not censored. The approach to modeling is as follows.

Step 1: Determine covariates that may be predictive of switching. Decide the rule to drop or keep covariate (e.g. if p-value >> 0.05, drop)

Step 2: Model the probability of switching (using a logistic regression) and for each patient estimate the predicted probability of switching. For those patients who have not switched calculate the inverse of these predicted probabilities.

Step 3: For each patient that has not switched adjust the survival times by the inverse of the probability weights.

Step 4: Fit a survival model to the data using the original randomization allocation and censor patients who switch (as in a PP analysis) on the date of switching.

Step 5: Compute mean survival and QALY.

4.8.4.4 RPFSTM

This method uses the accelerated failure time model (AFT) (see Table 4.9) form of a survival model with the objective of presenting a measure of treatment effect by adjusting for those who cross over.

The approach of the RPFSTM is to consider the total survival time T_i consisting of two parts (using Jonsson's 2014 notation): T_i before crossover on the control arm, referred to as T_i^{on} and survival time after switching T_i^{off}:

$$T_i = T_i^{\text{on}} + T_i^{\text{off}}\ [\text{Overall Survival Time}] \tag{4.3}$$

TABLE 4.9

Summary of Survival Analysis Methods

Model	PH	Useful for Extrapolation	Statistic	AFT
Kaplan-Meier	No	No	Median, Mean, Survival rate	No
Exponential	Yes	No	HR	Yes
Weibull	Yes	Yes	HR, Survival rate	Yes
Gompertz	Yes	Yes	HR, Survival rate	No
Log-normal	No	Yes	HR, Survival rate	Yes
Log-logistic	No	Yes	HR, Survival rate	Yes
Generalized gamma	No	Yes	HR, Survival rate	Yes

In addition we have something called the 'unobserved' survival time, U_i – or the survival time that *would have been observed* on the control arm after progression if the patient had not switched plus a measure of effect, ψ (called the acceleration factor, which is considered to be a causal factor; values of $\psi < 0$, suggests a beneficial treatment effect).

$$U_i = T_i^{\text{off}} \exp(\psi) * T_i^{\text{on}} \text{ [Unobserved Survival Time]} \tag{4.4}$$

If $\exp(\psi) = 0.7$, for example, this is like saying that 1 year taking the study treatment (control arm) is equivalent to 0.7 years of not taking the treatment. The value of ψ is iterated until a value is found for which a statistical test (e.g. log-rank) yields the highest p-value. The process of estimation is carried out through G-estimation – a flexible semi-parametric approach tor estimating effects of exposure in non-randomized studies (Robins, 1986; Faries et al., 2010). Assumptions for RPFSTM include assuming a common treatment effect: i.e. the treatment effect from progression onward (until death) in the control group is similar to the treatment effect from randomization until death in the experimental group. In addition U_i is considered to be independent of the randomized treatment group and there is an explicit assumption that switchers and non-switchers are comparable (or need to be comparable). Further details of this method can be found in the references in the bibliography (e.g. Li et al., 2015; Faries et al., 2010; Dukes, 2018).

There are several core assumptions in the model:

(a) The treatment effect is the same regardless of when experimental treatment is initiated (common treatment effect).

(b) The randomized arms are properly balanced, this implies that the average survival time in the two groups (control vs. experiment) would have been equal if none had received the experimental treatment (i.e. $S_{\text{control1}} = S_{\text{control2}} = S_{\text{control}}$).

(c) Patients have no other choice of being on or off treatment, so if multiple treatment switches are possible, further assumptions about these 'treatment effects' are needed also.

The U_i values are used instead of the T_i values for the switching cases in further survival analysis. So basically, this is a technique that adjusts or shrinks the post-switching times of the crossover patients. But extra censoring (referred to as 're-censoring') is required to maintain the assumption of independent random censoring (which results in a loss of information at the end of the survival curve and thus reduces the precision of the estimates) (Latimer, White et al., 2018).

4.8.4.5 Two-Stage Adjustment Model

A simplified two-stage method was developed by Latimer et al. (2016) for situations in cancer where the switching occurs at or close to disease progression. For this, one must define a secondary baseline time to progression (instead of randomization time as usual). The post-progression survival is then estimated with an accelerated failure time (AFT) survival model for non-switching control patients versus switchers at the time of the secondary baseline, with prognostic covariates similar to those in the IPCW approach but measured only at the time of progression.

Finally, the additional treatment effect associated with switching (based on the estimated AFT factor) is 'shrunk' toward the survival times for similar non-switching control patients. This alleviates the need to collect time-varying data throughout the trial period but still needs to respect the 'no unmeasured confounding' assumption for the covariates. Compared to the IPCW method this method does not, however, capture changes in covariates occurring post-progression.

It is also possible to re-censor the survival times in order to correct for the fact that when we shrink the survival time for switchers we also shrink the administrative censoring time for those of who did not die during the trial, but re-censoring then entails a loss of information. Generally, it is then advised to present results with and without re-censoring (Walker et al., 2004; White et al., 1999).

4.8.4.6 Other Approaches: Structural Nested Mean Models (SNNM)

When marginal structural models are not applicable, a structural nested model (SNM) may be used (Yamaguchi & Ohashi, 2004; Greenland et al., 2008). This has been proposed by Robins (1994) in the context of causal effect estimation in the time-varying settings where both the treatment T (the cause) and a set of (pre-treatment) moderator variables M vary over time when assessing the effect of T on the outcome Y. In this context the moderators may themselves be dependent or influenced by the outcome of earlier treatment (Almirall, Ten Have, & Murphy, 2010). These have mostly been studied in the presence of non-compliant, fully sequential treatments but rarely for switching (Yamaguchi & Ohashi, 2004).

The underlying assumptions used for any analyses involving switching will be difficult to demonstrate. An analysis that adjusts for crossover/treatment switching will not salvage a trial that has shown to be negative prior to adjustment. If the ITT population does not show treatment benefit, adjustment is unlikely to be considered as strong evidence of treatment benefit from the experimental drug. The regulatory questions as to what would have been the treatment benefit without the presence of crossover cannot be totally separated from a reimbursement question.

One last consideration for treatment switching relates to how probabilistic sensitivity analysis (PSA) is conducted in the presence of switching. Where switching is of concern, the PSA and ICERs should be presented by taking into account the above methods. Estimates of ICERs and PSA from both the standard (not taking into account switching) PSA and from those that result from adjusting for switching should be reported. The issue also extends to extrapolation of survival curves, since switching may continue well beyond trial follow-up has completed.

4.9 Data Synthesis and Network Meta-Analyses

This section introduces an important area related to health technology assessment covering two broad areas: mixed treatment comparisons (MTCs), sometimes called network meta-analysis (NMA), and evidence synthesis, which concern pooling together data from several randomized trials (or other studies) and estimating a type of average treatment effect directly or indirectly.

4.9.1 Mixed Treatment Comparisons

Randomized controlled trials (RCTs) that have two or more treatments are an effective yet expensive and lengthy method of comparing treatment effects. In some cases there is simply not enough time or enough resources to perform additional trials to compare a new treatment with existing comparators. In such situations an alternative method is to carry out an MTC, which uses existing data in a summarized form. The International Society of Pharmacoeconomics and Outcomes Research (ISPOR) describes an MTC as a network in which some of the pairwise comparisons have both direct and indirect evidence (Hoaglin et al., 2011). This means that some pairwise comparisons can be carried out in a given trial (direct comparisons), but using additional data can help to obtain more precise estimates. For example, in an

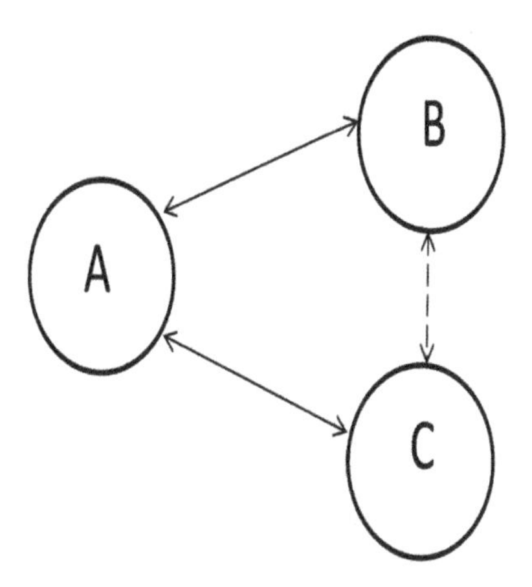

FIGURE 4.14
Diagram representing direct comparison for A versus B and A versus C (solid lines) and the indirect comparison for B versus C (dashed line).

RCT comparing A versus B and another separate trial comparing A versus C, the comparison of B versus C can be made indirectly.

There are two pieces of information for treatment A (A vs. B and A vs. C), and a single piece of information for each of B and C (Figure 4.14). Treatment B versus C is the indirect comparison.

Pharmaceutical companies may not be able to conduct a direct comparison of a new treatment against the standard or 'best' treatments for practical or commercial reasons. This may be because there is no standard treatment, or because it is commercially risky or expensive. Therefore, an MTC can be the only way to compare treatments for estimating effects that may otherwise not be possible. MTCs can be described as an extension of the models for pairwise meta-analyses. They are slightly more complex in that they can be applied to connected networks of arbitrary size and complexity. Some definitions of interrelated concepts when conducting MTCs are now provided:

4.9.1.1 Direct Comparison

A direct comparison is described as a head-to-head randomized controlled trial (RCT) of pairs of treatments under investigation; for example treatment A versus treatment B, as in Figure 4.14.

4.9.1.2 Indirect Treatment Comparison (ITC)

An indirect comparison occurs when two or more treatments of interest are compared using a common comparator. For example, in Figure 4.14, treatment A is the comparator in common that facilitates an indirect comparison between treatments B and C. Indirect comparisons are also commonly referred to as adjusted or 'anchored' indirect comparisons.

4.9.1.3 Meta-Analysis

A meta-analysis is carried out when there is more than one trial involving the same pairwise comparisons. It combines the treatment effects (or other results) from these trials and presents one overall or pooled measure of effect size.

4.9.1.4 Network of Evidence

A network of evidence is a description of all the trials that include treatments of interest and/or trials including the comparator treatments. A network diagram (Figure 4.14) gives a visual representation of all the direct comparisons that have already been made between the treatments, and can make it easier to determine the potential for indirect comparisons. It can be as detailed or as simple as required, i.e. it need not include all the treatments in the network but just the ones that are of interest. A network meta-analysis (NMA) is a more general term for describing MTCs and indirect comparisons, and can be defined as an analysis where the results from two or more trials that have one treatment in common can be compared. Jansen et al. (2011) provide a useful summary of these.

4.9.2 Assumptions for Carrying Out MTCs

There are several assumptions to take into consideration when carrying out an MTC analysis. First, it is important to bear in mind that randomization only holds within the original trial and not across the RCTs. Unlike meta-analyses, where results might be pooled despite strong differences in patient characteristics as well as differences in the circumstances in which outcomes were collected, MTCs assume homogeneity across trials for (indirect) effects to be plausible. Hence, the homogeneity assumption must be satisfied.

The similarity assumption (Jansen, 2011) states that if trials differ among the direct comparisons (e.g. a trial comparing A vs. B differs from a trial comparing A vs. C), and these differences are due to 'modifiers' (see examples listed below) of the relative treatment effects, then the estimate of the indirect treatment effect is biased. To explain this, consider two trials where one trial involves a comparison of treatments A versus B (Trial 1) and the other compares A versus C (Trial 2). If Trial 1 includes patients within the age range 20–30 years and Trial 2 includes patients within the age range 60–80 years, then age is an effect modifier. Hence, any indirect comparison will produce a result where potential confounding can bias the indirect estimate of B versus C. Thus, to avoid violations of the above two assumptions, trials must be comparable on effect modifiers such as:

- Patient characteristics
- The way in which the outcomes are defined and/or measured
- Protocol requirements, such as disallowed concomitant medication
- The length of follow-up

In summary, with regard to NMA, it is important to check whether the trials are sufficiently similar to yield meaningful results for the ITC and MTC. A further assumption, the consistency assumption, must also hold. This means that trials must be comparable in effect modifiers *and* there must be no discrepancy between the direct estimates and the indirect estimates. Due to the way it is defined, this assumption can only be, and need only be, verified when there are direct and indirect comparison data available for particular pairwise comparisons. If the consistency assumption does not hold, then the indirect estimates may be biased. In MTC analysis, however, since there is always a sampling error, a strict evaluation of consistency based on point estimates would not be appropriate.

Lastly, an assumption of *exchangeability* should be satisfied. Exchangeability means that the relative efficacy of a treatment would be the same even if it were carried out under the conditions of any of the other trials that are included in the indirect comparison. In practice, this assumption cannot be verified conclusively, though verification of the similarity assumption would give more reason for the exchangeability assumption to hold.

All the above assumptions must be considered very carefully when selecting studies for inclusion in any sort of network meta-analysis because the validity of indirect comparisons depends on both the internal validity and the similarity of the trials conducted or reported.

Example 4.9: An MTC Comparing Gefitinib with Erlotinib for NSCLC

A simple MTC was planned to compare erlotinib versus gefitinib. Erlotinib versus placebo was compared in one trial (Lee, 2012) and gefitinib versus placebo was compared in a separate trial (Thatcher, 2005). Further details can be found in Khan (2015).

In order to determine whether the assumptions above were likely to hold, attention was paid to ensuring that, where information was available, the trials were comparable on the effect modifiers mentioned above. In particular: the male to female ratio was checked and the median age was compared between the three treatment groups; all the primary outcomes were measured in the same way; and outcomes for all studies were measured by progression-free survival (PFS) and overall survival (OS). Other factors such as whether the trials were double-blinded multicenter trials and patient recruitment per region were also checked. However, there are often factors such as adherence to the research protocol, quality of staff conducting the study, and other contributing factors that might increase heterogeneity between studies. A summary of results from seven trials is shown in Table 4.10.

Using the data from Tables 4.10 and 4.11, we now conduct an MTC to estimate the treatment effect for gefitinib versus erlotinib. Three additional studies could also have been included (one Phase II study, one retrospective multicenter study, and another single center retrospective

TABLE 4.10

Summary of Results from 7 Published Trials of Lung Cancer Treatments

Study	Author (year)	Treatment	Comparator	OS HR	PFS HR
GP1	Thatcher (2005)	Gefitinib (n = 1129)	Pl. (n = 563)	0.89	0.82
GP2	Zhang (2012)	Gefitinib (n = 148)	Pl. (n = 148)	0.84	0.42
GP3	Gaafar (2011)	Gefitinib (n = 86)	Pl. (n = 87)	0.81	0.61
EP1	Shepherd (2005)	Erlotinib (n = 488)	Pl. (n = 243)	0.70	0.61
EP2	Capuzzo (2010)	Erlotinib (n = 438)	Pl. (n = 451)	0.81	0.71
EP3	Herbst (2005)	Erlotinib (n = 526)	Pl. (n = 533)	0.99	0.94
EP4	Lee (2012)	Erlotinib (n = 332)	Pl. (n = 332)	0.93	0.81

Notes: G: gefitinib; Pl.: placebo; OS HR: hazard ratio for overall survival; GP: gefitinib vs. placebo comparison; EP: erlotinib vs. placebo comparison. Studies 1, 2, 3 compare gefitinib vs. placebo, whereas 4, 5, 6, and 7 compare erlotinib vs. placebo. HR = hazard ratio.

TABLE 4.11

Lung Cancer Data for Example 4.11

Study	Treatment	OS HR [95% CI]	PFS HR [95% CI]
[1]GP1	Gefitinib (n = 1129)	0.89 [0.77–1.02]	0.82 [0.73–0.92]
[2]GP2	Gefitinib (n = 148)	0.84 [0.62–1.14]	0.42 [0.33–0.55]
[3]GP3	Gefitinib (n = 86)	0.81 [0.59–1.12]	0.61 [0.45–0.83]
[4]EP1	Erlotinib (n = 488)	0.70 [0.58– 0.85]	0.61 [0.51–0.74]
[5]EP2	Erlotinib (n = 438)	0.81 [0.69–0.94]	0.71 [0.62–0.82]
[6]EP3	Erlotinib (n = 526)	0.99 [0.85–1.15]	0.94 [0.85-–1.03]
[7]EP4	Erlotinib (n = 332)	0.93 [0.93–1.10]	0.81 [0.68–0.95]

[1] *Notes:* Thatcher et al. (2005).
[2] Zhang et al. (2012).
[3] Ghaffar et al. (2011).
[4] Shepherd et al. (2005).
[5] Cappuzzo et al. (2010).
[6] Herbst et al. (2005).
[7] Lee et al. (2012).

study could also have been included as RCTs). However, only the seven Phase III RCTs in Table 4.11 are used.

A network diagram for the data in Table 4.11 is shown in Figure 4.15.

Rather than use just the pooled estimates as in a meta-analysis, the treatment effects from each study are used in the MTC to avoid loss of information.

Step 1: Identify the measure of effect. In this case it is the hazard ratio and, therefore, we will work on the log hazards scale.

Step 2: Determine whether a Bayesian fixed effects or random effects model is to be used. We will choose a random effects model.

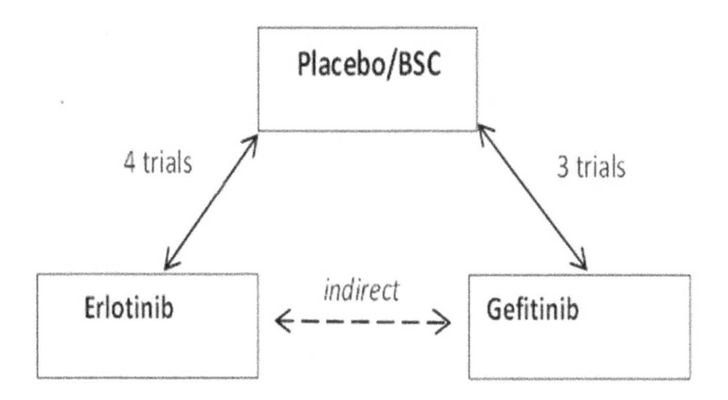

FIGURE 4.15
Network meta-analysis diagram for Table 4.11.

Step 3: Identify the network structure. This also depends on whether pooled estimates are used or the individual effect sizes from each trial. For example, a meta-analysis (see Khan, 2015) generated pooled effects of the direct pairwise treatment effects. These could be used, but as noted earlier we use the 'raw' effects (treatment differences) available from Table 4.12.

Step 4: Specify the model assumptions.

Let the log hazard ratio for a study be pooled from a distribution that has a normal distribution with mean μ_i and a precision that is determined by the standard errors (SE*i*) of the studies (subscript *i* is for each study). Let y_i be the log hazard ratio for study *i*, and t_i the precision of the distribution for the log hazard ratios, then the likelihood for the model is as follows:

$$y_i \sim N(\mu_I, t_i)$$

where t_i is: $1/[SE_i * SE_i]$

There are 3 treatment effects: TE(1), TE(2), and TE(3) associated with the treatments placebo, erlotinib, and gefitinib respectively, each with the following identical non informative priors: Therefore:

- TE(1) ~ N(0, 0.00001)
- TE(2) ~ N(0, 0.00001)
- TE(3) ~ N(0, 0.00001)

Step 5: Identify the data to be used in the MTC.

These data include 7 hazard ratios (in Table 4.11) and the 7 standard errors. It is important to ensure the direction of the comparison is correct. For example, in Table 4.11 the HR for gefitinib versus placebo in study 1 is 0.89. The HR for placebo versus gefitinib would be 1/0.89 = 1.12 and log (HR) = 0.11653, which would be used in the analysis.

Step 6: Write the code (WINBUGS or SAS).

```
                    WINBUGS CODE:
# MODEL
model {
for (i in 1:N) { # indexes studies
t[i] <- 1 / SE[i]*SE[i]
y[i] ~ dnorm(mu[i], t[i]) # Likelihood function
mu[i] <- (TE[t[i]] - TE[t2[i]])
} # end i loop
# OUTPUTS
for (base in 1:(NT-1)) { # indexes treatments
for (comp in (base+1):NT) { # indexes comparators
theta[base,comp] <- exp(TE[base] - TE[comp])
}} # end base, comp loops
# PRIOR DISTRIBUTIONS
for (k in 1:NT) {
TE[k] ~ dnorm(0.0,0.00001)
} # end k loop
} # END MODEL
#DATA
list(N=7, NT=3, HR=c(0.1165338163, 0.1743533871,
0.2107210313,
0.3566749439, 0.2107210313, 0.01005033585,
0.07257069283),
SE=c(0.072, 0.155, 0.164, 0.098, 0.079, 0.077, 0.088),
t=c(1, 1, 1, 1, 1, 1, 1), t2=c(3, 3, 3, 2, 2, 2, 2))
```

The indirect comparison of erlotinib versus gefitinib results in a very slight advantage (likely to be clinically irrelevant) for erlotinib. However, the PFS effect from gefitinib suggests it would offer a potentially more cost-effective treatment. One would also expect HRQoL during the progression-free period to be better with gefitinib compared to erlotinib, which would influence the cost per QALY.

4.10 Summary

It is not possible to cover all the statistical methods used for modeling survival and other data for cost-effectiveness analyses in this book. We have not discussed subjects such as, for example: hurdle and dispersion models (for

TABLE 4.12

Summary of Main Statistical Issues Relating to Economic Evaluation of Cancer Drugs

Issue	Costs	HRQoL		Survival	
Distribution	Normal Gamma	Any justifiable (normal, beta, etc.)	Normal Beta (EQ-5D) Other justifiable	Nonparametric (e.g. Cox PH)	Exponential, Weibull or suitable justifiable
Other assumptions	Normal Gamma Over-dispersion	Possible over-dispersion	Possible over-dispersion	Proportional hazards (PH)	PH or non-PH
Statistics of choice	Mean costs	Mean Median Any justifiable	Mean	Mean survival Hazard ratio (survival rate) median	Mean Truncated / restricted Mean
Missing data	Multiple imputation methods	Multiple imputation, depending on mechanism of missingness assumption (e.g. MAR, MCAR, MNAR) Worst case Impute using placebo	Multiple imputation, depending on mechanism of missingness assumption (e.g. MAR, MCAR, MNAR)	Right censoring or similar	Right censoring or similar
Extrapolation	Model -based	None	Model-based (e.g. post progression HRQoL)	none	Model-based (Weibull, exponential or suitable)
Treatment switching	Included in mean costs	Not typically adjusted for	Not typically adjusted for May assume that HRQoL improves or deteriorates depending on nature of switching Mean statistic will be used regardless	Censoring at crossover IPCW RPSFT Two-stage methods As a sensitivity analysis since regulatory question is what would have been the effect on OS without switching	Censoring at crossover IPCW RPSFT Two-stage methods See section above Important to harmonize estimands for efficacy and effectiveness wherever possible

ITT: Intent to treat population.

TABLE 4.13

Results from WINBUGS

Comparison	OS HR	PFS HR
Erlotinib vs. placebo	0.855	0.777
Gefitinib vs. placebo	0.874	0.419
Erlotinib vs. gefitinib	0.996	0.544

cost data); joint modeling of costs and effects; landmark analyses; propensity modeling (for real-world data) for non-randomized data; mixed modeling for analyses of utilities; and multiple imputation. This would require an entire book in itself. Nevertheless, we presented at the end of this chapter Table 4.13 that summarized the types of statistical methods that could be relevant for modeling data for economic evaluation of data collected in cancer patients.

4.11 Exercises for Chapter 4

1. Distinguish between variability and uncertainty.
2. Explain the following terms in the context of survival analysis: rate, hazard rate, risk, proportion, and probability.
3. What is a hazard ratio? interpret a hazard ratio of 0.80.
4. What distribution would you expect costs to follow and why?
5. What is a transition probability matrix in the context of healthcare?
6. How might parametric survival models be used in an economic evaluation?
7. Distinguish between the different types of switching and their implication for cost-effectiveness analyses.

5

Collecting and Analysis of Costs from Cancer Studies

5.1 Types of Costs Typical of Cancer Trials

To estimate costs of healthcare in treating cancer, we need first to distinguish between unit price and health resource use (in physical units). Health resource includes items such as number of visits to the hospital, number of nights spent in hospital, number of milligrams of drug, and so forth. The conversion of these healthcare resource items into costs requires a unit price (P) associated with each resource. The quantity of the resource (Q) is then multiplied by the price to derive a cost: $C = P \times Q$. Since there are lots of different types of resources, we can reference each type by a subscript *i*, so that the cost of each resource used is: $C_i = P_i \times Q_i$.

For each patient, we can compute the total cost of health resource consumed (with an additional subscript *j*, for each patient): $C_{ij} = P_i \times Q_{ij}$. The unit price of a health resource is likely to be the same for each patient. The cost will change depending on how much of the resource use is used. The 'unit price' is the expense incurred by the purchaser/provider of the resource and will depend on the decision-maker's perspective of the analysis.

The individual patient-level costs are then added up to get a total cost per patient over a given follow-up period. If the patient is followed up for 1 year, the total costs over a 1-year period will be computed for that patient. Another patient might have died after 6 months, and hence total costs will be computed over 6 months. The above approach allows us to compute the average (mean) cost per patient per time period (e.g. monthly, yearly, by cycle), the average cumulative cost over time, and the overall average total cost, and compare these between treatment groups. These costs could be plotted to get an idea of the distribution of costs between treatment groups. Furthermore, the total costs could also be categorized. It may be useful to know what the breakdown of costs is, because some particular resource use might be used more (e.g. hospitalization costs if there are severe toxicities). Costs could be categorized as drug costs, surgery, radiotherapy, laboratory, imaging, post-treatment surveillance, etc.

5.1.1 Categorization of Health Resource Use

In general, resources directly related to treatment or the consequence of treatment may be categorized as shown in Table 5.1.

Some resource acquisition costs and resource use are published or easily accessible. For other resource use, such as those involving complicated procedures (for example, surgery, radiotherapy, and imaging), primary research may be needed to collect this data.

Typical health resource use in a breast cancer trial might include: first-line chemotherapy, radiotherapy, additional (subsequent lines) chemotherapy, treatments for adverse events, genetic testing (e.g. for the BRCA gene, whether mutant positive or negative), surgical procedures (e.g. initial lumpectomy or mastectomy, perhaps also reconstructive plastic surgery), duration of hospital stay, and hospital outpatient appointments or day care. It is therefore important to identify at the study design stage all the health resources that will be monitored and where data will need to be collected during and possibly beyond the trial (for real-world data, see Chapter 8).

5.1.2 Resource Use Monitoring

Health resource use monitoring is particularly important in cancer trials where a patient can undergo several lines of treatment between periods of stable disease (SD) and progressive disease (PD). Consequently, one should include health resource use from the whole patient pathway – from the start of treatment until cure or death. That is, an economic evaluation over a lifetime horizon should be considered. This implies health resource use should be collected even beyond protocol study follow-up. For example, for long-term recurrence (sometimes several years after the end of the intervention) of either the disease or adverse events, any costs of palliative care or longer-term management, if required, need to be considered (and monitored).

A key consideration is to determine how in the future, downstream costs associated with an experimental cancer treatment compare to those in the

TABLE 5.1

Categorization of Health Resource Use

Resources Related Directly to the Drug	Resources Related to the Consequences of Administering the Intervention
• Nurse time for administering an infusion • Drug amounts (mg per tablet or infusion) • Materials and equipment (single-use and also multiple-use equipment) (compare for example a throw-away plastic syringe and the use of an infusion pump)	• Treatments for side effects, intensive care unit admission (e.g. due to a serious toxicity for example) • Additional visits to the hospital, length of stay in hospital, visits to the doctor • Social or personal services (carer support, physiotherapist, psychologist support), cost of parking at the hospital, cost of not going to work by either carer or family member

control arm. For example, if the type of palliative care and its duration is expected to be the same in both groups (assuming a two-arm study) then there is likely to be little benefit in monitoring these health resource costs for an economic evaluation because we are usually interested knowing about those health resource items where the difference in mean costs (incremental costs) is likely to be larger.

It may be difficult to know beforehand which health resources items are likely to be used more in one particular group than the other. It may be possible to postulate a hypothesis that a new treatment is associated with more or less healthcare resource use at the trial design stage. For example, a new chemotherapy might be expected to have a better safety profile, and so we may expect costs from additional treatments for toxicities to be lower, meaning fewer hospital or doctor's appointments. In such cases we might focus on specific health resource use at study design. Similarly, where there are higher numbers of follow-up CT scans (i.e. additional CT scans after treatment has been completed) between experimental and control arms, this not only biases some outcomes such as PFS, but the costs may also be overestimated – the issue here relates to inadequate trial design. Taking more scans on one arm compared to the other offers greater opportunity to detect (and shorten) PFS, while increasing the costs of scans (not to mention the risks of radiation exposure).

5.1.3 Baseline Characteristics and Health Resource Use

Baseline characteristics are sometimes relevant to clinical outcomes. The typical approach is to adjust treatment effects for factors such as age, gender, ECOG, and disease stage (to name a few). However, these (risk) factors (see Chapter 1) may also be related to post-baseline costs. Patients who have poorer ECOG, or are elderly, may well be the same ones with later post-baseline health resource use. For statistical analyses of costs, not only are clinical or demographic covariates used to adjust and control the variability of the ICER, or the incremental costs, the baseline costs will also be important for this adjustment. Baseline measures of medical resource use can be used to reduce the variance in incremental cost estimates (Ramsey et al., 2005; 2015). For example, some costs such as carer costs, concomitant medication, and visits to hospitals will occur prior to randomization. These costs may or may not be different between treatment groups (it is something we might check). When computing the mean incremental costs, the baseline costs would be included in any statistical model. Patients with high baseline costs often have high post-baseline costs. The mean incremental costs will be based on modeling the correlation between post-baseline costs and baseline costs (along with other factors). This usually provides shorter confidence intervals for the incremental costs (depending on the type of analyses).

Baseline costs might be presented following categories as in Table 5.2 overall and by baseline characteristics to show the relationship between baseline costs, post-baseline costs, and baseline characteristics. Note that in Table 5.2,

TABLE 5.2

Example of Mean Costs Collected at Baseline and Post-Baseline

	Treatment A (Mean)		Treatment B (Mean)	
	Baseline (£)	Post-Baseline (£)	Baseline (£)	Post-Baseline (£)
Gender				
Male	4,000	7,000	2,000	4,000
Female	2,000	4,000	1,000	1,500
ECOG				
0	2,500	2,400	2,450	1,890
1	2,000	2,100	1,980	1,400
2	4,000	3,800	3,800	2,200
Stage				
I-II	3,000	6,000	3,000	3,000
II-IV	1,500	5,000	1,450	2,500

age is not included. Age would need to be categorized for presentation (however, it can be incorporated as a continuous covariate in statistical analyses without categorization).

Table 5.2 shows that mean baseline costs for ECOG and stage are similar between groups. Treatment B appears to have lower post-baseline mean costs compared to treatment A. There seem to be differences in costs at baseline for males and females between treatments: males in particular have lower baseline costs (£2,000 vs. £4,000) for treatment B, reflected in post-baseline costs. Here baseline adjustment would result in a different mean incremental cost compared to when baseline is ignored (raw mean difference).

5.1.4 Costs Determined by a Study Protocol

An important factor that can be overlooked is the fact that an economic evaluation does not seek to estimate the costs of a trial or study. Rather, it is the *value* of the intervention that needs quantifying. Such costs are derived from health resource identified in a clinical or study protocol. Since controlled clinical trials do not reflect real-world practice (as they are experimental settings), it is important to capture those costs related to the intervention during the experiment and beyond it. A study protocol may restrict the use of a number of resources that might otherwise be used in a real-world setting (e.g. restrict the use of some concomitant drugs or subsequent treatments). On the other hand, a protocol might increase the use of other resources (like imaging or genotyping procedures and laboratory tests) – perhaps to capture PFS better. Several issues require consideration.

(i) *Differences in hospital sites from which patients are recruited.*

Most clinical trials recruit a selected sample of patients (through application of inclusion/exclusion criteria). The trials are conducted in a nonrandom sample of hospital sites or other health settings (often larger or academic hospitals).

(ii) *Identifying unit prices and costs of health resource use from different hospitals.*

This can be challenging because one would need to have access to the billing data located in the finance departments of hospitals, or information from insurance claims, or one may need to perform primary research to find out these unit costs. An expert panel could be used to elicit expected unit prices. However, opinions may differ widely.

(iii) *Changes to the trial.*

Where a substantial protocol amendment is carried out such that the trial design is altered in some way, or additional assessments are collected, this will impact health resource collection. Prior to the amendment, different costs may have been collected compared to post-amendment resulting in health resource data from two different types of experimental conditions.

(iv) Using early phase data. In Phase II trials, an early ICER might be derived to inform Phase III trial design and future economic evaluation. However, a Phase II trial may have more exhaustive protocol-defined assessments, such as more scans to determine the optimal time when disease progression occurs, more laboratory tests and HRQoL data assessments. These are likely to be optimized in a Phase III trial and hence an ICER from a Phase II trial will need to be treated with some degree of caution when informing trial design for cost-effectiveness for a later Phase III trial.

5.2 Perspective of Analysis and Costs Collection

It is the study perspective that will define which costs will be included and which unit cost (price) will be used to value the resources used. Two extreme situations can exist: one where all the costs are borne by the patient (full out-of-pocket expenses) or by private health insurance in situations/countries where a public healthcare system is not available; and, at the other end, full coverage of all healthcare expenses by a central government, or other agency, or administration.

Most developed countries have a healthcare financing system that falls somewhere between these two extremes. For example, although the UK has a fairly centralized National Health Service (NHS) with widespread responsibilities over the whole healthcare spectrum, there are some interventions or drugs that are not covered by the NHS, or not recommended by NICE.

Moreover, in many countries, for some interventions or treatments such as dental treatments or (certain) drugs, a patient contribution (co-payment) may also be expected (Burau, 2015; Wendt et al., 2009).

Most countries have a mix of partially/fully covered or reimbursed interventions depending on the status of the patient, their income, disease, type of intervention, and/or perceived efficacy of the intervention or drug. Such systems of healthcare can result in complex approaches to payment for treatment for patients and can often result in patients paying out-of-pocket expenses. In such cases there may be an argument for cost-effectiveness analyses to be conducted from a societal perspective. In the majority of cases, the main perspective will be that of the public payer for the healthcare in a restricted budgetary perspective. In the UK, for example, cost-effectiveness analyses are conducted mainly from an NHS (and sometimes Personal Social Services (PSS)) perspective.

In several countries there are special budgets for drugs with their own coverage and reimbursement rules. This results in the so-called 'silo' effect where, historically, decision-makers sitting on drug committees did not feel that non-drug expenses were important when considering the financial impacts of new drugs. For the same reason costs borne by patients or organizations outside the health budget (societal costs) will often be overlooked. Many national economic evaluation guidelines have an explicit statement regarding their perspective choice. Therefore, many studies use only the country official fees or tariffs as unit cost (see Section 5.5).

5.3 Collecting Health Resource Use Across the Treatment Pathway

Table 5.3 shows how collecting health resource use information can be separated by periods of time. Each time period has a specific emphasis. Some costs may be irrelevant (e.g. the pre-staging process) whereas others are clearly important.

Pre-staging: The health resource use required for assessing asymptomatic disease, screening tests, or symptomatic visits to a GP or specialists before cancer definitive diagnosis is related to costs. These costs cover the pretrial period generally and are often either unknown or not relevant for the trial objectives. Such costs are not 'treatment emergent' and therefore can be ignored for an economic evaluation in the context of a clinical trial.

Staging: Cancer suspicion is high, and a number of tests, imaging, and surgical procedures (biopsies) are undertaken to get a final diagnosis and cancer stage. Although health resource use takes place, these costs should not be confused with the costs of the intervention. Sometimes the costs of a performing a clinical trial can get tangled up with the costs related to the

TABLE 5.3

Health Resource Use Categorized by Time Periods for a Clinical Trial

Pre-staging	Staging	Start of Treatment	Post-treatment	Post-trial	Palliative Care
Definitive diagnosis of condition No health resource use relevant as not 'treatment emergent'	Imaging Biomarker tests Resource use for confirming diagnosis not relevant for economic evaluation Only tests that are considered predictive of treatment (e.g. EGFR testing) Collect any baseline costs – such as care, support, family help at baseline as this could increase or decrease post-treatment	Chemotherapy Radiotherapy Surgery Concomitant medication Laboratory testing Pathology Hospitalization for adverse events Administration costs of delivering intervention (e.g. infusions) Scans/imaging	Maintenance therapy Additional scans Subsequent treatments	Additional medical care Hospital, doctor, nurse visits Social care (carer support) Family support Treating long-term or lifelong toxicities	End-of-life care Equipment and aids for self-care Palliative radiotherapy Specialist nurses (e.g. Macmillan or Marie Curie nurse)

consequences of delivering the treatment. Since patients entering a clinical trial already have a diagnosis of cancer, any health resource use related to establishing their diagnosis, eligibility for the trial or part of inclusion/exclusion criteria are unlikely to be relevant for an economic evaluation. Some health resource use that occurs just prior to randomization or baseline might be useful and can help to manage the variability in post-baseline costs (after adjusting for baseline).

Start of treatment: Health resource use after randomization is usually the most important, often covering the entire spectrum of treatment options including chemotherapy, concurrent chemotherapy with radiotherapy, surgical procedures, and any laboratory and/or pathology testing, as well as any other costs likely to be incurred when the treatments are taken (or administered) in a 'real' or 'natural' setting beyond protocol follow-up time. In some trials there is an open label (or extended follow-up) period where the 'real-world effects' (see Chapter 8) can be observed, which will also include costs.

Post-treatment period: After treatment has concluded, follow-up continues (e.g. 6 cycles of chemotherapy have been taken but follow-up continues for 2 more years) and an observation period is scheduled where the response status (i.e. any progressive disease in terms of tumor growth, metastases or additional malignancies, still alive or dead) of the patient is assessed and monitored. In case of relapse/recurrence generally, a new treatment line will be started depending on whether the patient is able to sustain it. This may depend on the previous treatment and, in some cases, the patient's genetic profile where targeted therapies are concerned.

Post-trial period: For patients who are alive or even cured of their cancer at the end of the trial, further medical care could still be needed. This can be either lifelong treatment such as when definitive sequelae (e.g. remaining symptoms related to the cancer, but not the cancer) are present (such as lymphoedema in breast cancer, permanent stoma in bowel cancer, etc.). The associated costs could therefore be higher or lower on a given arm, depending on the initial trial therapy choice (arm).

Palliative care: This is sometimes referred to as the 'end-of-life' stage and is associated with failure of all previous treatments or if the patient has deteriorated to an advanced metastasis, where the cancer has spread at multiple sites in the body. Palliative care may also include chemo- or radiotherapy, without intention of cure. Apart from the costs of chemo- or radiotherapy, the costs of the carer and specialist palliative nurse, as well as additional societal costs play a role here.

5.3.1 Time Horizon

An important consideration for collecting health resource use data follows on from the above in terms of the time horizon. In cancer trials, at the end of the maximum follow-up period (it would be expensive to conduct a trial that follows all patients until death, if some patients lived for a long time), some patients may still be alive. For these patients, their costs are censored at the last time point known alive. Hence, future costs are unknown for those patients still alive and would need to be estimated. In Section 5.8, an example is provided on how to adjust for censored costs.

Example 5.1

In a trial in newly diagnosed glioblastoma patients comparing two treatments (experimental E and control C), after 3 years of follow-up, 35% of patients are alive on E and 25% on C. The mean costs for E over the 3-year period were $21,000 and $35,000, respectively.

To estimate future costs (ignore discounting for now), we first need to predict the proportion of patients alive after 3 years for each group. We can do this by using a special type of statistical model called a parametric survival model (introduced in Chapter 4). Assume that the survival model predicts no patient to be alive by year 8 and beyond. Once this is done, we need to make one of several possible assumptions about the behavior of future costs.

The simplest method is to assume that the average per patient costs over the previous 3 years or over the last year would be constant over the next 5 years. This is known as last observation carried forward (LOCF). This assumption of constant costs will need to be evaluated separately. Table 5.4 shows the computations for future costs assuming an average (mean) constant cost of $3,000. If we assume 1,000 patients were enrolled and the average cost per patient for E in year 3 is equal to $3,000, then if we also assume costs are constant from year 4 and beyond, we can compute future expected costs.

The assumption of constant mean future costs however may not be realistic. There is no reason to believe that once further away from the start of treatment, a patient would have the same level of care and therefore costs for several reasons:

- If a patient is still in remission, then patient monitoring will be less intensive over time and therefore less costly
- Conversely, if disease progression has occurred, then treatment costs would increase significantly because the patients may even be removed to an intensive monitoring unit or moved to palliative care.
- Cancer is associated with deteriorating health and disease progression (and related health states), hence from a physiological perspective it is unlikely that the assumption of constant costs over time is tenable. In the same way that we identified the problem of extrapolation of utilities in Chapter 3, it is possibly better to extrapolate the behavior of future costs using appropriate modeling techniques, rather than assume constant costs. Markov or multistate survival models identified earlier could be used for this purpose (Chapter 4 and Chapter 7).
- Patients that relapse later may be treated differently to those who relapsed earlier in the trial because medical practice and

TABLE 5.4

Example of Future Cost Estimation

	% Alive	% Alive (Predicted)					
	Year 3	**Year 4**	**Year 5**	**Year 6**	**7**	**8**	**Total (Y4–Y8)**
E (% alive)	35%	25%	10%	5%	2%	0%	
C (% alive)	25%	15%	12%	3%	1%	0%	
E (costs)	3,000	750	300	150	60	0	1,260,000[a]
C (costs)	3,000	450	360	90	30	0	930,000

[a] *Note:* Calculated as $3,000 × 0.25 + $3,000 × 0.1 + $3,000 × 0.05 + $3,000 × 0.02 = $1,260 × 1,000 patients.

technology change over time – the so-called 'technological drift.' The nature of the 'shift' is, however, unknown since all estimated costs are calculated using current technology,

Actual and future healthcare costs unrelated to the disease under study are normally ignored in the cost analysis although there has been some discussion about this in the literature (Versteegh et al., 2016; Hoefman et al., 2013; Rapange et al., 2008; Van Baal et al., 2017, Van Baal & Wang, 2011)

5.4 Costing Methods: Micro versus Macro Approach

There are two main approaches to calculating costs: a macro approach and a micro approach. The macro or gross-costing approach uses a 'top-down' approach for breaking down the costs borne in a traditional accounting way, resulting in estimations such as, for example, the average (mean) cost per case, or per diagnostic-related group (DRG) or average cost per hospital day.

The micro approach uses a bottom-up methodology by tracking down the individual resources and activities performed during an intervention or treatment and aggregates the intermediate costs up to a total cost. The advantage is its precision and level of detail. The disadvantage is that the level of detail with which costs are collected is time-consuming, and sometimes may not be worthwhile because differences between groups in terms of some of these cost items may be negligible, although they might be collected for interest. In practice, a mixture of both (macro and micro) approaches might be used by collecting drug costs in more detail (e.g. drug name, drug dose, number of days or cycles given, dose reductions, or amount of wastage), whereas the cost of chemotherapy administration as an outpatient in a given cancer hospital would be determined from the average cost per visit, either at that hospital or, eventually, at a national level.

5.4.1 Average versus Marginal and Incremental Cost

The average total cost (ATC) is the sum of average variable costs and average fixed costs; thus, the ATC is equal to the total cost divided by the number of units produced. At the patient level, this is equivalent to computing, for each patient, the total cost across all subcomponents (drug cost, cost of treating adverse events, cost of hospital visits, etc.) incurred for their care. The average or mean total cost is subsequently calculated for all patients in a given treatment group.

Marginal cost is the *change* in the total *cost* that arises when the quantity produced is incremented by one unit, that is, it is the *cost* of producing one more unit of a good. In general terms, *marginal cost* at each level of production includes any additional *costs* required to produce the next unit. Therefore, the marginal cost will tend to decrease most when production is increased in cases where fixed costs are large compared to the variable costs. An example is a proton therapy machine or robotic surgery that needs high-cost equipment, and possibly investment in buildings that need to be renewed/upgraded over a relatively short time period (8 to 20 years)

Example 5.2

In this (simple) example, we will show that when there are high fixed costs, such as expensive equipment (e.g. imaging equipment, biomarker/DNA extraction machines), the average cost of using the equipment will decrease if they benefit a large number of patients.

Assume a family practitioner with a secretary where both are paid on a per patient visit basis. Assume a fee for service of €25 per visit for the practitioner and €10 for the secretary, and no other costs for the time being. On day 1, 30 patients are seen and on Day 2 31 are seen. We now can calculate the cost for the service for these 2 days

	Day 1	**Day 2**
Number of patients	30	31
Practitioner	25 * 30 = 750	25 * 31 = 775
Secretary	10 * 30 = 300	10 * 31 = 310
Total cost	**1050**	**1085**
Average cost	1050/30 = €35	1085/31 = €35
Marginal cost		1085 – 1050 = €35

We see in this case that the average cost is constant and that the marginal cost equals the average cost. Let us now assume the practitioner bought some IT equipment for both of them to use for a total of €3,000 and that it will have to be replaced in 3 years' time (without depreciation). Assuming 200 working days per year at 30 patients per day, we can now recalculate the average and marginal cost.

	Day 1	Day 2
Number of patients	30 * 200 = 6000	6001
Practitioner	25 * 6000 = 150,000	25 * 6001 = 150,025
Secretary	10 * 6000 = 60,000	10 * 6001 = 60,010
Equipment	€3000/3 = 1000	€3,000/3 = 1000
Total cost	**€211,000**	**€211,035**
Average cost	€35.16666	€35.16663
Marginal cost		–€0.0002

We now see that the average cost is only slightly higher, but the marginal cost is negligible given the large number of patients seen. This is because fixed costs are still low compared to variable costs and are spread out over a large number of patients. Had the practitioner invested much more in equipment, say €180,000, then the average cost would be much higher because the influence of fixed costs becomes greater. It also means that the average cost for the same procedure with similar technology may vary widely between institutions according to their operating level at full or less than full capacity. We leave it to the diligent reader to calculate the different costs for this case.

The above implies that when two alternatives are compared they should be compared at the same capacity level. In general, at the overall hospital level about 70% of costs are labor costs but this proportion varies widely between departments and procedures. Compare for example radiotherapy with psychiatry or a visiting nurse service.

5.4.2 Inflation

Some clinical trials take several years to complete. Health resource use consumed by patients earlier in the trial, say in 2008, may have a different price by the end of the trial, which might be completed in, say, 2013. The unit prices, or rather their value due to inflation, may have changed. Dvortsin et al. (Dvortsin, Gout-Zwart, Eijssen, Van Brussel, & Postma, 2016) noted that drugs such as cetuximab, bortezomib, and bosutinib had different prices: "Treatments in the late stage were found to be more expensive per QALY by a factor ranging from 1.5 to 12" (this may be explained by the fact that patients' health changes over time, e.g. deteriorates from Stage I to Stage IV cancer, and therefore costs of care later on are likely to be higher). Hence, price differentials will need to be adjusted. Dvortsin et al. reported that late stage treatment was more expensive by a factor 10, and could lift the ICER over the threshold, potentially rendering a new treatment as not cost-effective.

We would need to inflate or deflate the prices by bringing them to a standard year and either report the mean costs at 2013 prices (usually the reporting takes place using later prices at the end of the trial or at the time of analysis). In some countries a national statistics office or some other public agency publishes a price index for healthcare services. When using these price indices attention should be paid to check whether the indices published relate to a healthcare industry, or other retail goods. If no healthcare price index can be found, then we would need to rely on the more general cost-of-living or macroeconomic GDP price deflator. The drawback is that healthcare prices grow more rapidly than in other sectors of the economy.

Example 5.3

A clinical trial was conducted between 2008 and 2013. The unit prices for hospital stays are reported as £400 per night using 2008 prices. The final analyses will be performed using 2013 prices. First, we need to find an inflation index (which is published somewhere). We need one for the year 2008 *and* one for the year 2013. Assume the 2008 index = 105 and the 2013 index = 125.

The formula for inflating prices is:

$$\frac{\text{price index current year }(2013) - \text{price index base year }(2008)}{\text{price index base year }(2008)} * 100$$

$$= (125 - 105)/105 = 20/105 = 0.19 \times 100 = 19\% (\text{a } 19\% \text{ increase})$$

The cost of £400 per night in 2008 is now (400 × 1.19) = £476 in 2013 prices.

A caveat here is that this applies only when the healthcare resource is fixed and does not change over time in the construction of the index (a so-called chained price index). This could become particularly problematic when using a disease-specific price index with rapid technological change (Dunn et al., 2018; Hall & Highfill, 2013).

5.4.3 Time Preference and Discounting

Time preference refers to the idea that people prefer to receive benefits sooner and pay costs later. Some people may exercise today in the hope that they live longer later; others may or prefer to enjoy their leisure time through smoking or watching TV now. Individuals are considered to have a positive time preference in the sense that they might have a preference for health benefits earlier rather than in some distant future even when the inflation rate is zero (which may or may not always be the case for a specific individual).

The current practice is therefore to discount both future costs and future benefits (e.g. QALYs or life-years gained) by a discounting factor after the first year to estimate the present value. Generally, a constant discount factor (between 1.5% and 5%) is used and fixed by the national guidelines for economic evaluation. In some countries, a different discount factor for costs and outcomes is used (e.g. 3.5% per annum in the UK).

The net present value (NPV) is the sum over a number of years (*n* years) of the present value of the cost incurred in each year $\text{NPV} = \sum \text{FV}/(1+\text{r})^{\text{n}}$ where *n* is the year and *r* is the discount factor. Reporting using undiscounted and discounted results is useful because the discount rate can have an important impact on the conclusions of an analysis. In cancer trials, the proportion of patients who remain alive at the end of the trial is not often zero. Hence the future survival rates for each treatment group is a future benefit from which future QALYs are generated. It is these future benefits that are subject to discounting. Discounting is not applied when the cost-effectiveness analyses take place over a time horizon of less than 1 year (for a general discussion on discounting see Claxton et al. (2011) and Drummond et al. (2015).

Example 5.4

The total costs for a patient in each of years 1, 2, and 3 are £3,000, £7,000, and £5,000 respectively (total of £15,000). Discounting starts at year 2, hence, we will discount at 3.5% in each of years 2 and 3. After discounting, the value of £15,000 received by year 3 is £14,045

	Year 1 (2015) (£)	Year 2 (2016) (£)	Year 3 (2017) (£)	Total (£)
Cost	3,000	7,000	5,000	15,000
Discounted	3,000	6,535[1]	4,510	14,045

[1]£7,000 × $1/(1 + 0.035)^2$ = £6,535.

5.5 Charges

Unit costs should not be confused with charges. Charges are the amounts paid by insurers, or national/local health systems, or similar public agencies, or private insurers to individual care professionals or organizational healthcare providers, including hospitals. These can be defined at the diagnostic-related group (DRG) hospital episode-level for hospitals, or in fee-for-service reimbursement systems, down to individual care procedures, drugs, and laboratory tests, and so on. The reimbursement in this case is based on official positive reimbursement lists such as the 'Red Book' in the US for drugs, the NHS drug tariff list in the UK, and other similar sources for other countries (Truven, 2018).

In some countries (e.g. Canada, Spain, Italy), tariffs are decentralized, to a greater or lesser extent, by region or province. Many countries, especially for hospital reimbursement, use a combination of fixed daily fees, DRG or episode-based fees, and for-service fees, making cost estimations quite complex. However, in these cases the diffusion of electronic billing systems, whether hospital-based or those of (national) insurers, makes it, in principle at least, easier to retrieve billing data either for groups of patients or individually tagged ones. Access to such data is, however, governed by national privacy laws and access can be restricted for external parties.

5.5.1 Cost-to-Charge Ratios

Charges rarely reflect the actual costs of the goods or services provided. In the US, through its Medicare Cost Reports, the Center for Medicare Services (CMS) publishes cost-to-charge ratios that represents the total amount of money required to operate the hospital, divided by the sum of the revenues received for patient care and other operating revenues. These are hospital averages, however, and are difficult to apply to specific bundles of procedures therefore (Brent, 2002)

For clinical procedures, the Center for Medicare and Medicaid Services (CMS) has also developed the resource-based relative value system (RBRVS) approach that is used to calculate reimbursement fees through the Medicare Physician Fee Schedule (MPFS). Each current procedural terminology (CPT) code in the MPFS is assigned a relative value unit, which is then multiplied by the annual conversion factor (a dollar amount) to yield the national average fee. These are further adjusted according to geographic indices based on provider locality. Payers other than Medicare, such as private insurers, may also adopt these relative values and apply their own conversion factor(s).

5.5.2 Other Non-Medical Costs (e.g. Societal Costs)

When taking a societal perspective in a welfarist approach, productivity losses and related costs, which measure the cost of the 'time of ill health' of the patients (and possibly their informal caregivers) should also be assessed because unwell individuals are no longer partially or completely 'productive' in a broad sense (see Drummond et al., 2015; Drummond & McGuire, 2002).

The traditional approach called the human capital approach (HCA) is to value productivity losses by the patients using the average gross wage (including the employer's tax share and overheads). This has the advantage of being an easily accessible information source – the only information to be collected is time out of 'productive work.' However, for non-employed individuals (e.g. students, retirees, stay-at-home parents) this amount may be different but is certainly not equal to zero. For example, the average net income replacement ratio for retired individuals is generally in the range of 40% to 60% of the average salary in developed countries.

5.6 Distribution of Costs

In this section, we discuss several issues in the statistical modeling of patient-level cost data. We will first assume *non-zero and complete cost data* (no censoring or 'missingness') for each patient. These assumptions will then be relaxed and discussed separately to allow situations where missing data is possible.

It is important to note that the key objective of a cost estimation model in an economic analysis is to provide estimates of the *mean* cost, and the difference in mean costs between treatments is used for cost-effectiveness analysis (the mean incremental cost), regardless of whether the distribution is skewed or not. What this implies in practice is that a suitable statistical model needs to be determined that will allow an estimate of the mean costs for each group and then calculate the mean incremental cost. There are several features of cost data that are worth noting:

(i) In general, cost data are strictly positive $(C > 0)$. It would be difficult to justify the costs of patients in a clinical trial for a cancer treatment as 'true' zeros. This is because they are likely to have used some health resource after having been randomized to treatment. In some non-cancer trials, it may be possible that patients are cured (e.g. pain relief, reflux) and there may be zero future costs. However, this could only happen after treatment (which incurs costs).

(ii) Cost data are most likely to be right-skewed (positive skew) and have no theoretical fixed upper limit. They are termed a 'leptokurtic' distribution with excess kurtosis (with a tall peak). In some cases the distribution of costs may even be multimodal (have more than one peak). The reason for this is because, inevitably, some patients are more ill than others and therefore usually have high costs due to higher comorbidities or lengthier hospital stays.

(iii) In clinical trials, there are varying time periods of observing costs, so that we have repeated measures. However, in general, it is the total mean cost cumulated over all periods and resource items that is primarily of interest.

(iv) The mean costs may depend on a number of covariates such as age, gender, comorbities, cancer stage, baseline health status, etc., which therefore need to be taken into account when calculating mean incremental costs. For example, if a clinical trial is stratified by ECOG status, those with poorer performance status (ECOG > 2) may have different (higher) mean costs compared to those with a better prognosis. These differences could be reflected in the ICER.

(v) There will inevitably exist costs that are missing. This is not the same as the zero costs discussed earlier. Missing health resource use can happen due to patient withdrawal from the study because of disease progression, death, or for other reasons. It is worthwhile taking into account the burden one is placing on patients for the collection of health resource as this can contribute toward the amount of missing data. A commonly used collection tool in the UK is the client services receipt inventory (CSRI), which collects health resources over many aspects of care (e.g. hospital stays, therapists, social services costs). However, these can be excessive and time-consuming to collect, especially when the incremental differences are likely to be negligible. Hence, careful thought needs to be given before subjecting cancer patients to this level of data completion. Excessive amounts of time and energy expended on cleaning this type of data (as well as finding the associated unit costs), which is unlikely to have an impact on the ICER, should be avoided. Medications is a good example of this. In a reported database for a non-cancer trial in dementia (e.g. the dementia and physical activity (DAPA) trial; Khan et al., 2018) the medications ran into over 5,000 individual records, which took a very long time to clean, yet showed little difference between treatments in terms of costs and impact on the ICER.

5.6.1 Transforming Cost Data

Often costs are not normally distributed showing a combination of skewness and over-dispersion (e.g. where lots of patients have zero costs or many patients have a specific high cost), and, therefore, a transformation might be considered appropriate. One common transformation is logarithmic (natural logs), when data are positively skewed in order to make the distribution more normal. Figure 5.1 shows costs that were skewed and transformed resulting in greater normality. Note in Figure 5.1 how the numbers (scale) change with a quite marked impact on the high costs. Some special statistical tests exists to check the degree of non-normality in the data. Some commonly used tests are the Kolmogorov-Smirnov, the Shapiro-Wilks (SW), or Shapiro-Francia (SF) tests. For the data in Figure 5.1a, normality is rejected (the data are not normal) prior to transformation; after the transformation in Figure 5.1b, especially the square root transformation, the data are now more normal.

An important consideration in transformation is when costs are zero. Zero costs cannot be transformed using a logarithmic function. An arbitrary small constant (e.g. 0.01) is sometimes added to whenever a zero cost occurs, as this allows a log transformation. However, this could be misleading when computing mean costs because the logarithm of very small numbers is negative. For example, $\log(0.001) = -6.91$ and hence causes the mean costs to be lower.

A second important consideration is that after logarithmic transformation, the mean after logging values is called the 'geometric mean.' It is well known that this value is in fact an estimate of the median and not the arithmetic mean. The variance too, after log transformation, is not an unbiased estimate of the variance of the original cost data prior to transformation. This is important for interpreting incremental costs on the original scale. Hence, for this reason, statistical models for costs analyses might be preferable to the use of a transformation for estimating the mean incremental cost. Some cumbersome corrections can be used to derive the unbiased estimates

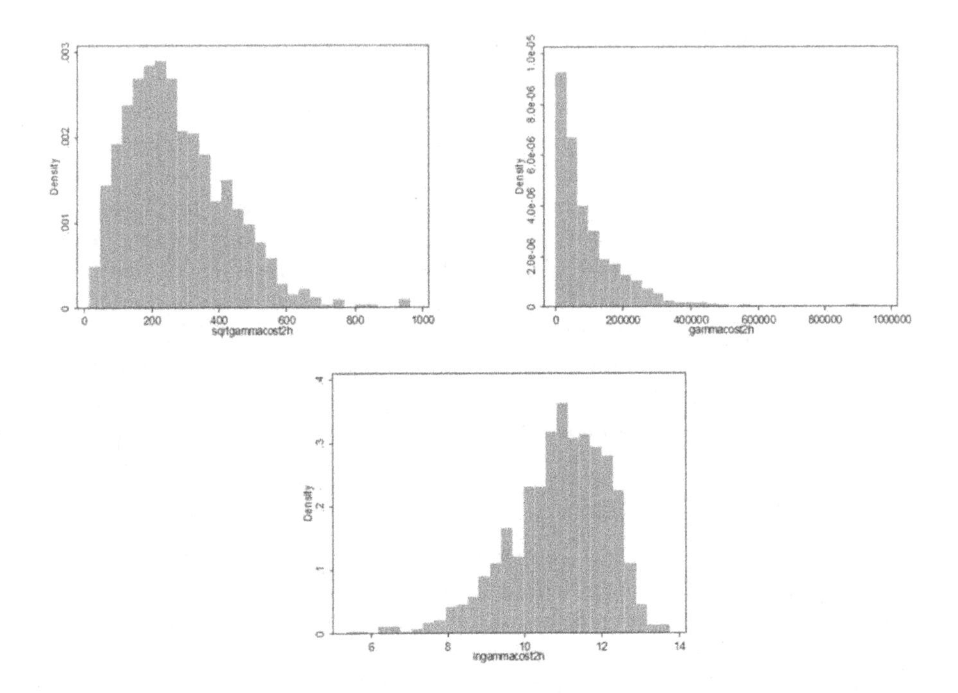

FIGURE 5.1
Example of transformation of a gamma distribution before and after square root and logarithmic transformation.

of mean costs (after transformation). A so-called 'smearing factor' was proposed by Duan (1983) for when the treatment groups have a common variance; Khan (2015) gives details of other transformations.

5.7 Handling Censored and Missing Costs

We distinguish between two types of missing data:

(i) Missing in the sense that the patient missed the visit, or a page from the case report form (CRF) was lost or the health resource was used, but the quantity was unknown (for example, the date of hospital admission was recorded in the CRF, but the duration of stay was unknown). Another example might be where a health resource use page from the CRF is lost, but the data lost are similar between treatment groups. An important issue for this type of missing data is that missing is not the same as zero cost; and a resource use set to zero is not the same as saying the resource use is missing

(ii) An incomplete record of health resource use because the patient was either lost to follow-up or the study was 'complete' before the primary outcome was observed. This type of 'missing' is known as censored data – censored at the last date of contact. In this case, the total costs for that patient represent a minimum (because, if followed up, the costs might turn out to be larger if the reason why they dropped out was because they were more ill). Consequently, calculating a simple mean cost would be biased. It has been suggested (Willan & Briggs, 2006) that patients who are censored are likely to have lower costs. This will impact the mean costs across patients.

One reason for missing resource use (cost) data is when patients withdraw from the trial early, due to lack of effect, adverse events, early death (due to a competing event), or when the study has ended before the outcome of interest can be observed. Missing data are problematic in any clinical trial when this occurs, whether the outcome is resource use or any other clinical endpoint, and it is more likely to occur in clinical trials where the primary outcome of interest can occur several years after randomization (e.g. survival endpoints). There is often little or no plan to collect any additional data after study withdrawal or adverse events.

Missing data of type (i) can be handled through well-established analysis methods such as multiple imputation and other complicated approaches (e.g. shared parameter models) involved in testing assumptions about the mechanism of missingness, such as: missing completely at random (MCAR), missing at random (MAR) and missing not at random (MNAR). A detailed discussion of these would require a separate volume, and so they are not elaborated on further here. References in the bibliography can be consulted for interested readers (e.g. Carpenter & Kenward, 2013; Farclough, 2010; Van Buuren, S. (2018). F). Most literature on missing data in economic evaluation tends to focus on censored costs. The focus here is less about estimating missing health resource (e.g. number of GP visits for a particular patient), but on the monetary value itself of the missing resource. Therefore, attention will be paid to missing data of type (ii) for the purposes of deriving the incremental costs.

In many clinical trials the ITT population is often the primary population for analysis. This means that regardless of any violations, compliance, or early withdrawal from the trial, if the patient was randomized, their data should be analyzed. If data are missing at some point after randomization, or midway through treatment, strategies are needed to deal with how to handle such missing data. What makes this issue particularly relevant to the analysis of costs is that patients who have missing data might well be the same patients who also have higher costs (because the missing values might be associated with problems with side effects and ultimately the treatment).

Patients who drop out from the trial due to toxicity from the experimental medicine may go on to receive additional medication or treatment for their adverse events. If the patient has been lost to follow-up then the costs are likely to be underestimated. Although it is difficult for patients to recall their pain response over the last 7 days, the patient is less likely to forget they went to visit a GP or saw a nurse. Therefore, if the CRF was ticked as 'Yes' to a question regarding whether a GP visit had been carried out, but the date of the visit was missing, this would not necessarily be considered a missing data problem.

5.7.1 Strategies for Avoiding Missing Resource Data

There are several approaches to preventing missing or censored cost data:

- Design clear and well understood CRFs, with clear instructions, when collecting resource use.
- Think carefully whether assessment time points are adequate. Assessments that are too far apart, for example 1 month and 6 months, may result in costs being missed between these months; the recall period may also be too long. For example, a question at 6 months "Did you have any other medication for your pain since your last assessment?" requires the patient to remember everything that happened between the first and sixth month.
- Continue to collect all or some data after the patient has discontinued from the study or has discontinued from the trial (if possible).
- Select outcomes that are easily ascertainable.
- Use those clinical sites that have good experience with following up (not just the ability to recruit).
- Train trial staff on how to communicate with the site staff so that follow-up data can be obtained. It is not helpful when a trial coordinator or clinical research associate (CRA) *demands* (possibly rudely) that site staff obtain the missing data. There would not be much motivation to obtain follow-up data when communication is a problem.
- Pay site investigators for the quality of follow-up and the completeness of CRF data or use other types of incentives.
- Inform patients why collecting resource use data is important: because it will help determine whether the new experimental treatment offers value for future patients (this may not go down too well with all patients!)

5.7.2 Strategies for Analyzing Cost Data When Data Are Missing or Censored

Several analysis strategies can be suggested if data are missing or censored.

(a) Complete case analysis
(b) Imputation methods

(c) Model-based methods
(d) Complete case analysis

When there are complete cost data, any method can be used to analyse the costs. When patients who do not have complete cost data are excluded from the analysis, not only would this violate the ITT principle, but would lead to biased estimates of mean costs (Huang, 2009; Wijeysundera et al., 2012). Although data from patients who are censored are omitted, leading to loss of information, the associated loss of power for statistical inference is less of a practical concern because differences in mean costs are not powered for statistical significance. What is more important is the resulting bias in the estimate of the mean and standard errors of the incremental cost.

5.7.3 Imputation Methods

Single imputation methods such as last observation carried forward (LOCF) should generally be avoided. Just as in clinical endpoints, when the disease severity deteriorates over time, the LOCF is not realistic; similarly, with cost data, as the disease progresses the costs might increase over time. Other imputations, such as using the mean costs, worst case, or baseline carried forward, sometimes used for clinical endpoints (and suggested in some clinical regulatory guidelines, EMA, 2012) also result in biased estimates of mean costs and are not appropriate for costs. For example, the worst case for a clinical endpoint involving pain on a scale of 0 to 10, might be 10; but the 'worst' or 'maximum' cost could be anything; similarly, baseline carried forward might be a way to determine a conservative treatment effect, but using baseline costs carried forward can result in lower mean costs, because as the disease progresses, costs are likely to increase.

Multiple imputation methods on the other hand might be suitable for handling missing data of type (i) above (Section 5.7) to improve estimates of the mean cost. Whereas the single imputation approaches are effectively guesses for the data that are missing, multiple imputation is a slightly more complicated method that results in a 'better' estimate of the missing data compared with the above methods (e.g. such as LOCF). These methods are discussed extensively elsewhere (Rubin, 2004; Carpenter & Kenward, 2013). An important point concerning multiple imputation is that it is important to state what is being imputed from where. For example, it makes no sense to impute missing costs from the control arm for the experimental arm. In addition, patients who dropped out are likely to be different in some way to those who remain on the trial and have data. Hence imputing costs from a group who did not drop out for those who did (even if on the same arm) is likely to lead to biased estimates of mean costs. To generate the mean incremental cost when using this approach, an imputation model is assumed and the missing costs are predicted several times (meaning several complete data sets are generated). Consequently, the mean cost is determined for each treatment group for each of the data sets. Finally, algorithms are used to derive the final point estimates of mean costs for each treatment group and the mean incremental cost is derived.

5.8 Handling Future Costs

Future costs related to the intervention are always to be included in a cost-effectiveness analysis. An example of a future-related cost might be anticipated longer-term costs of side effects from radiotherapy and the consequent costs of treating them. Depending on the perspective one takes, such costs may include medical or healthcare system costs and even wider societal costs (e.g. direct out-of-pocket costs sustained by the patient, informal care, productivity loss). Unrelated medical and non-medical costs can be ignored as these can be assumed to be similar between treatment groups.

In cancer trials where overall survival is often the primary outcome, and patients survive longer in the experimental arm, future costs may also accrue for a longer period since an increased mean life span for a number of individuals over and above that of the control arm is likely to be a direct consequence of experimental intervention, and such future costs should therefore be included. For example, if patients incur non-cancer-related medical costs after 33 months (say for arthritis) one should also take these into account because these are directly linked to the patients living longer. Some others (Weinstein & Fineberg, 1980; Weinstein & Manning, 1997; Garber and Phelps, 1997) take an opposing view. This is a complex decision-making problem because it seems contradictory: on the one hand, a new groundbreaking cancer treatment is efficacious and offers a longer survival benefit, while on the other hand, for patients with comorbidities, the associated costs of treating the comorbidities are increased resulting in more expensive treatment that may possibly render the new treatment to lack cost-effectiveness, because it is 'so good.'

To date, there seems to be no clear-cut answer or consensus on how to handle this problem, and often the choice is left to the health economist. One (simple) way to incorporate these costs is to add gender-age average overall population-wide medical costs (eventually corrected for cancer costs) from national health expenditure data. In fact, this aspect would perhaps be more important for budget impact predictions (a budget impact relates to the affordability of new treatment by a health system) than for trial-based cost-effectiveness analysis (for a discussion see Drummond & McGuire, 2001; Drummond & Sculpher, 2015).

A further complexity is the definition of cancer-related and non-cancer-related (future) costs. Cancer treatments have numerous, sometimes long-lasting side effects that impact other organs (e.g. central and peripheral neuropathologies, cardiac toxicity, dermatology) where the causality cannot always be clearly established, even during the trial observation period, let alone beyond the trial.

Example 5.6: Simple Extrapolation of Costs

A common situation occurs where at the end of the trial there are patients still alive. In this case one would need to extrapolate the long-term survival after the trial ends, together with the corresponding costs, until the last surviving patient dies. For example, assume a trial with a follow-up duration of 2 years and a maximum survival of 3 years in the control arm, and 5 years in the experimental arm (after extrapolation of the survival curves). During the trial the cancer treatment costs are collected (see Table 5.5); the non-cancer medical expenses are however considered irrelevant and are therefore set to zero. The new treatment is more expensive partly due to drug costs and partly due to increased toxicity, but it yields improved survival for some patients.

At the end of the trial (post-trial), the average (estimated) annual medical cancer care cost per surviving patient is equal to €50 in the control arm but somewhat higher (€60) in the experimental arm because of long-term treatment adverse events. This cost is a mix of care and follow-up for patients with no sequelae, for patients with sequelae needing more intensive follow-up, and for patients who die in that interval (year) and therefore receive possibly a further treatment line and palliative care. In the year following the end of the trial, non-cancer costs are still limited in both arms. Since the experimental arm patients survive longer and are therefore aging further, their care costs for other comorbidities increase as well. Hence, the total lifetime costs are due to the complex interplay between the proportion of patients surviving over time, until all are deceased. The time profile of their medical care costs follows a typical bathtub (U-shaped) profile (i.e. high cost during active therapy at the start, decreasing after the end of the treatment, increasing slowly with age, and finally increasing rapidly in the last year of life.

TABLE 5.5

Example of Costs During and After the Trial

Period	Year	Cancer-Related Costs (€)		Non-Cancer-Related Costs (€)	
		Control	Experimental	Control	Experimental
During trial	Year 1	100	120	0 (NC)	0 (NC)
During trial	Year 2	80	100	0 (NC)	0 (NC)
Post-trial	Year 3	(50)	(60)	(20)	(20)
Post-trial	Year 4	0	(60)	0	(30)
Post-trial	Year 5	0	(60)	0	(40)
Post-trial	Year 6	0	0	0	0

Notes: ( ) = estimated amount; NC = not collected.

In this simplified example, we see that the per patient cumulative trial cancer treatment costs are respectively equal to €180 and €200 but over the lifetime can be substantially higher (€250 for control vs. €490 for experimental) because patients who survive longer incur both medical costs for their cancer and for their other comorbidities, and this would possibly change the ICER (Faria, 2014; Clement, 2009). This was observed in the recent study (Olchanski et al., 2015) who reported that by including all medical costs, that is, cancer-related medical costs plus cancer-unrelated medical costs, the ICER drastically increases (i.e. worsens) and may reverse the cost-effectiveness decision. Therefore, inclusion of unrelated medical costs during added years of life may "implicitly penalize therapies that add expensive life years."

5.9 Case Report Forms and Health Resource Use

An important aspect of cost analysis is data collection and how we collect data for health resource use. In clinical trials the case report form (CRF) is a critical document that is reviewed by several professionals to ensure that clinical data can be collected accurately. This is no less true of CRFs designed for health resource use. In this section we give several examples of CRFs that can be used in clinical trials. These CRF designs are examples and modifications can be made to accommodate specific trial needs. One important consideration when collecting resource use data in a clinical trial are unscheduled visits, such as additional GP visits. Not all unscheduled visits are direct treatment costs. For example, a repeat visit for a laboratory test is not necessarily a direct treatment cost. Therefore, a distinction needs to be made between collecting the resource use associated with treating patients and the costs of running the clinical trial. Where adverse events data are collected for reporting incidence rates, the treatment emergent adverse events (TEAE) are more important because these again are associated directly with costs of treatment (these adverse events emerge after treatment has been taken). Figures 5.2 through 5.5.

▸ **RESOURCE USE SINCE LAST ASSESSMENT** (please enter '0' if none) - **INCLUDE THIS VISIT**

How many nights has the patient spent in hospital?

Medical General/Acute ☐ Date of admission __/__/____ *(dd/mm/yyyy)*

Surgical General/Acute ☐ Date of admission __/__/____ *(dd/mm/yyyy)*

Hospice/Respite ☐ Date of admission __/__/____ *(dd/mm/yyyy)*

HDU/ICU ☐ Date of admission __/__/____ *(dd/mm/yyyy)*

How many days has the patient attended hospital as an: Outpatient ☐ Day Case ☐

FIGURE 5.2
Example CRF from a lung cancer trial.

CRF: SITE OF CARE IN HOSPITAL

Admission to Hospital or Unit	Unit (*)					
	ICU	CCU	Step-down	General care	OTHER	
						Specify Unit

CRF: IMAGING STUDIES IN THE HOSPITAL

	Pretreatment		Posttreatment					
	Day -2	Day -1	Day 1	Day 2	Day 3	Day 4	Day 5	
	__/__	__/__	__/__	__/__	__/__	__/__	__/__	
Imaging studies	Enter number of images per day							
X-rays (#)								
CT Scans (#)								
MRI scans (#)								
Ultrasound (#)								
Other Specify (#)								

CRF: SITE OF CARE IN HOSPITAL

	Pretreatment		Posttreatment					
	Day -2	Day -1	Day 1	Day 2	Day 3	Day 4	Day 5	
	__/__	__/__	__/__	__/__	__/__	__/__	__/__	
Type of Bed (at noon)								
Intensive care unit								
High care unit								
General care unit								
Other care unit								
Discharged								

CRF: PHYSICIAN SERVICES IN THE HOSPITAL

	Pretreatment		Posttreatment					
	Day -2	Day -1	Day 1	Day 2	Day 3	Day 4	Day 5	
	__/__	__/__	__/__	__/__	__/__	__/__	__/__	
Physician Services	Enter # of minutes or use (*) to indicate a visit when number of minutes are unknown							
Cardiologist								
Neurologist								
Infectious disease								
Nephrologist								
Surgeon								

FIGURE 5.3
Example CRF for a general cancer trial.

5.10 Statistical Analyses of Costs

Statistical analyses of costs data can be determined using a variety of methods, from simple univariate (i.e. just calculating the total mean costs for each group using complete cases), to complex model-based methods. In cancer trials, it is important to take into account the full trial design features so that estimates of mean incremental costs take into account features such as heterogeneity, over-dispersion, censoring, and other features (e.g. repeated measures or clustering, where each patient has costs at several time points). In general, the types of statistical analyses of patient-level costs may take the shape of the following statistical models:

(i) Linear regression (ordinary least squares, OLS)
(ii) Generalized linear models (GLMs) that allow one to specify the distributions of costs as:
    a. Gamma distributed for skewed data (or log-normal)

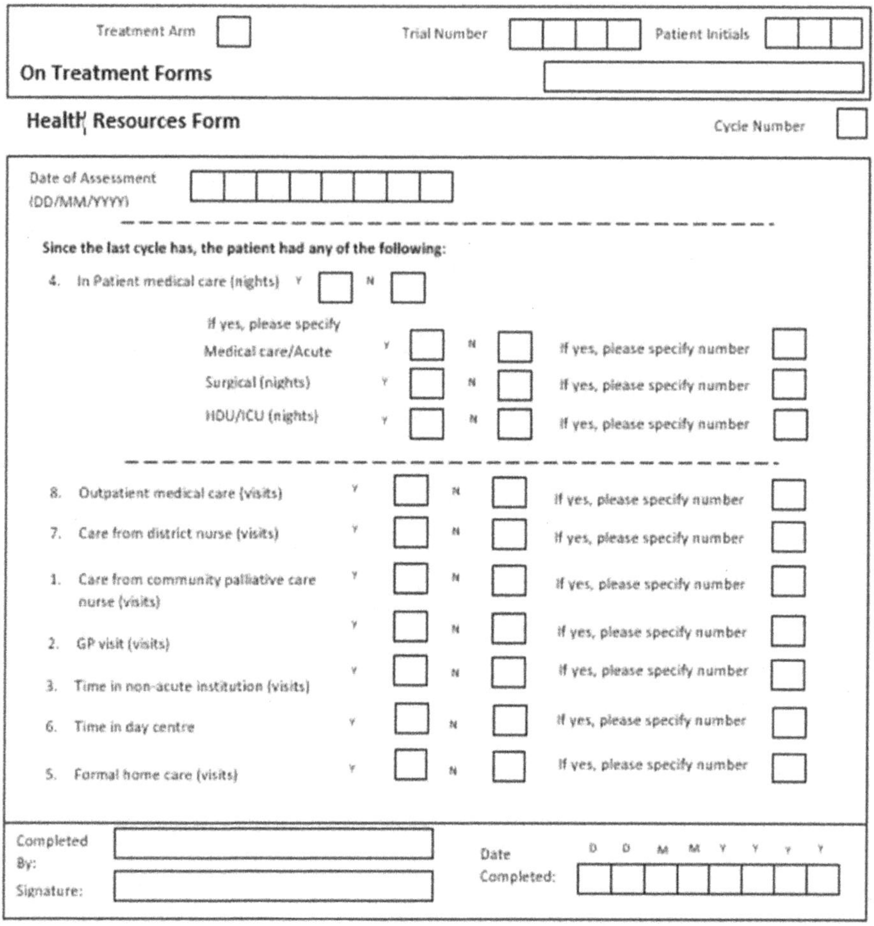

Treatment Arm Trial Number Patient Initials

On Treatment Forms

Health Resources Form Cycle Number

Date of Assessment (DD/MM/YYYY)

Since the last cycle has, the patient had any of the following:

4. In Patient medical care (nights) Y N

If yes, please specify

Medical care/Acute	Y	N	If yes, please specify number
Surgical (nights)	Y	N	If yes, please specify number
HDU/ICU (nights)	Y	N	If yes, please specify number

8. Outpatient medical care (visits)	Y	N	If yes, please specify number
7. Care from district nurse (visits)	Y	N	If yes, please specify number
1. Care from community palliative care nurse (visits)	Y	N	If yes, please specify number
2. GP visit (visits)	Y	N	If yes, please specify number
3. Time in non-acute institution (visits)	Y	N	If yes, please specify number
6. Time in day centre	Y	N	If yes, please specify number
5. Formal home care (visits)	Y	N	If yes, please specify number

Completed By:

Signature:

Date Completed: D D M M Y Y Y Y

FIGURE 5.4
Example CRF from a sarcoma cancer trial.

b. Poisson or negative binomially distributed where there is over-dispersion (for count data such as number of hospital visits)

(iii) Using models (i) and (ii) above, but also including a random subject effect, where the difference between each patient's individual cost (effect) and some average cost (e.g. average of all patients at one site) is taken into account in the analyses (often known as mixed effects models)

(iv) Two-part models (such as hurdle models) that first model the chance of zero resource use, and then use a second model that computes the expected (mean) intensity of the resource use.

A. PATIENT ACCOMODATION		
1. Usual place of residence during the last three months?	Owner occupied house/flat	
	Privately rented house/flat	
	House/flat rented from housing associated/local authority	
	Sheltered housing/warden control	
	Extra care housing	
	Care home **providing nursing care**	
	Care home **providing care**	
	Dual Registered home (providing both personal and nursing care)	
	Acute psychiatric ward	
	Rehabilitation ward	
	General medical ward	
	Other:	
2a. Has the participant lived anywhere else in the last three months?	Yes (Go to Q2b)	
	No (Go to Q3a)	
2b. Please state the approximate number of nights spent in this accommodation in the last three months:		No. of nights
	Owner occupied house/flat	
	Privately rented house/flat	
	House/flat rented from housing associated/local authority	
	Sheltered housing/warden control	
	Extra care housing	
	Care home **providing nursing care**	
	Care home **providing personal care**	
	Dual Registered home (providing both personal and nursing care)	
	General medical ward	
	Rehabilitation ward	
	Acute psychiatric ward	
	Other:	
3a. Has the individual been in receipt of direct payments during the last three months?	Yes	
	No	
3b. If yes please state the total weekly value	£ ☐☐☐☐.☐☐	
4a. Has the individual been in receipt of individual budgets during the last three months?	Yes	
	No	

FIGURE 5.5
Extract of CSRI inventory of broader societal health resource use.

(v) Models used to estimate the mean health resource use (and not the costs). Once the mean health resource use is estimated by using, for example, two-part hurdle models, the unit costs can be applied to estimate the costs. This is different from modeling derived costs.

Example 5.5: OLS Model after a Square Root Transformation

In this example, a simple regression model of the form:

$$C_{ij} = \mu + \beta * \text{Treatment}_j + \varepsilon_{ij}$$

where C_{ij} is the cost for patient i on treatment j, μ is the common intercept (the overall mean ignoring treatment) and ε_{ij} is the error term (the difference between each patient's cost and the overall mean cost for a given treatment); and β is the rate of increase (or decrease) in costs.

For the purposes of this example, an OLS model is used after a square root transformation. The square root transformation involves taking the square root of costs first and then analyzing the data. Since costs are positively skewed, then this transformation can work well. A log transformation would have problems with costs equal to zero whereas the square root transformation does not (the square root of zero is zero).

Table 5.6 gives the mean cost difference between the two groups equal to 1.02 (4.00 vs. 2.97) after a square root transformation. After a back transformation (by squaring), the mean costs are 16.01 and 8.88 respectively or a mean incremental cost of 7.13 (17.37 vs. 10.05) between the two groups. On the raw, non-transformed scale, this mean difference was 7.32, which is quite close to 7.13.

Example 5.6: Modeling Costs with and without Covariates (Normally Distributed)

The following example of 48 patients with patient-level total costs is used to generate the mean incremental costs before and after adjusting for age and country effects. In this example only costs are modeled (ignoring effects). The INMB is estimated using a suitable value of λ, the willingness to pay, in order to generate the base case estimate of the INMB. If the correlation between costs and effects is also included (modeled), a more complicated bivariate model (two response variables) will be required (see Table 5.7 and 5.8).

TABLE 5.6

Results of Mean Costs after Transformation (Square Root)

```
Mean estimation                    Number of obs   =      2,000

            0: group = 0
            1: group = 1
```

Over	Mean	Std. Err.	[95% Conf.	Interval]
gamma_all				
0	10.05558	.2259303	9.612495	10.49866
1	17.37788	.3107348	16.76848	17.98728
sqrtgamma				
0	2.979869	.0343094	2.912583	3.047155
1	4.001552	.0369706	3.929047	4.074057

TABLE 5.7

Data for Example 5.6

Patient	Treatment	Country	Age	Cost (£)	Patient	Treatment	Country	Age	Cost (£)
1	A	UK	34	5,268	25	B	Germany	63	8,126
2	A	UK	26	1,535	26	B	Germany	34	6,535
3	B	UK	58	8,261	27	A	Germany	30	12,111
4	A	UK	64	526	28	A	Germany	59	4,236
5	A	UK	44	3,126	29	B	Germany	54	7,126
6	A	UK	32	2,671	30	B	Germany	71	7,671
7	B	UK	66	4,319	31	A	Italy	66	4,151
8	A	UK	42	2,111	32	A	Italy	34	4,213
9	B	UK	34	8,881	33	B	Italy	31	5,481
10	B	UK	68	9,123	34	B	Italy	54	3,923
11	A	France	74	18,146	35	A	Italy	78	22,146
12	A	France	59	5,111	36	A	Italy	34	25,111
13	B	France	34	5,998	37	A	Italy	57	8,199
14	B	France	62	4,129	38	B	Italy	34	12,129
15	A	France	48	3,112	39	A	Italy	32	13,199
16	A	France	61	2,189	40	B	Italy	34	23,489
17	B	France	34	3,777	41	A	Spain	57	13,797
18	B	France	34	6,453	42	B	Spain	58	16,111
19	A	France	29	7,268	43	A	Spain	33	7,658
20	A	France	44	9,121	29	B	Spain	44	9,311
21	B	Germany	34	4,321	45	B	Spain	79	1,321
22	B	Germany	61	4,139	46	B	Spain	35	1,590
23	A	Germany	34	5,912	47	B	Spain	69	12,917
24	A	Germany	34	3,998	48	B	Spain	34	9,654

TABLE 5.8

Summary Output for Example 5.6

Model	LS Mean	Incremental Cost	95% CI	p-Value
Without Covariates	A 7,705	6[a]	(–3356, 3367)	0.997
	B 7,699			
With Covariates	LS Mean[b]	Incremental Cost	95% CI	p-Value
	A 7,844	180[a]	(–3090, 3450)	0.912
	B 7,664			
Age				0.596
Country				0.029
Country*Treatment				0.549

[a] *Notes:* Difference between A versus B: treatment A has higher mean costs.
[b] After adjusting for covariates (age *p*-Value = 0.596; country *p*-Value = 0.029).

TABLE 5.9

Summary Treatment by Country Mean Costs

Country	Treatment A Cost (£)	Treatment B Cost (£)
France	7,491	5,089
Germany	6,564	6,320
Italy	12,837	11,256
Spain	10,728	8,484
UK	2,540	7,646

Interpretation:

- The mean incremental cost is £6 without accounting for covariates and increases substantially to £180 when accounting for age and country.
- Age is not associated with higher (or lower) mean costs, but country is associated with costs (i.e. there are significant differences in mean costs between countries). The treatment*country interaction *p*-value is 0.549, suggesting that on the whole (across all countries) the incremental cost does not differ significantly.
- We should be careful about the interaction terms, because trials are often not powered to detect interactions (for clinical effects, let alone costs), especially for a sample size as small as this. Table 5.9 shows the country-specific mean costs for each treatment. There is large variability in incremental costs, which partly explains the lack of significance; in addition, in the UK the costs of treatment B are much higher than those for treatment A. Local payers (e.g. NICE) may be more interested in this aspect of incremental cost than the overall much smaller incremental cost. The mean differences in costs between treatment in Germany are smaller (£244).

Example 5.7: Missing Costs due to Censoring
Method of Lin et al. (1997)

When patients drop out of the trial due to disease progression (or other reasons), the full costs are unknown because the patients' survival (or follow-up) times are censored. For patients who have died, future costs are sometimes set to zero, which would bias estimates of mean incremental costs. Several methods are available to take into account censoring for estimating costs. One method is Lin's method (Lin et al., 1997).

The method shown in this example provides an estimate of the mean cost by taking into account patients who are followed up to a particular time point and then are lost to follow-up (censored). The estimate of mean costs uses the survivor function (Kaplan-Meier) to generate weights that are multiplied by the mean costs for specified intervals. For endpoints that do not have a mortality endpoint, the event of interest might be time-to-dropout. In a 12-week study where mortality is not the primary endpoint of study, almost all patients are likely to remain in the study and most patients would be censored.

The calculations for mean costs can be broken down into the following steps:

(i) Divide the follow-up period into smaller (not necessarily equal) time intervals. For example a follow-up of 1 year could be split into 12 equal intervals (1 month apart).
(ii) Calculate the mean costs within each interval (i.e. for each of the 1-month intervals) only for those patients alive at the start of the interval. For example if 100 patients are alive at the start of month 1, then the mean 1-month cost will be determined for the 100 patients.
(iii) Compute the survival rates at each interval (every month in this example) using survival methods (typically a Kaplan-Meier plot). For example, the OS rates at 1 month might be 90% (after 1 month, 10% have died).
(iv) Calculate the expected monthly cost by multiplying the monthly survival rates by the monthly costs.
(v) Add up the mean costs for each of the 12 months (i.e. month 1 + month 2 + … month 12) to get the total mean costs (total of the means).
(vi) Repeat for each treatment group.

One limitation of this method is that it does not adjust for covariates when estimating the mean cost. However, Lin (Lin, 2000) provides an extension of this that can adjust for covariates.

Table 5.10 shows a table of costs and mean costs calculated for each treatment over a 12-month follow-up period using the Lin (1997) approach. Firstly, we split the 12 months into 2-monthly intervals and derive the costs (treatment costs, nurse visits, etc.). One might think of each interval as a cycle of 8 weeks (roughly 2 months) of treatment for a particular cancer corresponding to months [0–2], [2–4], [4–6], [6–8], [8–10], and [10–12].

TABLE 5.10

Adjusting for Censored Costs

		Interval					
Patient	Treatment	1 [0–2]	2 [2–4]	3 [4–6]	4 [6–8]	5 [8–10]	6 [10–12]
1[a]	A	5,000	3,000	4,000	7,000	6,000	5,000
2	A	7,000	6,000	2,000	300	0	0
3 Etc.	A	Etc.	Etc.	Etc.	Etc.	Etc.	Etc.
51[b]	B	7,000	2,000	0	0	0	0
52	B	5,000	3,000	4,000	8,000	4,000	0
53 Etc.	B	Etc.	Etc.	Etc.	Etc.	Etc.	Etc.
	Mean B	5,300	3,900	1,200	4,650	6,170	3,195
$S(t)_A$	A	90%	85%	80%	40%	20%	10%
$S(t)_B$	B	90%	75%	65%	20%	5%	2%

[a] Patient censored.

[b] *Notes:* Patients 2 and 51 died during interval 4 and 2 respectively.

In Table 5.10, for each interval, the mean costs are computed taking into account whether patients have complete cost data in the interval. Cost calculations are based on patients alive at the beginning of the interval. The survival rates are obtained by plotting the survival times (assuming the endpoint is mortality) and using the observed product limit estimates (i.e. KM estimates). For each group, the cumulative (i.e. total) mean cost for treatment A is computed as (£6,300 × 0.9) + (£4,900 × 0.85) + (£4,200 × 0.8) + (£3,650 × 0.4) + (£4,520 × 0.2) + (£5,450 × 0.1) = £12,744. The same is then performed for treatment B; and then the incremental cost can be calculated. Note that this method is based on patients alive at the beginning of the interval. An alternative method is also available (see Lin, 1997, method 2), which computes the mean costs of those patients who die within an interval and then multiplies these costs with the probability of death within the interval (from the KM survival estimates). Adjustment for covariates when estimating mean costs in the interval is also possible (Lin, 2000). Whatever method is used, care should be taken to check the assumption that censoring within the interval is not somehow systematically related to treatment groups.

5.11 Summary

Chapter 5 described the different costs that need to be tracked and how the analysis perspective drives their choice. We also described the type of costs in relation to the treatment pathway and showed some examples.

Micro-costing (bottom-up) and macro-costing (top-down) cost collection methods were discussed and compared as well as the difference between cost and charges. A number of statistical features of cost data were described such as distributions, transformations, and the handling of censored and missing cost data. We also discussed some analysis methods and strategies to minimize missingness. The handling of future costs and their extrapolation beyond the trial horizon were introduced, and, finally, we presented examples of economic case report forms (CRFs) that can be used for collecting data on health resource use in cancer trials.

5.12 Exercises for Chapter 5

1. Distinguish between the types of costs one might expect in a cancer trial. How different might they be compared to a trial in epilepsy?
2. What are the distinct stages of collecting health resource use in a cancer trial?
3. Explain the difference between inflation and discounting.
4. Design a case report form for collecting health resource use data in a lymphoma trial.
5. In a cancer trial, health resource use data were observed to be heavily skewed with censored and missing data. Distinguish between censored and missing data; and discuss how you might analyse such data.

6

Designing Cost-Effectiveness into Cancer Trials

6.1 Introduction and Reasons for Collecting Economic Data in a Clinical Trial

There are several reasons for designing the cost-effectiveness of a clinical trial prospectively. First, it is often cheaper and easier to collect health resource use data alongside a clinical trial rather than having to design separate retrospective studies of costs and effects (Drummond 1993). In some cancer trials where the follow-up period can last for many years, it may be costly to follow patients extensively (e.g. until death) to collect relevant data. Delaying publication of important clinical findings on the efficacy of a new treatment in order to collect additional 'real-world evidence' for cost-effectiveness may also not be considered ethical.

Second, several reimbursement agencies require economic data to be collected alongside clinical trials to demonstrate value of new treatments. With several new treatments given market authorization showing 'small' or 'modest' treatment effects, the burden of proof is on the claimant to demonstrate why any healthcare system should finance one treatment over the other. In the UK, NICE makes specific reference to clinical trial data being used in assessing cost-effectiveness. When government agencies make specific requests, especially where it concerns payments for the provision of new drugs, such requests are not to be taken lightly – which might alone justify why designing the economic component carefully in a clinical trial is important.

In Chapter 1, it was shown how an early decision to reimburse a new treatment can influence future revenue. Reimbursement authorities may request economic evaluation of new cancer treatments closer to (and sometimes before) a decision is made for licensing. Some reimbursement agencies may prefer to have an early review of the value argument (submission dossier) put forward. This may be in the interests of both the sponsor and the patients. In the UK, the early access to medicines scheme (EAMS) gives a promising innovative medicine (PIM) the possibility to have an accelerated route to licensing (see Medicines and Healthcare products Regulatory Agency

(MHRA) website for details). Similar schemes may exist in other European countries. Any delay in a recommendation from reimbursement authorities can unnecessarily restrict access to treatments by patients and healthcare professionals – despite receiving market authorization. This is not entirely the same situation in all countries. For example, in Germany, a period of free pricing is offered where the manufacturer/pharmaceutical company is offered an agreed price for the new treatment, while value is assessed.

The economic value of a new treatment, however important, is unlikely to trump the clinical reasons for patient access to it – either privately or through the local health system. Many HTAs are conducted after marketing authorization has been provided (although pharmaceutical companies may generate evidence for both efficacy and effectiveness in tandem). It is possible that the future relationship between the regulatory and reimbursement procedures may be altered to take into account the overlap and (sometimes unnecessary) duplication that takes place. In several HTAs there have been concerns from manufacturers that questions raised by payers belong to the domain of licensing authorities (there is no reason why this should be case). Some of these questions had no apparent consequences on licensing during the initial assessment only to be raised later by reimbursement agencies For example, in the HTA review of ofatumumbab for chronic lymphocytic leukemia by NICE (NICE, HTA TA202, 2010) it appeared that evidence review experts were critical as to why interim OS results were not made available, not appreciating that reporting unplanned interim analyses has huge implications for bias and future trial conduct. The potential for contradictory advice from two agencies whose objectives are different is of concern. If, for example, NICE offer advice on trial design that might compromise licensing, this is clearly a cause for concern and government agencies need to align more closely to avoid such situations.

In academic clinical trials, where licensing is not relevant, reasons for collecting economic data are associated with evaluating the impact of the proposed health technology from the National Health Service (NHS) and government policy perspective. In some grant award application forms, there is a desire to know from a funder perspective (e.g. National Institute for Health Research (NIHR), Cancer Research UK (CRUK) whether the planned trial will impact future national healthcare resource use. The new health technology proposed need not be a new drug. For example, in a grant application, a new treatment might propose to compare patients followed up intensively for tumor progression (e.g. >4-monthly scans) compared to patients with a less intensive follow-up schedule (3-monthly scans). The main objective might be to determine whether more intensive follow-up results in the earlier detection of disease progression. More intensive follow-up may lead to more efficient health resource use in the long term compared to less intensive follow-up. Treatments are not compared in this type of trial (both take the same treatment): the effects of differences in PFS between the follow-up schedules is compared.

A further reason for collecting economic (health resource) data in a clinical trial is because clinical trials provide strong internal validity of estimates of average costs and effects, although they may lack external validity. Additional evidence is sometimes needed to make informed decisions about the cost-effectiveness of new treatments, particularly in a real-world setting (Sculpher, 2006). If a decision cannot be reached regarding the cost-effectiveness of a new treatment based on data from one or more clinical trials, the impetus for collecting economic data loses some force. If the 'weight of evidence' from clinical trial data is considered too 'weak' to offer a robust conclusion for cost-effectiveness, then it becomes debatable whether the economic data collected alongside a clinical trial adds to a demonstration of the value of a new treatment. Gheorghe et al (2015) suggest operationalizing the idea of generalizability and incorporate it into trial design – such as trials designed for the real-world setting – with a view to getting market authorization. It may be argued that despite the lack of external validity in RCTs, they remain the optimal recognized framework to derive unbiased, or at least less biased, estimates of treatment effects.

Evidence from nonrandomized trials (single arm Phase II trials) has been acceptable in certain settings such as unmet needs or rare tumors (the licensing of gefitinib is an example in NSCLC). Therefore, it could be possible to use nonrandomized evidence as a basis for a cost-effectiveness decision. This might involve combining data from the trial with external data. The question of mixing data from controlled and noncontrolled sources to provide unbiased estimates of treatment effects is a challenging one. Cost-effectiveness analysis is not necessarily an inferential problem like that of efficacy analyses in a regulatory setting, where there is a need to provide an unbiased estimate of effect; it is a decision problem with an objective of reducing uncertainty with more information (external and internal) around measures of effectiveness and value.

For example, if we wish to carry out an economic evaluation comparing a new treatment with a standard, it is not straightforward to extract costs and HRQoL effects from published sources and combine this data with clinical trial data (efficacy data) as inputs into an economic model. Costs and effects from randomized and nonrandomized trials will be handled (combined) separately by trial type; the nonrandomized evidence may be pooled with the randomized evidence for sensitivity analyses in some situations where there is limited data, using perhaps some special meta-analyses methods (e.g. network meta-analyses).

Some of the above issues relate to the magnitude of the differences between clinical trial and nonclinical trial conclusions. (Kunz et al., 2007) conclude:

> On average, non-randomized trials and randomized trials with inadequate concealment of allocation tend to result in larger estimates of effect than randomized trials with adequately concealed allocation. However, it is not generally possible to predict the magnitude, or even the direction, of possible selection biases and consequent distortions of treatment effects.

There are differences in the way costs (resource use) are collected in a study that is nonrandomized compared to a clinical trial (Hltaky, 2002). For example, side effects on a placebo arm in a randomized trial may not translate into real costs in practice. It is not unusual to collect data on resource use that are of highest monetary value (bias), or that are likely to show differences between treatment groups. Not every item of health resource use in a trial is likely to be captured and hence data collection forms (case report forms (CRFs)) are often designed to collect selected treatment-related health resource use data.

One important reason for collecting economic data in a clinical trial is because it is considered unethical to conduct a trial purely for the purposes of demonstrating value for money (although arguably, it is also unethical to waste resource where it could be put to better use elsewhere). If bias is to be minimized, then the RCT framework may still be the only framework that accommodates *both* efficacy and effectiveness. The idea of a balance between internal and external validity was proposed earlier, (Drummond, 1993).

More than twenty years later the argument has somewhat shifted from the idea that a pragmatic clinical trial with minimal inclusion/exclusion might be acceptable for showing cost-effectiveness, to a situation where a single clinical trial may no longer be admissible for demonstrating the value argument (see for example Sculpher, 2006). We shall see in Examples 6.1 and 6.2, that evidence from smaller trials can be used to demonstrate value arguments. Combining clinical trial data with 'other' evidence to demonstrate value using complex methods (with not always realistic assumptions) appears to be one way of showing the value of new treatments through combining evidence and cross-trial comparisons. If researchers are led to believe that the RCT framework does not have 'enough' external validity for a conclusive reimbursement decision, then the impetus for collecting economic data may be lost in the trial. This puts control of the value argument into the hands of the payers and not the manufacturer. A further question here is how internal or external validity can be quantified. When is a lack of external validity so serious that a cost-effectiveness decision no longer becomes valid?

It remains important to design a clinical trial for cost-effectiveness in addition to efficacy, noting the lack of external validity from RCTs. We discuss some of these trial design aspects below.

6.2 Clinical Trial Designs for Cancer Studies

6.2.1 Clinical Trial Designs

(i) *Parallel Groups and Crossover Designs*

Where an economic evaluation has been or is required for a clinical trial, some knowledge of trial design is useful. In general, cancer trials are designed to compare the effects of treatments in different groups of patients with the same condition. In a randomized parallel group design, two (or more) independent groups of patients receive experimental treatment or a control treatment (e.g. the current standard of care). The responses from these patients are compared *between* the groups. These designs are typical of cancer trials.

In some situations, a patient may receive both drugs, the experimental and the control. This is usually a crossover design. Trials with respiratory drugs for example may involve giving each patient both drugs in two separate treatment periods. Here, the patient acts as his/her own control (crossover trial). Treatment effects are determined within patients. Crossover designs (not to be confused with switching) are very unusual and unsuitable for cancer trials for several reasons (e.g. if the outcome is death, some patients cannot be treated in the second period).

Figure 6.1 shows a parallel and a crossover design. The arguments for and against crossover trials can be found in Jones (2014).

(ii) *Single Arm Phase II Designs*

A single arm trial is designed such that a single cohort of patients receive the same treatment. There is no randomization. The trial is designed with a comparison against a historical (control) response or survival rate. These are typically conducted in Phase II trial designs, where *preliminary* evidence of efficacy is required, in contrast to Phase III, where *confirmatory* evidence of treatment benefit is determined. Variations of this design are:

(i) Fleming's (single stage) design (Khan, 2012). Here, for example, 20 patients could be treated and a criterion is derived such that if 10 patients or more out of 20 (≥50%) achieve a complete or partial response (i.e. the tumor has been reduced), then the new treatment is considered worthy of further investigation. When there are no other treatments available and the cancer is very rare, it may be possible to get a license based only on a surrogate outcome such as PFS or tumor response. If follow-up is too short for OS, economic evaluation will involve the extrapolation of survival data.

(ii) A variation of the single stage design in (i) is a two-stage design. An example of this is Simon's two-stage design, which is further classified as either minimax or optimal design (Khan, 2012). The decision to either investigate efficacy further (or declare efficacy) is conducted in two stages. As an example, a sample size could be required to demonstrate a difference in PFS rates between an experimental drug and a historical control, let us assume $n = 50$ for the total trial. The criteria to proceed are based on two steps:

(a) If after the first $n = 20$, we observe 10 or more patients (50% response) who are alive and progression-free at 6 months (since starting treatment), then recruit a further $n = 30$.

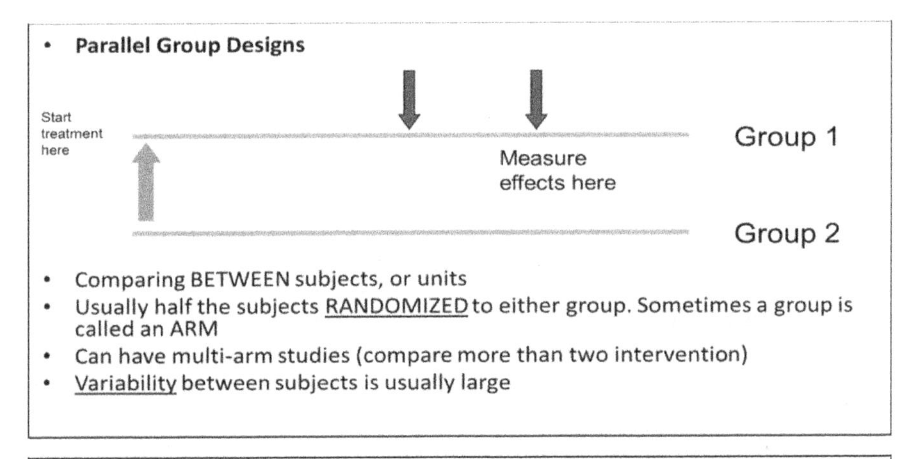

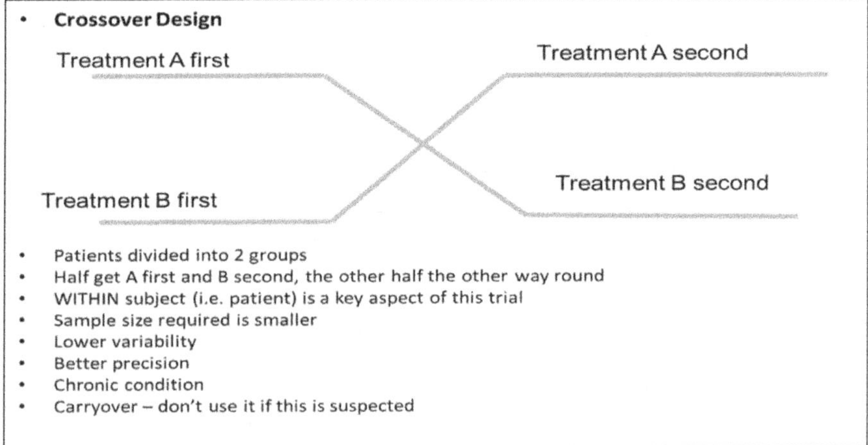

FIGURE 6.1
Parallel and crossover designs.

(b) After observing the full 50 patients, if 25 out of 50 are alive and progression-free at 6 months, then the treatment is a good candidate for further evaluation or possibly even registration.

Clearly, if only 3 patients are alive and progression-free at 6 months out of the first 20 (15%), the likelihood (probability) of 22 being alive without progression in the next 30 (73% PFS rate) will be very low. Thus, a low number that are alive without progression can lead to an early decision to stop the trial. As far as economic evaluation is concerned, one should still plan for collecting health resource use data assuming the trial will continue to $n = 50$ (unless evidence suggests otherwise) in the second stage. All patients will be valuable for a cost-effectiveness analysis and not just those in Stage 2. Further variations of these designs include single and two stage designs for dual outcomes (safety and efficacy) such as Bryant and Day (1995) and Yap (2013).

Recently, several trials using data from a single patient cohort have been used to provide evidence for efficacy. Moreover, an economic evaluation has also been performed using data from the experimental observed trial and compared against a historical (rather than a concurrent) control. We present below two examples for the same indication, with different drugs resulting in two different decisions (one recommended and one rejected for reimbursement). In Section 6.6, we will present a more detailed exposition of the design implications for HTA assessments and point out in practical terms how these need to be considered. For now, the point is that Phase II evidence alone may be used for economic evaluation, but it must be robust and substantial.

Example 6.1: Single Arm Trial in Patients with Ofatumumab for Chronic Lymphocytic Leukemia

BACKGROUND

Ofatumumab (Arzerra, GlaxoSmithKline) is a fully human, high-affinity, monoclonal antibody that is targeted against the CD20 cell surface antigen of B-lymphocytes. Ofatumumab received marketing authorization for the treatment of chronic lymphocytic leukemia in patients who are refractory to fludarabine and alemtuzumab. It is delivered by intravenous infusion. Further details are to be found in HTA TA202 (NICE, 2010) This was an uncontrolled (nonrandomized) trial in $n = 154$ patients. The primary outcome was tumor response rate; secondary outcomes included time to onset of response, duration of response, progression-free survival, time to next therapy for chronic lymphocytic leukemia, overall survival, reduction in tumor size, safety, and pharmacokinetic endpoints.

EFFICACY

After an interim analysis from 59 patients, an observed response rate of 58% (34/59) [99%CI: 40–74%, $p < 0.0001$) was compared to a planned target of 15%. All responses were partial remissions (i.e. partial response). The ERG (NICE Economic Review Group) comments from an economic evaluation perspective can be summarized as:

(i) Absence of robust evidence from randomized controlled trials. It was not possible to accurately assess the impact of bias on the outcomes, including adverse events.
(ii) Limited data because of small sample size ($n = 59$) and an absence of recent data.
(iii) No HRQoL.
(iv) Differences in baseline characteristics existed between groups who responded and did not respond (e.g. the patients who responded might have been younger compared to the ones who did not respond: possibly older and with worse prognosis).

(v) The drug was not considered cost-effective despite European Marketing Authorization approval for a license.

One issue following point (v) is that efficacy is determined on the tumor response rate but the economic evaluation was based on the OS. This difference in approach between two agencies is related to the different decision-making problems – one of efficacy and one of cost-effectiveness. The relationship between response and OS should have been examined further. Indeed, the assessment report states:

> The Committee concluded that, based on expert evidence, it was plausible that ofatumumab may offer clinical benefits to patients, but that that it was not possible to determine the magnitude of the effect from the evidence presented.
>
> The Committee recognized the difficulty of conducting randomized controlled trials in small populations of patients with limited life expectancy, as highlighted by the clinical specialists. However, the Committee concluded that such difficulties could have been addressed more effectively than they had been in the manufacturer's submission.

The Committee further discussed the potential for using data from historical controls, for example from retrospective observational Ofatumumab data for the treatment of chronic lymphocytic leukemia refractory to fludarabine and alemtuzumab.

The Committee also noted that the manufacturer had not provided more recent data from the Hx-CD20-406 study (the interim analysis was from May 2008, with no further data expected before 2011). The Committee heard from the manufacturer that this interim analysis was planned in the study protocol and that an unplanned analysis would not be possible, in accordance with best statistical practice in clinical trials, which discourages unplanned interim analyses.

This appears an unusual statement in that the magnitude of the overall response rate was 58% – 15% = 43%. Unless there was no correlation between ORR and survival, it is hard to see why a plausible benefit should not exist. This drug was not approved for reimbursement.

Example 6.2: Single Arm Trial in Patients Treated with Venetoclax for Chronic Lymphocytic Leukemia

Venetoclax was approved for the treatment of chronic lymphocytic leukemia (CLL). Prior to marketing authorization, venetoclax was designated a promising innovative medicine and was available to patients in the NHS through the EAMS (a scheme whereby patients may have the drug available at a given price because it has shown promising effects and is innovative). Details can be found in the HTA TA 487 (NICE, 2017).

The evidence of efficacy came from a single Phase I (n = 67) and two single arm Phase II trials (n = 158 and n = 64). The primary outcome was overall objective response rates (ORR). Secondary outcomes included OS. The ERG concluded:

> *The committee was concerned that the single-arm design of the trials made it difficult to assess the efficacy of venetoclax (that is, there was no comparator arm of patients having best supportive care) …*
> *The committee concluded that interpreting the results from the venetoclax trials was challenging without a direct comparator, and that this was compounded by the small patient numbers in the trials.*

Nevertheless, it was recommended for reimbursement. We now present a side-by-side summary of the evaluation of evidence from two different ERG committees for a drug for the same indication with opposite decisions.

A summary of Table 6.1 showing two reimbursement decisions from Phase II trial data indicates that the evidence from the venetoclax is considered to be:

(a) More substantial in quantity (i.e. more data).
(b) Appears more effective.
(c) However, the evidence was criticized for several reasons such as:

  (i) Whether rituximab was the best choice of comparator, or BSC, or a drug called idealalisib in combination with rituximab.
  (ii) The choice of utility for progression-free survival (0.71 vs. 0.853).
  (iii) Lack of comparative data (no randomized trials).
  (iv) Whether the end-of-life (EoL) criteria were met; there is a possibility to increase the cost-effectiveness threshold to £50,000/QALY if EoL criteria apply.
  (v) Most patients are diagnosed at age >65 and there are consequences for affordability, intolerance to treatment, and side effects.
  (vi) Improvements in HRQoL should affect the whole family and not only the patient.

(iii) *Adaptive Designs*

(a) Group Sequential

Where a decision to stop a trial early due to efficacy is considered, an adaptive trial may be used. There are various forms of adaptive design. The Phase II designs mentioned earlier (single and two stage designs in Section 6.3) are also a type of adaptive design (for single arm trials). In the two-stage design earlier, the decision to stop or continue after Stage one is based on availability and strength of efficacy data in the first $n = 20$ (if >10 out of 20 are alive and progression-free at 6 months, one may continue and recruit more subjects). An example of a group sequential design is shown in Figure 6.2.

TABLE 6.1

Two Reimbursement Decisions

Year	Venetoclax [TA487] November 2017	Ofatumumbab [TA202] October 2010
Recommendation (NICE)	**YES**	**NO**
Recommendation (License)	**YES**	**YES**
Drug company	AbbVie	GSK
Price	£4,789.47/28 days	£182.00 per 100 mg vial Dosing is 300 mg for 1st infusion plus 2,000 mg for 8 weekly infusions
Duration of treatment	Treat until PD (£58,752.23/year)	8 weeks
Number of patients planned	N = 67 (Phase 1)[a] N = 158 (Phase II)[b] N = 64 (Phase II)[c]	154
Number of patients for evidence	283	59
Interim analyses	Yes (n = xxxTBD)	Yes (n = 59)
Trial design	One Phase I and two Phase II[a]	Single arm
Primary efficacy outcome	ORR (RECIST)	ORR (RECIST)
Target effect (primary)	60% (Phase II single arm)	15% ORR
Observed effect (primary)	77% (Phase II single arm)	58%
Median (mean) OS	Not reported/available	13.7 months
Median (mean) PFS	27.2 to 41.4 months	5.7 months
Median (mean) PPS	Not reported	
Grade 3–5 toxicity	Not reported/ available	64%
Time horizon	10 years	10 years
Comparator	BSC (ritiximab/inappropriate) ERG used idelasilib (study 116)	BSC (inappropriate/not optimal)
HRQoL (EQ-5D)	Collected in trials (EQ-5D-5L)	None – externally used
Utility	0.853 company, 0.71 (ERG) and agreed at 0.748	0.65 for PFS and 0.47 for PD
Incremental QALY	Not reported/available	0.353
Incremental cost	Not reported/available	£13,565
ICER	£47,370	£38,421/QALY
ERG revised ICER	£57,476 to £77,779	£50,300 to >£81,500/ QALY

[a] *Notes:* One Phase II was a two-arm nonrandomized trial, and the other Phase II trial was a single-arm design.

[b] Study M12-175 (n = 67, Phase I dose escalation).

[c] Study M13-982 : two-arm nonrandomized (n = 158).

[d] Study M14-032 (n = 64 single arm) plus (n = 41 open label safety extension).

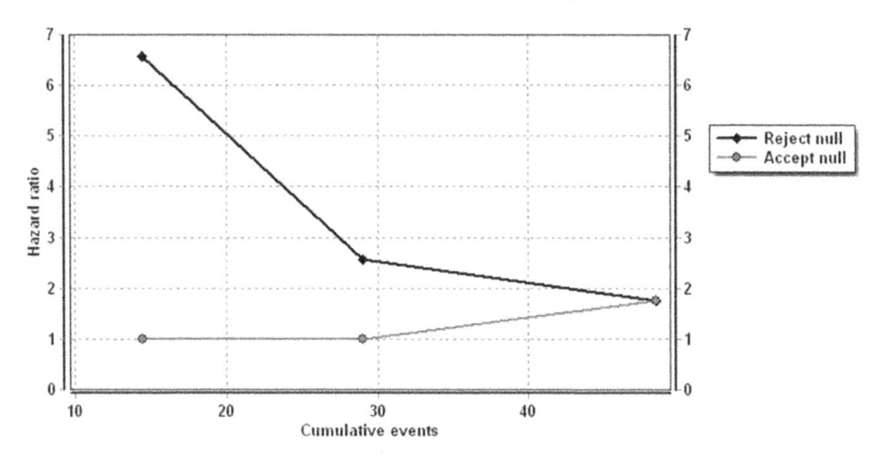

FIGURE 6.2
An adaptive group sequential trial with two interim analyses.

Figure 6.2 shows the decision procedure for stopping a trial early for efficacy or futility. The Y-axis is the observed hazard ratio related to the observed treatment effect and the X-axis is the number of events of interest. The two boundaries (lines) relate to stopping early for efficacy (top line) or futility (bottom line). There are 3 points, one at 15 events, another at about 29 events, and the final at around 49 events. These have been computed mathematically and relate to the 2 interim analysis time points (1 interim analysis occurs when a total of 15 events have been observed and the other at around 29 events). The final analysis occurs at around 49 events. If, after 15 events, the observed HR is around 6.5 (this compares control vs. experimental, so the HR for experimental vs. control would be 1/6.5 = 0.15, a very strong efficacy signal), there is an option to declare early efficacy and stop. If the decision is to continue, then after 29 events have occurred and the HR is around 2.5 (or 0.4), another opportunity to stop the trial early for efficacy is possible. In contrast, if after 15 or 29 events the observed HR is 1, the trial may be stopped for futility.

Figure 6.2 relates to a trial with two groups that was designed to detect an HR of about 1.78 (or 0.56 for experimental vs. control), using 80% power and an overall 2-sided significance level of 5%; a total of 120 patients (60 per group) and about 30 death events in total were needed. Two interim analyses were planned: the first at 25% of the total events (15 out of 60 events) and the second at about 50% (29 out of 60 events). A stopping rule for futility was considered (i.e. stopping the trial if evidence appeared there was unlikely to be benefit for future patients). The top line in Figure 6.2 is a boundary for the effect size for stopping early and the bottom line is for stopping for futility. If the observed HR crosses either of these boundaries, the trial may be stopped for either efficacy or futility. A rule called the O'Brien and Fleming rule was used to take into account the multiple interim analyses (number of times analyses are conducted). If we wish to stop early and declare the treatment to be efficacious, this is very difficult earlier on because the HR ratio would have to be around 6.5 or 1/6.5 = 0.15 (depending on the direction of comparison), which is a very large clinical effect.

If the trial does happen to stop early because the drug shows promising benefit, evidence for effectiveness may nonetheless be limited. Adaptive designs are designed to stop based on efficacy endpoints, but cost-effectiveness calculations do not appear in the derivations of the stopping rules. These can be incorporated, but is beyond the scope of this book. For a more practical demonstration see Bartha et al. (2013) and Chabot et al. (2010). Bartha et al. (2013) report an instance where payers were receptive to the idea of using immature survival data for their decision.

It is very important that statistical principles are followed and the integrity of the trial is not compromised by requests for additional data to assess effectiveness. In Example 6.1, the ERG noted an absence of interim data and the manufacturer was criticized for not providing sufficient OS data, meaning that a cost-effective judgment could not be made. The wording of the response from the ERG to the manufacturer appears to suggest a criticism for not performing an unplanned analysis. However, such unplanned interim analyses can lead to bias and can compromise the entire trial. Hence, requests for data for the purposes of cost-effectiveness needs careful consideration before it is provided.

b) Multi-Arm, Multi-Stage (MAMS)

The so-called MAMs design (Royston, Parmar, & Qian, 2003) allows multiple arms to be compared against one or more controls in a single trial. The nature of the adaptation allows comparisons to be made between multiple treatments and a control at multiple time points (i.e. at several interim analyses). Treatments that do not show sufficient promise in terms of an intermediate outcome (such as PFS or ORR) may be discontinued. Recruitment to the control and remaining experimental arms continues to determine evidence for efficacy. Currently, only efficacy outcomes (whether mean, proportion, or time-to-event) are considered in the decision rules for assessing benefit. What is likely to be important is whether specific arms are likely to be cost-effective, not just efficacious. This implies that the methodology of MAMs designs may need to be extended to several outcomes that include costs and effects. Decisions on whether arms should be dropped or future patients (who were initially randomized to treatments that were not efficacious) should be randomized to more promising arms should also take account of information on whether in the real-world they are likely to offer value. In other words, continuing the trial on the basis of efficacy alone may not be

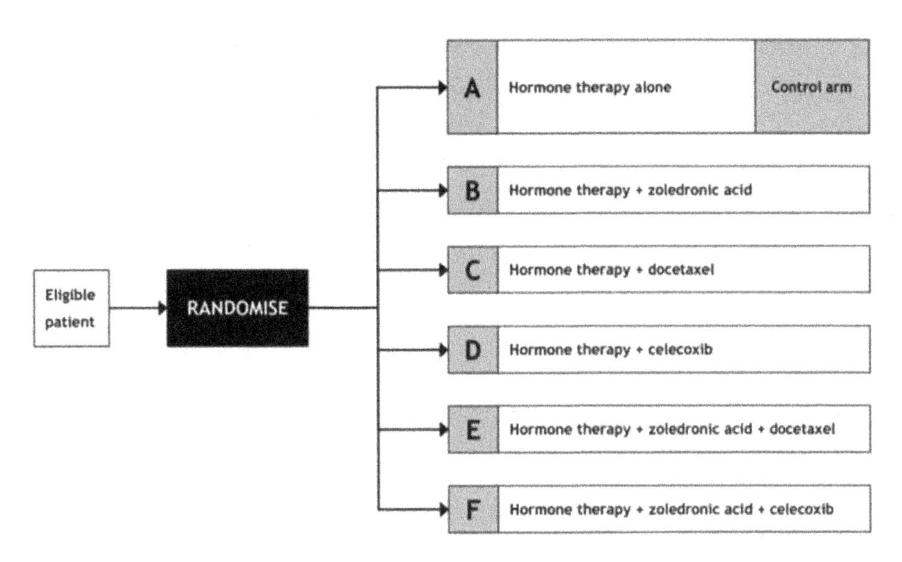

FIGURE 6.3
Example of the STAMPEDE MAMs design. (Sydes et al., 2009.)

sufficient guarantee patients will have access to these treatments if they are later found to lack cost-effectiveness (Figure 6.3).

In summary, novel designs such as adaptive, response adaptive, and group sequential designs for demonstrating early benefit, may limit the possibility of observing medium- to longer-term costs and benefits if the trial stops for early efficacy. The treatment benefit in such trials would need to be large to stop early. Such designs can rely on *statistical significance* (p-values) or posterior probabilities for decisions on efficacy, rather than the clinical effect size, which is important for economic evaluation. The driver for cost-effectiveness is related to the clinical effect size and not the p-values. For example, a trial can be stopped early for a modest clinical effect with a smaller than expected variability, but that may not be cost-effective.

Longer-term measurements for economic evaluations may not be a priority in a sequential/adaptive framework and therefore another separate trial might be needed to demonstrate longer-term benefits/effects, which not only raises ethical issues (e.g. why should a trial be run for economic considerations when there is no longer clinical equipoise), but also risks invalidating the conclusions of the first trial (e.g. ensuring additional follow-up measures), especially if it was positive (although one would expect consistency in the results between trials for the same population, endpoint, drug, conditions, etc.). Where trials are stopped early, some additional evidence may be sought from observational (real-world evidence) studies or retrospective evaluation of databases (like the Hospital Episode Statistics (HES) data or audit data such as the National Lung Cancer Audit (NCLA)).

6.2.2 Interim Analyses and Data Monitoring Committees (DMC)

A related issue is that of independent data monitoring committees (IDMC), on which health economists are increasingly playing a more active role, particularly in some academic trials in the UK. The reasons for this are essentially to evaluate how the opportunity costs for continuing a trial are reflected in the decision-making.

A small treatment benefit that is likely to result in a nonclinical yet statistically significant difference may not result in a positive cost-effectiveness conclusion. In order to ensure public expenditure is used in an optimal way, funds could be directed to other trials that do show promising benefit. While one may argue that such a decision could be made purely on clinical grounds without using cost-effectiveness arguments, the two are likely to be inextricably linked. The challenge for health economists here is that while arguing that cost-effectiveness from a lifetime perspective needs to be evaluated to reduce uncertainty (as is often stated in ERG reports), the interim data do not provide for such decision-making.

Several important considerations need to be taken into account with interim analyses, especially where a cost-effectiveness component is included.

(i) All relevant major health resource use data are adequately collected (e.g. to ensure the IDMC has sufficient information to make a decision).

(ii) Data collected does not compromise the trial design. For example, where PFS is used as a surrogate, the desire to also look at OS should not constitute an unplanned interim analysis that renders both the final efficacy and cost-effectiveness analyses to be biased (or even invalid).

(iii) The ongoing conduct of the trial is not compromised. Where the trial is analyzed blind (even the IDMC will not know treatment group allocation), health resource use data collected does not provide the opportunity to make a good guess as to which arm patients are allocated to.

(iv) Data are not shared, or information is not shared between people appointed as members of the IDMC because they are colleagues. Many academic trials work with in groups of collaborators who are often familiar with each other's work (they might meet at conferences or be joint investigators); information from one arm of a trial could be shared to influence the conduct of a separate trial where there is a common comparator. Whereas there may be legal consequences in industry trials where financial interest exists if confidentiality is compromised, such penalties are not known in academic trials (Sartor & Halabi, 2015). We believe that if such a practice can happen in an industry-sponsored trial, the impetus and pressure to secure grant funding may be equally as great, hence a more robust approach is needed. Clinical trial units that conduct academic trials need to be much more robust to ensure such practice is removed, to avoid the credibility of published results being open to question.

(v) *Open Label Extensions*

Open label extensions (OLE) occur where, at the end of the randomized phase, patients can be followed up outside the randomized protocol-defined conditions. An open label extension after an initial double-blind phase can be helpful for understanding real-world effects. During the open label extension, longer term costs (e.g. for later adverse events, effects of maintenance of new treatment, etc.) can be evaluated. Sometimes after the double-blind phase of a trial, all patients are switched over to the experimental treatment (despite the benefits of the new experimental treatment remaining unproven). In that case, longer-term effects and costs can become available for the experimental arm only, and not for the comparator.

The importance of an open label extension should not be underestimated or glossed over, in terms of both design and statistical analysis. The emphasis is often placed on the double-blind part of the trial. The open label part can often be used more efficiently to maximize the value argument because this part of the trial reflects real clinical practice better than the controlled phase. For example, patients might take concomitant medication, additional patients might be entered who were not previously allowed, or longer-term effects can be assessed. This would suit an economic evaluation that is usually performed after the results of the clinical effects are made available (although the planning of economic models would be much earlier). An OLE may be conducted in a separate protocol (one protocol for the double blind and one for the open label), or as a single protocol. A clear definition of the starting and stopping between the two stages needs to be carefully determined.

(vi) *Observational Studies*

Not all clinical evaluations can be performed through RCTs. For example, we could not (ethically) randomize one group to tobacco and other to placebo to determine if they developed lung cancer. Similarly, it will be challenging to randomize a group of children to the MMR vaccine and another group to no vaccine to see if they developed autism (following the Wakefield controversy on MMR related to autism, see Maisonneuve & Floret, 2012).

An observational study provides data on the natural history of a condition where data are collected in a representative population from the disease of interest. Clinical trials may not provide the data needed for a decision due to limitations in the selected population (e.g. due to inclusion criteria), choice of comparator (new treatments licensed after the main trial results submitted), limited length of follow-up (e.g. with OS, may be able to have longer follow-up to determine rare outcomes), limited sample size, and absence of HRQoL data. This limits the generalizability of the trial results.

Observational studies can therefore provide an important source of data and may be the only source of evidence for collecting cost-effectiveness data in some cases. In observational studies, patients are not randomized, and the timing of measurements and other procedures is not controlled. These are often conducted in real-world (naturalistic) settings. One major issue is the presence of selection bias. For example, if we select patients in one group who have the risk of an expected outcome of interest (e.g. PD) and in the other group, patients are those with the outcome, this type of comparison or 'case mix' is likely to be problematic. Ways to account for the selection bias will be discussed in Chapter 8 (RWD) through the use of propensity scores and other adjustment models, Guo and Fraser (2014).

In an observational study, the estimate of the treatment effect (or 'drift') may be subject to considerable selection bias; it will be important to control the data quality with complete histories and patient characteristics. Baseline characteristics data will be needed such that adjusting treatment effects for potential selection bias can be adequately determined. Observation studies are particularly useful for evaluating the often-needed longer-term consequences of treatments not observed during clinical trials. This also includes data on HRQoL, utilities, and health resource use.

(vii) *Retrospective Case Control Studies*

Case control studies are used to retrospectively (data collected on past events) determine if there is an association between an exposure and a specific health outcome. Patients are selected in a case control study based on their known outcome status (e.g. died, progressed). For example, we might collect data from hospital notes about incidence of disease (e.g. a particular cancer) after being exposed to a number of variables (explanatory variables, e.g. smoking, age, gender, disease history, prognostic markers). We wish to investigate whether these variables explain or are related to the outcome of the disease. Consequently, explanatory variables are subject to variability and outcomes are known. This type of data is easier (and faster) to collect and usually cheaper than an observational study or conducting an RCT.

A case control study might be useful where the disease (and/or outcome) is rare because investigators can intentionally search for the cases. A cohort study in a rare disease requires a large number of patients with the outcome of interest (exposed) to get an adequate number of cases. 'Cases' and 'controls' should be clearly defined prior to commencing the data collection. Data on health resource use, too, needs to be determined *a priori* to avoid biased conclusions.

6.3 Planning a Health Economic Evaluation in a Clinical Trial

6.3.1 Important Considerations When Designing a Cancer Study for Economic Evaluation

One key aspect of planning a health economic evaluation is to identify:

(i) What data will be collected for economic evaluation?
(ii) How will the data be collected?
(iii) When will the data be collected?

The answer to these three questions is closely related to the overall objectives and the design of the trial, in particular whether the economic evaluation is prospective or retrospective. Whereas in almost all cases clinical trial data are collected prospectively, cost and quality of life data are not always collected prospectively. Some possibilities are summarized in Table 6.2 below which outlines the type of economic evaluation that could be undertaken (last column).

(a) Costs/Resource Use and Effects Collected Prospectively

In the context of a clinical trial, costs and resource data are collected at the patient level prospectively. For each patient there are several measures of effects and several measures of resource use (such as hospital visits, consultations, scans, number of doses, etc.). The trial is typically designed for a clinical endpoint, but the economic component is accommodated or added on. In some cases, both clinical and economic endpoints are formally designed (including sample size calculations) into the trial. For example, sample size is likely to be based on the clinical endpoint, as will timing of the main primary and secondary endpoints. However, the data collection forms (also called case report forms (CRFs)) might be designed to capture resource use and specific adverse events in detail, especially those associated with important

TABLE 6.2

Collecting Data in a Trial for an Economic Evaluation

Costs collected	Clinical Endpoint (Primary)	Other Outcomes (e.g. utility)	Possible Economic Evaluation Method
Prospectively	Prospectively	Prospectively	Stochastic (patient level)
Retrospectively	Prospectively	Prospectively	Stochastic/decision tree/ Markov
Retrospectively	Prospectively	Retrospectively	Decision tree/ Markov
Retrospectively	Retrospectively	Retrospectively	Decision tree/ Markov

costs. Extended patient follow-up time may allow for collection of data in the form of an open label extension with relaxed inclusion criteria (whereas in a trial without an economic component, the follow-up period might be restricted).

An economic evaluation is usually performed after the results of the clinical effects are made available (although the planning of economic models will be much earlier). There is unlikely to be any benefit in carrying out an economic evaluation if there is no clinical benefit (unless value is shown in some subgroups). The economic evaluation is usually carried out using stochastic methods, that is, using patient-level observations for the statistical analysis of costs and effects. Another approach to analysis is to summarize the individual cost and efficacy data (e.g. means and/or frequencies) and use these as 'inputs' into a health economic simulation model to estimate the ICER.

(b) Clinical Effects are Collected Prospectively but *Some* Health Resource and Quality of Life Data is Collected Retrospectively

The clinical trial in this scenario is designed only for the clinical component, and costs and utility (HRQoL) are extracted from external sources or published literature. For example, in an oncology trial the clinical effects might be a measure such as progression-free survival (PFS) time – calculated from the time from randomization until disease progression. The health resources involved with the new treatment, along with HRQoL data, are extracted from the clinical trial database (from compliance, exposure rates and HRQoL modules of the CRF), but concomitant medication use might be taken from published sources. Collecting concomitant data in a CRF can be an arduous task in a clinical trial because the data often needs to be queried for items such as missing dates, details of mode of administration, converting names from active ingredient to either brand or generic name (brands are more expensive), and so forth. In practice, the percentage of patients who take a specific form of concomitant medication might be determined from literature rather than using data collected in the trial.

Patient-level safety data will also be collected (e.g. specific adverse event grades for each patient), where the average cost of treating each adverse event can be extracted from external published sources using reported duration of adverse events. The duration of adverse events in the trial give an idea of *actual* resource use to treat adverse events in real clinical practice. For example, rash is a well-known side effect of the drug erlotinib (Lee et al., 2012) that is treated with some topical ointment; the incidence of rash can be collected but details of the treatment for rash can include information such as frequency, dose, name, and route of administration, which may not be collected in the CRF. If the time to rash disappearance could be determined from the CRF, this might provide a useful estimate of the duration of concomitant medication use. However, unless the duration of an adverse event is a critical clinical or cost outcome, one generally restricts computation of duration for the most important adverse events (usually most costly) to minimize database and programming time. To compute duration, the start and stop times of adverse events will be necessary to compute and these are not always available. Lewis et al. (2010) estimate the costs associated with the duration of an adverse event by using concomitant treatment from published data. Data managers and clinical programmers would need to ensure that important data such as the dates of onset and termination were available for this type of calculation.

In some situations, clinical effects may need to be extrapolated from the clinical trial, even where effects are measured prospectively. For example, 5 years of follow-up time may not be long enough to monitor PFS (progression might occur at 6 or 7 years after the start of treatment) in some cancer trials. Estimates of PFS times in the specific patient population could be made at year 6 and beyond based on literature data. Alternatively, Dukhovny et al. (2012) modeling and simulation might be used to estimate PFS effects beyond the fifth year of follow-up; The follow-up period could also be extended (more costly) during the design stage of the trial so that extrapolation and therefore uncertainty can be minimized. Having observed data (outcomes) available is always less uncertain compared to extrapolating data, no matter the complexity or ingenuity of the models used.

(c) Clinical effects and outcomes are collected retrospectively

If no clinical trial data are available, data are likely to be extracted from published sources. An important feature of the data here is that cost-effectiveness analyses are usually determined from summary data (e.g. mean costs or effects). These (inputs) are often used for simulation in a cost-effectiveness model. The key difference compared to prospectively collected data is that since data collection is retrospective the inputs for an economic model are based on whatever data has been collected previously. The quality of the economic evaluation, therefore, depends on *where* the data were extracted from, their quality, and their consistency with the population under study. In many cases the retrospective data are extracted from published clinical trials such as in Dukhovny et al., 2012 or O'Connor et al. (2012). Dukhovny et al. (2012) described their economic evaluation as being 'retrospective,' however, the trial was designed prospectively for an economic evaluation. In this book, when we consider retrospective analyses, we take this to mean that the clinical trial did not plan for an economic evaluation or collect economic data prospectively – not that the analysis was carried out at some much later time. If the former were true, all analysis would be retrospective (economic evaluation and statistical analysis) because analyses are almost always done after the trial has been completed (except perhaps in some sequential (or

Bayesian) type of trial designs, where analysis is conducted while the trial continues).

In some situations, prospectively collecting data may be too risky commercially or may just not be the most efficient way (e.g. comparing head-to-head with a competitor drug, such as nivolumab vs. pembrozulimab, see NICE, 2017 on nivolumab). In Examples 6.1 and 6.2, the company withheld the OS rates from public view during the review of its economic model by NICE. The details of cost or utility data may also be withheld for commercial sensitivity. Consequently, in such cases the use of retrospective data may be the only option available.

One common scenario is to compare a new treatment A with the current standard of care S. In a three arm trial of A, S, and best supportive care (BSC), reimbursement assessors may argue for including S as the third arm to address value for money in terms of superiority (A vs. S). A pharmaceutical company may have its own commercial (or regulatory) reasons to avoid a direct comparison of A with S (e.g. to minimize impact on market share). One possibility is to carry out a comparison of A versus S in some indirect way (Section 4.9) (Ades et al., 2011):

(a) Treatment A (the new treatment).
(b) BSC (needed to demonstrate efficacy).
(c) Treatment S (needed to demonstrate efficiency and effectiveness).

Suppose treatment S has nonetheless been compared with BSC in a separate trial and a comparison with treatment A results in A being on average worse than S (A < S). It may therefore be commercially risky for the manufacturer of A to compare A with S.

Notwithstanding, an indirect comparison would allow an estimate of treatment benefit between A and S that would otherwise not be made – or even known. The so-called mixed treatment comparison allows for the possibility of avoiding direct comparisons, albeit in a noncontrolled setting. A mixed treatment comparison would use published data from a trial that compares treatment S with treatment BSC and A versus BSC as a way to compare the efficiency of A versus S. Figure 6.4 shows an indirect treatment comparison between A versus S through a common arm BSC.

6.3.2 Integrating Economic Evaluation in a Clinical Trial: Considerations

Integrating a health economic component into a clinical trial has been discussed previously (Haycox, 1997; Drummond, 2005; Glick et al., 2011, 2014; O'Sullivan et al., 2005; Petrou & Gray, 2011; Ramsey, 2015). We now expand further on the major aspects of trial design for economic evaluation below and summarize these in Table 6.3 (Figure 6.4). More details can be found in Khan (2015).

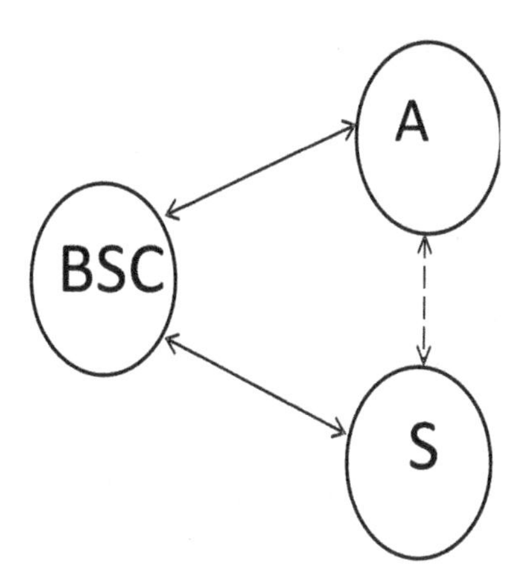

FIGURE 6.4
Diagram representing direct comparison for A versus B and A versus C (solid lines) and the indirect comparison for B versus C (dashed line).

TABLE 6.3
Summary of Key Clinical Trial Design Issues for a Health Economic Evaluation

Key Issue	Key Considerations
Endpoints and outcomes	• Identify which endpoints are truly clinical, which are economic, and which may be both
Choice of comparator	• Standard of care or another comparator • Direct vs. indirect comparison
Timing of measurements	• Open label extensions • Duration of follow-up • Capture later and early costs
Trial design	• 3-arm trial or 2 separate trials (efficacy and CE) • Adaptive designs may have limited follow-up
CRF design	• Identify resources to collect • Focus on big cost items
Power and sample size	• Number of patients required to demonstrate CE • Power-specific subgroups where CE most likely • Value of information
Treatment pathway	• Identify costs and benefits in the treatment pathway
Generic entry/ patent expiry date	• Identify dates for project management and speed of preparing reimbursement argument
Compliance	• Compliance may be related to side effects and hence more costs
Subgroups/heterogeneity	• Identify subgroups *a priori* defined where treatment benefit is more likely and greatest
Early ICER/INMB	• An early ICER helps to work out where the new treatment is in the CE plane
Multicenter/multinational trial	• Country-specific CEAC or ICERev • Multilevel modeling techniques

6.3.3 Endpoints and Outcomes

Those endpoints that are clearly clinical, clearly economic, and that have potential overlap should be identified as early as possible. The primary endpoint is often thought to be unambiguously clinical, whereas HRQoL may be considered 'somewhere in the middle' between an economic and clinical endpoint (Figure 6.5).

Compliance endpoints may be relevant to both clinical (e.g. for per protocol populations) and economic evaluations (cost of actual drug use). The type of HRQoL measure is also an important consideration: should the HRQoL measure be disease-specific, like the QLQC-30 for cancer, or should it be a generic one such as the EQ-5D? Careful thought needs to be given as to how important secondary endpoints can be used to add to the value to a new treatment. Demonstrating value of a new treatment should take into account more than just one endpoint alone. If the endpoint is rare such as chondroma of the mandibular condyle (a benign tumor in the head and neck) then perhaps a clinical trial is not the best design.

The QALY discussed earlier is not an endpoint but a composite of 2 endpoints (HRQoL and survival, but not necessarily limited to OS). This metric is considered to be a preferred choice in some countries to demonstrate the value argument, although not accepted universally (e.g. Germany and some other countries do not consider the QALY as the primary basis for demonstrating value). The value argument should not be dependent on a single outcome, even if it is a key measure. In situations where a primary endpoint is positive but all secondary endpoints are negative (worse effects), a decision

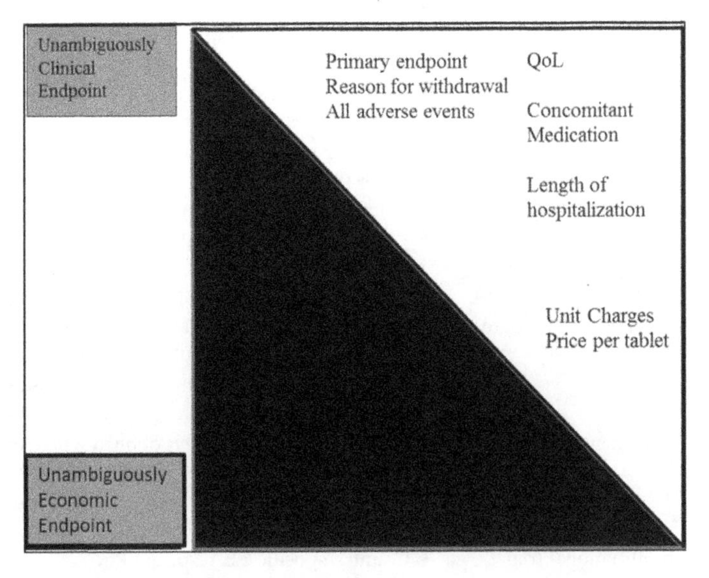

FIGURE 6.5
Relationship between clinical and economic endpoints in a clinical trial.

in support of cost-effectiveness may be difficult compared to the case where the secondary endpoints are, on average, not worse (no difference).

Some generic HRQoL measures lack the sensitivity to detect treatment benefit, such as the EQ-5D in lung cancer patients (Khan, 2015). A cancer-specific HRQoL measure, such as the QLQ-C30, can have greater sensitivity to detect treatment effects. It can be incorrect to conclude an absence of cost-effectiveness, when the problem itself lies in the measures used to assess cost-effectiveness. Other outcome measures, such as Quality of Time Spent Without Symptoms of Disease and Toxicity (QTWiST), a special type of QALY (Gelber et al., 1996) that subtracts from the overall survival the period of time during which either treatment or disease reduces HRQoL, may be considered as an alternative to the QALY in some cases. Disability-adjusted life-years (DALYs) and other measures may be considered as outcomes.

The failure of an economic evaluation to demonstrate a cost-effective QALY difference is not sufficient evidence to conclude an absence of an overall value argument. Indeed, in Germany, IQWiG does not consider QALYs as a prominent measure (or the only measure) that demonstrates the value of the new technology, but any measure that captures a combination of mortality, morbidity, and QoL. A translation of the text from IQWiG is shown:

> As the benefit of an intervention should be related to the patient, this assessment is based on the results of studies that have investigated the effects of an intervention on patient-relevant outcomes. In this context, 'patient-relevant' refers to how a patient feels, functions or survives. In this context, consideration is given to both the intentional and unintentional effects of the intervention that allow an assessment of the impact on the following patient-relevant outcomes, in order to determine the changes related to disease and treatment:
>
> 1. Mortality
> 2. Morbidity (complaints and complications)
> 3. Health-related QoL

(IQWiG, version 3.0, 27/05/2008)

A comparison between a new treatment and the standard of care is often needed in an economic evaluation. If a *potential* comparator has not been approved for licensing because it is undergoing a review by the EMA, this does not mean that a new experimental treatment cannot be compared with this potential (future) comparator. For example, at the time of submission of lenalidomide for licensing (NICE TA171, 2008), bortezomib was undergoing review by the EMA. Later bortezamib became the standard of care while lenalidomide was under review. The sponsor argued that a comparison for economic evaluation with bortezamib was not possible because at the time bortezamib was not the standard of care. The assessors (for reimbursement) argued by noting that although this may be true for licensing, such an argument did not apply to economic evaluations and the sponsor should have considered a comparison with bortezamib (see NICE TA171, ERG Report). The method of indirect or mixed treatment comparisons may be used in such situations.

6.3.3.1 Timing of Measurements

The primary efficacy endpoint is usually the main focus of a trial with collection occurring at some 'optimal' set of time points (e.g. for PFS, scans taken at some ideal time points). For other (secondary) endpoints, such as HRQoL, the assessment times of collecting data are important. Ensuring enough pre- and post-disease progression HRQoL measurements are available will allow more precise QALY estimates. If the median PFS is 6 months, for example, then HRQoL might be collected every month. However, if median PFS is only 3 months, more frequent HRQoL assessments might be made prior to 3 months. For other endpoints, extended follow-up for monitoring compliance, end-of-life care, long-term efficacy, and safety might also be needed.

In many trials HRQoL is often collected until disease progression (e.g. cancer trials), although in theory it could be collected until death or to the onset of palliative care. However, it might be felt that collecting HRQoL after disease progression is very difficult because patients will deteriorate rapidly. If some patients continue to take some treatment even after he/she has progressed, time to second progression might be a useful endpoint. In such cases, having information about HRQoL between the first and second progression will help inform decision-makers about the value of treatment over a longer period of time (and justify treatment with the new drug beyond first progression). The period between first and second progression (or death) is essential to estimate the value of a new treatment over the lifetimes of patients. Moreover, during the post-progression period, patients tend to take additional concomitant/anti-cancer treatments, which may have a noticeable impact on HRQoL, because many of these are third- or fourth-line treatments with higher toxicity burdens.

In some cancer trials, all patients may not be followed until death, so costs are censored for some patients, whereas complete costs are available for others. Adequate follow-up is needed to capture all the later as well as the earlier costs. Follow-up time should not be so long that demonstrating cost-effectiveness and reimbursement is delayed or becomes too imprecise.

6.3.3.2 Trial Design

Trial design was discussed earlier in Section 6.1. In this context, trial design refers to the experimental design of the trial and not the broader aspects of trial design such as blinding, choice of comparator, timing of measurements, etc. Parallel group designs are the most common in cancer clinical trials.

6.3.3.3 CRF Design

In clinical trials, data is recorded on a case report form (CRF) or a data collection form (DCF). Until relatively recently, CRFs were designed without considering resource collection. Resource use was estimated from surveys or based on external publications. In a clinical trial designed prospectively for economic evaluation, resource data, especially for ambulatory care, is generally captured through interviewing patients using nurses or trial staff during scheduled clinic visits (note: this applies only to community outpatient care; for in-hospital care, whether for a standard stay or otherwise, data are tracked by extracting data from the hospital's patient file either manually or electronically; in-hospital costs in a fee-for-service health system can be extracted from the hospital billing system). Questions such as: "When was the last time you visited the GP since your last visit to the clinic?" or "Was an outpatient visit to the hospital made?" are included in the CRF. The responses to such questions are then used to calculate the costs per patient. Resource use is entered into the CRF in physical units and not monetary value. The unit prices of each health resource are obtained from elsewhere (see Chapter 4).

Resource use cannot always be planned, unlike scheduled clinic visits. Often a patient might attend a protocol scheduled clinic visit and the question in the CRF might be "Since your last visit, did you see a GP?" in order to capture costs associated with GP visits. These unplanned visits could be captured in a patient diary. Recording data in a diary may be more suitable for health resource use (costs) because usually the total cost per patient can be derived in their personal real-world setting. Diary data however have a certain notoriety for being incomplete (missing data), unless electronic diaries are used, and this could result in unreliable health resource use being recorded. Compliance of medication might be captured through a diary, but the simplest option is to count the returned tablets. For intravenously (IV) administered infusions or radiotherapy given at hospitals, the CRF would be more appropriate.

Recording data in the CRF (or electronic CRF (eCRF)) involves patients being asked directly about resource use that has taken place. Sensible judgment is needed to determine whether a diary is needed or whether CRFs can be used to record resource use. It might be useful to run a test or pilot of the CRFs, especially if electronic data capture, such as eCRFs, are used. Chapter 5 provided some examples of CRF designs for health resource use.

6.3.3.4 Sample Size Methods for Cost-Effectiveness

Traditionally, sample size calculations are carried out to design clinical trials to detect clinically relevant differences between two treatments. In clinical trials designed for economic evaluation, it is usual to collect patient-level data on resource use (costs) in addition to efficacy and safety. While there may be arguments to power a clinical trial for demonstrating clinical benefit, the arguments for powering for cost-effectiveness have not been fully appreciated. There are several reasons why calculating a sample size for cost-effectiveness may not be considered relevant.

First, it is argued that without showing a clinical effect there is unlikely to be any cost-effectiveness argument – therefore efforts should be directed toward the clinical endpoint. Second, although the magnitude of a clinical effect can be justified, the size of a measure of 'effectiveness' may be less clear. For example, in trials where the endpoint is a combination of quality of life and quantity of life, the composite 'economically relevant' QALY difference is usually unknown. Third, ethics committees rarely query a trial protocol that has a cost-effectiveness objective but no sample size justification, whereas they would almost certainly query a protocol with no sample size justification for the primary clinical outcome. Finally, it may not be considered ethical to power a trial purely for demonstrating cost-effectiveness, because it is construed as an economic argument and not a clinical argument for the trial.

Despite the above reasons, the risks for a new experimental treatment that 'misses' the opportunity to demonstrate value either for reimbursement purposes or for national health policy reasons are real and should not be underestimated (many cancer drugs get rejected for reimbursement). This is akin to a 'false negative' where the likelihood of showing cost-effectiveness is real, but the trial may not have been designed appropriately to demonstrate i.e. it lacks power. It is perhaps for this reason that funding bodies such as CRUK or the NIHR have sections on sample sizes for cost-effectiveness objectives in their funding application forms.

In the UK, NICE offers an advisory service that provides advice to optimize designs of clinical trials aimed at demonstrating cost-effectiveness. The ability to power for cost-effectiveness, therefore, allows researchers, policymakers, funders, and drug companies to plan for another level of uncertainty toward the path of licensing and reimbursement or changing the standard of care in an economically viable way. A detailed exposition of sample size methods for cost-effectiveness in a frequentist and Bayesian framework is found in Khan (2015, Chapter 8) and Willan and Briggs (2006).

In the past, sample sizes for cost-effectiveness were calculated in different ways. One method was to calculate a sample size for clinical effects and costs separately, and then choose the maximum of the two. However, it is unclear what an important difference in costs between treatment groups is supposed to be. Moreover, this approach treated costs and effects as independent. In practice, patients with smaller treatment effects could have larger costs because they might be treated with other more expensive treatments, or might have stopped taking the treatment (e.g. for lack of effect) or side effects, which might also result in increased costs.

In clinical trials of efficacy, the sample size depends on several variables, including the hypothesized clinically relevant difference (e.g. measured using a hazard ratio) and the variability associated with the clinical effect. A sample size formula might look like the one below, used for continuous measures (as in a two-sample t-test):

$$n_E = \left(z_\alpha + z_\beta\right)^2 \frac{\left(\sigma_{E1}^2 + \sigma_{E2}^2\right)}{\Delta_{ER}^2} \tag{6.1}$$

In this formula, n is the sample size for each treatment group, σ_{E1}^2 and σ_{E2}^2 are expressions of the variability of the response in each of the two groups, Δ_{ER}^2 is the clinically relevant difference, and the values of Z_α and Z_β are special values taken from published tables (or a software) that express the risk of a false positive (often 5%) or a false negative (often 20%).

A sample size calculation for a cancer trial is calculated in a different way in that it is generally driven by the number of events (death or progression events) and the treatment effect (clinically relevant difference) is the hazard ratio (HR).

Sample Size Formula for Cost-Effectiveness

$$\begin{aligned} n_1 &= \left(z_\alpha + z_\beta\right)^2 \frac{\left[r\left(k^2\sigma_{E1}^2 + \sigma_{C1}^2 - 2k\rho_1\sigma_{E1}\sigma_{C1}\right) + \left(k^2\sigma_{E2}^2 + \sigma_{C2}^2 - 2k\rho_2\sigma_{E2}\sigma_{C2}\right)\right]}{r\left[k\Delta_{ER} - \Delta_{CR}\right]^2} \\ n_2 &= \left(z_\alpha + z_\beta\right)^2 \frac{\left[r\left(k^2\sigma_{E1}^2 + \sigma_{C1}^2 - 2k\rho_1\sigma_{E1}\sigma_{C1}\right) + \left(k^2\sigma_{E2}^2 + \sigma_{C2}^2 - 2k\rho_2\sigma_{E2}\sigma_{C2}\right)\right]}{\left[k\Delta_{ER} - \Delta_{CR}\right]^2}. \end{aligned} \tag{6.2}$$

For example, for a drug that is expected to improve OS by 20% (i.e. HR = 0.80) would be:

$$(1.96 + 1.28)^2 / 0.25^* \log(0.80)^2 = 845 \text{ death events needed}(90\% \text{ power})$$

The sample size here is driven by the number of events. If we assume the probability of an event is 0.75 (this is usually calculated in some complicated way) over the year (e.g. late stage lung cancer patients), the sample size is 1,127 or about 564 patients per group.

6.3.3.5 Sample Size Formulae for Cost-Effectiveness: Examples

In the above formula and calculations, there is no mention of costs for any of the treatment groups or a (co-)relationship between costs and clinical effects, nor is there detail of a cost-effectiveness threshold, nor anything about a cost-effectiveness ratio or benefit. When cost-effectiveness is also considered in the same trial (cost-effectiveness trial), the sample size formula needs to include additional factors:

(a) The way the effectiveness element is evaluated – i.e. using the ICER approach or the INB approach
(b) Costs in each group
(c) Variability of costs in each group
(d) Correlation between costs and effects in each group
(e) The cost-effectiveness threshold

Taking into account the above factors (a)–(e) makes the sample size formula more complicated. In some situations (such as using Bayesian methods), a formula (even if it is complex) might not be available. The sample size in these situations is calculated using simulation methods. Although, the sample size problem can be approached through simulation (see Khan. 2015), it is better (easier) to determine sample sizes by using a sample size formula rather than having to doing lots of programming. In a clinical trial for comparing two groups, where costs and effects are collected prospectively, we propose using the following sample size formula when patient-level data are available (see Khan, 2015).

In equation (6.2), the denominator of the expression $k\Delta_{\text{ER}} - \Delta_{\text{CR}}$ expresses the cost-effectiveness argument in terms of the desired incremental net benefit (INB) (see Chapter 1). We use λ= K to represent the cost-effectiveness threshold for the remainder of this chapter. Therefore, in reference to point (a) above, the measure of effectiveness is a single numerical quantity that combines separate measures of clinical efficacy and costs to form a measure of economic value worthwhile pursuing.

For example, if an existing treatment compared with the current standard of care offers an INB of £5,000 (measured in money terms), then we might want to ensure the new treatment has a sample size that can show INB values >£5,000. Sometimes, the measure of effectiveness might also consist of two separate measures: HRQoL and efficacy, to form a QALY. Therefore, the terms Δ_{ER} and Δ_{CR} in $\text{K}\Delta_{ER} - \Delta_{CR}$ are the mean difference in QALYs and the mean difference in costs between treatments, respectively. Therefore, the objective is to estimate the sample size that yields a specific INMB based on mean effects and costs. Table 6.4 summarizes the inputs for the sample size formula.

Example 6.3

In a two-group trial (treatment A vs. B) in a 1:1 allocation (r = 1), the following parameters are considered in order to calculate the sample size for showing an INB of at least £3,000.

We assume that the mean costs of the new experimental treatment averages to £20,000 per year (treatment A). The mean costs for treatment B, the current standard of care are £10,000, substantially cheaper. The new treatment will need to show a positive INMB, given that it is more expensive.

TABLE 6.4

Summary and Explanation of Terms for Equation (6.2)

Term	Definition
σ^2_{Ej}	Population variance for QALY measure in treatment group 1
σ^2_{Ej}	Population variance for QALY measure in treatment group 2
σ^2_{Cj}	Population variance for cost in treatment group 1
σ^2_{Cj}	Population variance for cost in treatment group 2
n	Sample size per group (multiply by 2 for the total sample size in a 2-group trial)
ρ_j	Correlation coefficient between efficacy (QALY) and cost for the treatment group 1
ρ_j	Correlation coefficient between efficacy (QALY) and cost for the treatment group 2
$K = \lambda$	The cost-effectiveness threshold unit cost the healthcare provider is prepared to pay to obtain a unit increase in effectiveness (in the UK, this is £20,000 to £30,000)
Δ_{ER}	Mean difference between group 1 and 2 in terms of (QALY) effects
Δ_{CR}	Mean difference between group 1 and 2 in terms of costs
r	Patient allocation ratio between two treatment groups (e.g. in 1:1 allocation takes value 1)
z_α	Value associated with false positive rate (typically 1.96 for 5% level)
z_β	Value associated with false negative rate (typically 1.28 for 20% (80% power) level)

The clinical effects in this (hypothetical) example are based on mean estimates of QALYs and survival rates from earlier trials. In the experimental arm, the HRQoL based on EQ-5D is estimated to be a mean of about 0.60 in each group. The mean survival for the new treatment was 17 months; for the standard treatment group it is expected to be around 14 months. The QALY is therefore about 10.2 (0.60 × 17) for treatment A and 9.4 (0.60 ×14) for treatment B. If the cost-effective threshold is £30,000, the number of patients required to show a positive INB (e.g. £5,000) on average assuming no correlation between costs and effects ($\rho_1 = \rho_2 = 0$) although in practice a positive correlation would be the rule.

We assume the variance of costs in the new and standard treatments are £10,000 and £6,000 respectively and for QALYs are 10.2 and 8.4 for treatments A and B respectively. The WTP value of $\lambda = K =$ £30,000, gives a value for the denominator in equation (6.2), $(\lambda^*\Delta_E - \Delta_C)^2$ of : £30,000 × (10.2 – 9.4) – (£20,000 – £10,000) = £24,000 – £10,000 = (£14,000)^2.

The value of £14,000 tells us that when the WTP = £30,000, the net benefit of the new treatment is at least £14,000. The sample size for each treatment group for a WTP of £30,000 in a 1:1 allocation, assuming a mean QALY difference of 0.8 and a mean cost difference of 10,000 using equation (6.2), : is computed as:

$$n = \frac{(1.96+1.28)^2 * \left[1*\left(£30{,}000^2 * 3.5+£10{,}000\right)+\left(£30{,}000^2 * 2.9 + £6{,}000\right)\right]}{\left[\ 1*£30{,}000\times(10.2-9.4)-(£20{,}000-£10{,}000)\right]^2}$$

$n = 605$

Therefore, a sample size of 605 per group (1,210 in total, allocated in a ratio of 1:1) is likely (80% power, 5% significance) to:

(i) Show an INB > 0.
(ii) Reject H_0: that the new treatment would offer no value to the (tax)payer – i.e. INB < 0.
(iii) Be unlikely to have sufficient power to show INB values < £14,000. From a payer perspective, the larger the INB, the better.

6.3.4 Treatment Pathways

In the same way clinical pharmacologists attempt to understand the mechanism of action of a drug, health economists seek to understand the mechanism of cost structures. This requires an understanding of the full treatment pathway. Without appreciating the pathway, key component costs could be lost. An example of a treatment pathway for diffuse large B-cell lymphoma is given.

Diffuse large B-cell lymphoma (DLBCL) is a fast-growing, aggressive form of lymphoma. It is fatal if left untreated, but with timely and appropriate treatment, approximately two-thirds of all patients can be cured. The standard treatment of advanced DLBCL is combination chemotherapy plus immunotherapy. The most common chemotherapy regimen for advanced DLBCL is called R-CHOP. R-CHOP includes rituximab, cyclophosphamide, doxorubicin, vincristine, and prednisone. The first four drugs are injected into a vein intravenously over the course of 1 day, while prednisone is taken by mouth for 5 days. Patients are treated with up to 8 cycles of this combination. Approximately one-third of the patients who fail to respond to this treatment regimen, receive more aggressive treatment, such as bone marrow transplant, if they are fit and young, or palliative treatment (Figure 6.6).

6.3.5 Time of Generic/Competition Entry

An entry of a generic drug onto the market has huge implications for demonstrating cost-effectiveness. If the reimbursement strategy is not planned adequately, revenue could be lost. Even with 6 months of patent exclusivity for an agreed price of €50 for a 28-day regimen, an estimated market of 20 million patients in Europe can yield in excess of €6 billion sales. For a drug receiving market authorization on 1 January 2010 and a reimbursement decision made on 1 December 2010 (because activities relating to health economics were delayed until after approval) with a generic entry date of 1 June 2011, about 1 year of potential sales revenue is lost. If the cost of the trial is £50 million and revenue in 1 year is £200 million, the impact of late preparation for reimbursement/ cost-effectiveness activities is not small.

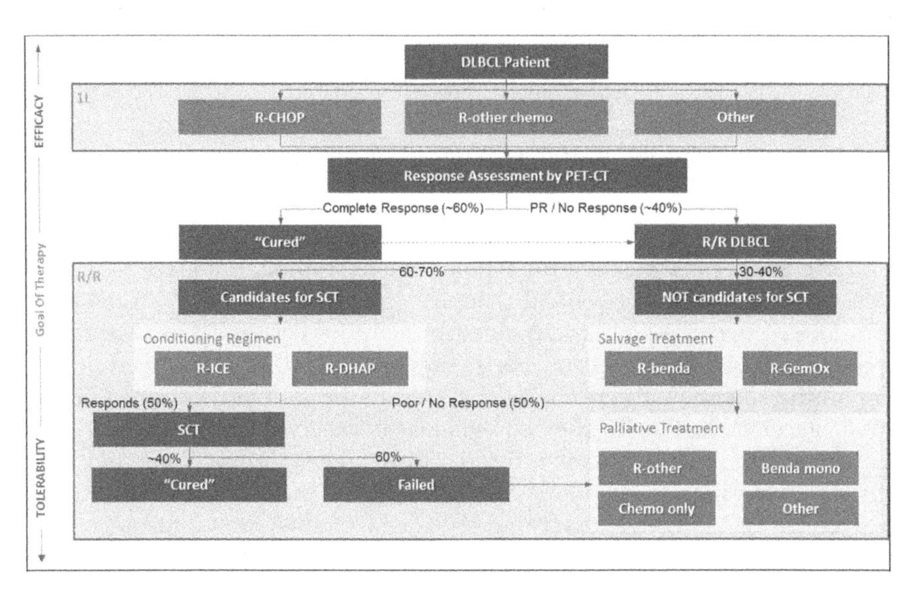

FIGURE 6.6
Example treatment pathway for diffuse large B-cell lymphoma (DLBCL).

6.3.6 Treatment Compliance

Treatment compliance (or lack of) is related to efficacy, safety, and efficiency. Lack of compliance may result in lack of effect, or even safety issues, particularly where the therapeutic window is narrow. Patients who take less medication or drop out of the trial are likely to be the same ones who have had more side effects.

Noncompliance in these patients is likely to result in greater costs. Patients who drop out also tend to be those who are more ill or where there is a lack of effect. Compliance during open label extensions is particularly important for monitoring (Hughes et al., 2001) as it may reflect what is likely to happen in real practice. Clinical trials often report trial results using per protocol population analyses that take into account both protocol deviations and treatment compliance. Only actual dosing needs be considered rather than planned treatment – which can contrast sharply with the ITT definition. In some ITT definitions, efficacy can be based on randomized patients (regardless of whether study medication was taken). Effectiveness should be based on those randomized patients who *took* study medication and therefore differ from usual clinical practice. Treatment compliance is likely to be higher in clinical trials because of the 'Hawthorne effect' as compared to real-life practice.

In some instances, not all the drug is administered and so some is subsequently wasted (sunk cost). For example, some intravenous infusions are very expensive (e.g. the cost of rituximab is $500 per infusion). If only 70% of the dose is used in the infusion, then the actual cost per mg used is $350 on the condition that the remaining 30% are used in another patient.

6.3.7 Identify Subgroups/Heterogeneity

Heterogeneity has been the subject of much interest (Claxton, 2011). It is often found that some (pre-specified) subgroups of patients in a clinical trial demonstrate greater benefit than the whole sample studied. If a large treatment effect is observed in a given subgroup of patients (e.g. those with the presence or absence of a biomarker), the argument for cost-effectiveness can be more forceful in this subgroup. For example, Lee et al. (2012) showed greater OS improvements with erlotinib compared to the standard of care in those lung cancer patients who showed evidence of rash within the first 28 days. There was no improvement in OS and only a modest improvement in PFS in the whole sample. An economic evaluation (Khan et al., 2015) demonstrated a stronger cost-effectiveness/value argument in this subgroup of patients with rash. However, rash is not a pre-randomization stratification variable and care should be taken with such subgroups for selection bias.

Reimbursement agencies (and regulatory agencies) may specifically look for effects/lack of effects in subgroups of patients. For example, in the comparison of lenalidomide with dexamethasone, several subgroups were considered; ICERs were presented for each of these subgroups (NICE HTA 171; ERG Report 2008). It is not uncommon to see a submission to reimbursement agencies where various subgroup analyses have been presented. In Examples 6.1 and 6.2, treatment benefit was highlighted for the chromosome 17p deletion biomarker for treatment with venetoclax (tested for prior-to-treatment initiation) for patients with lymphocytic leukemia (NICE HTA TA487, 2017). Addressing subgroup heterogeneity of treatment benefit is therefore important, not only for reimbursement requirements – but also to identify those subsets of patients who have a higher chance of receiving benefit (and showing cost-effectiveness) with a view to hopefully obtaining a premium price for these groups of patients.

The sources of heterogeneity might present through diagnostic testing, pre-specified genetic subgroups, or even differences in trial results. However, the INMB is unlikely to be >0 for every patient within a subgroup. The health benefits and effects are presented as averages (means), therefore, the INMB will be either higher or lower than the mean for some patients in that subgroup. At best we can say that the chance of an INMB > 0 is higher in the subgroup of patients compared to patients not in the subgroup. Subgroups should be predefined to avoid data dredging resulting in false positives.

6.3.8 Early ICER/INMB

There may be interest in generating an early estimate of the ICER/INMB to determine where the new treatment might fall in the cost-effectiveness plane, possibly using Phase II trial data. However not many Phase II trials collect health resource use data for cost-effectiveness purposes, although critical safety data and secondary endpoint data could be used from Phase II trial data to provide an initial estimate of the ICER. Costs and resource use in a Phase III trial may be different to those of Phase II trials however. For example, dosing may change, some endpoints may be dropped, or the target population to treat may change. The open label extension of a Phase II trial could, however, provide some insight into how patients respond to the new treatment in real-world situations, especially if the target populations between Phase II and III are the same. In Phase II trials, the selected dose may also be the same dose used in a larger Phase III trial; in some cases, it is hard to differentiate a Phase II trial and a Phase III trial, other than the sample size.

6.3.9 Multicenter Trials

One of the realities of clinical trials, particularly large Phase III trials, is that all patients are very rarely found in a single center (and sometimes a single country). For Phase I and small Phase II trials this might be true, but it is not the case for a large Phase III trial or a trial where rare tumor types are treated. Local reimbursement agencies may ask whether patients from their country were represented in the trial; and may raise an eyebrow if in a 10,000-patient multinational Phase III trial, patients from their country were absent. However, for some European countries, it is assumed that treatment effects are generalizable (Willke, Glick, Polsky, & Schulman, 1998).

Although generalizability might be true for clinical effects because the biology and mechanism of action of a treatment should be the same in a homogenous group of patients whether from Italy, Spain, or the UK, this may not be true for costs and other outcomes in an economic evaluation. Differences between costs of GP visits, for example, may just reflect underlying policy and societal differences between the countries. What is of particular interest is whether cost differences between treatments differ between centers (treatment by center interaction). Such interactions are not statistically powered (i.e. sample sizes are not large enough to determine whether cost differences between treatments depend on the country) and there is some concern that cost differences between centers are not being addressed properly in multicenter trials (Grieve, Nixon, Thompson, & Cairns, 2007; Thompson, Nixon, & Grieve, 2006) (Manca, Rice, Sculpher, & Briggs, 2005).

The specific question of an economic analysis in a multicenter trial is how the INMB varies between centers and how best to capture and then interpret this variability. One approach is to address this concern through statistical techniques such as multilevel modeling. The benefit of using a multilevel (or random effects) model is that an estimate of INMB can be generated for each center or country. While this may appear attractive and useful in some cases, several considerations should be noted before a multilevel or random effects approach is considered for multicenter analysis in an economic evaluation:

(i) First, it is assumed that centers are sampled at random and are representative of a population of centers. In practice, centers are selected based on competitive recruitment and other logistical reasons, therefore centers in a clinical trial are unlikely to be random. In some disease areas, we can be almost certain the centers were not selected randomly (e.g. only a handful of specialist centers may offer stereotactic whole brain radiotherapy).

(ii) Second, although modeling does allow for an estimate of the INMB across all centers and addresses the question of whether effects are generalizable across centers, the practical benefits of presenting cost-effectiveness results for each center for reimbursement purposes can be limited (as well as restricting use if only one subgroup is shown to benefit). For example, the UK BNF reports pricing for the UK in general and not by location. However, reporting the CEAC in a multinational trial by taking into account country-specific costs and effects may have some benefit for local reimbursement decision-making. Careful design considerations such as the number of patients within each country and demographic characteristics of each country should be examined so that reasonable values of the INMB and its precision can be estimated.

(iii) Third, a multilevel model or random effects model may not always be necessary. A fixed effects model with a treatment by center interaction will provide a simple yet robust conclusion as to whether the INMB differs between centers, especially when these were not chosen at random. Given the issues raised in (i), generalizability may be less of a concern because the centers in themselves are seldom randomly selected in a clinical trial. Although there is a loss of (statistical) degree of freedom if there are many centers, a loss of power to determine the statistical significance of an interaction may not be of great concern because clinical trials rarely power for cost-effectiveness, let alone interactions for showing cost-effectiveness.

The validity of any assumptions of multilevel models (MLM) needs to be critically evaluated before one can be sure about the conclusions (Grieve et al., 2007). For example, it is assumed that the parameters (e.g. mean costs) are exchangeable (Spiegelhalter & Best, 2003), that is, it is assumed there are no *a priori* reasons why mean costs in one center are higher than in another center, and further it is assumed that the variability of costs is constant between centers. Reasons for differences in INMB could be due to differences in demographics between centers or countries. For example, in a clinical trial where there are more patients with a disease diagnosis in one or two centers compared to the others, then the INMB is likely to be different between centers.

(iv) Multilevel models (MLM) might be valid where the data is clustered or correlated within a center such that the usual OLS estimates are biased and inefficient (Manca et al., 2005). But this can also be remedied using approaches such as weighted least squares or other approaches for the OLS estimates to remain valid so long as the other conditions of the Gauss Markov theorem hold. It has also been suggested that MLMs are more appropriate for determining why resource use (e.g. costs) vary between centers (Grieve, Nixon, Thompson, & Normand, 2005).

Figure 6.7 shows an example of clustered data where the INMB (Y-axis) shows considerable heterogeneity between centers (X-axis) and in particular varies for males and females across the 30 centers. One might expect the INMB across centers (the hospitals where the patients are recruited) to be similar (since there may be no real reason why a new treatment is more or less cost-effective in one center compared to another). In addition, for some sites, the INMB was markedly different between males and females – this might be expected, or again, have occurred by chance. A statistical test for differences in INMB between sites and also a center by gender interaction might (if there is sufficiently large sample size) help identify such differences in the statistical sense. One objective of MLM might therefore be to adjust observed differences in net monetary benefit (NMB) between treatments for the differences due to centers and gender.

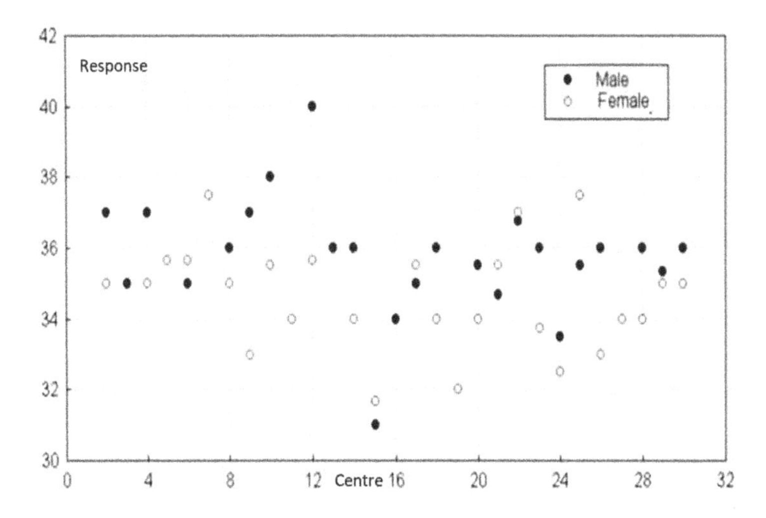

FIGURE 6.7
Clustered data within each center.

6.4 Case Study of Economic Evaluation of Cancer Trials

Table 6.5 compares design issues relevant to cost-effectiveness analyses from two recent cancer trials reported in an HTA (NICE HTA TA516, 2018). In Chapter 9, we will interpret in detail the results from both of these evaluations. For now, we briefly summarize the trial design features.

6.4.1 *TA516 Cabozanitib + Vandetanib*

Two Phase III RCTs of cabozanitib versus Best Supportive Care and vandetanib versus placebo (Table 6.5) were conducted in what appeared to be of good quality trials.

The trial endpoints were well defined (PFS and OS), and assessment time points for measures such as HRQoL were defined. However, HRQoL data were not collected in the trial and external sources were relied on (it is not mandatory for licensing to collect EQ-5D). A complicating feature of this trial was that four different data sets were defined, each varying on the labeling use and/or the specific subpopulation. The comparator was considered to be BSC for the licensing authorities, however for economic evaluation, vandetanib and cabozanitib should have been compared against each other. This had to be done using an indirect comparison, which was inadequate because of differences in the trial populations.

A further, important problem was that the OS was confounded because patients took vandetanib upon progression. This is likely to dampen the size of the effect between vandetanib and BSC for OS. The economic evaluation was based on the list price and not the purchasing discounted price. Hence the reason in the recommendation for discounted prices.

Results show that it is clear that price played a fundamental role in the calculation of the ICER. Even if the costs accruing from adverse events were lower, the ICER is unlikely to fall.

6.5 Summary

In this chapter, we have outlined the reasons for collecting economic data in a clinical trial, highlighting the importance for internal validity of RCTs. We discussed a number of trial designs including the challenges innovative trial design present for cost-effectiveness analysis, particularly during interim analysis. We presented the key trial design components important for cost-effectiveness and then summarized with a case study in the HTA literature. The next step is to discuss how these fit in the context of economic models.

TABLE 6.5

Comparison of Cost-Effectiveness Considerations from 2 Licensed Drugs

Detail of HTA	Cabozanitib + vandetanib TA516
Disease indication	Medullary thyroid cancer
Year	2017
NICE recommendation	**Recommended** *only if the company provides cabozantinib with the discount agreed in the patient-access scheme*
Population	Rare cancer (90 cases in 2014); **Cabozanitib**: progressive, unresectable locally advanced or metastatic medullary thyroid cancer **Vandetanib:** aggressive and symptomatic medullary thyroid cancer unresectable locally advanced or metastatic medullary thyroid cancer
Price	**Cabozanitib**: £4,800 (84 x 20 mg pack) **Vandetanib:** £5,000 (30 x 300 mg pack)
Duration of treatment	Until PD or no further clinical benefit
Comparator	Vandetanib vs. cabozanitib or BSC (including radiotherapy)
Design	Two Phase III trials (parallel group): double-blind RCT Cabozanitib vs. BSC (n = 330) Vandetanib vs. placebo (n = 331)
Sample size	N = 330 (EXAM Trial); 80% power N = 331 (ZETA Trial)
Time horizon	20 years
Multicenter	Yes
Multi-country	Yes (European)
Comparator in trial	BSC
Primary outcome	PFS
Secondary outcomes	OS, ORR, DoR, disease control at 24 weeks, RET mutation status, time to worsening pain
Observed PFS effect	C vs. P: 11.2 vs. 4.0 mo (HR = 0.28) [n = 330] V vs. P: 30.5 vs. 19.3 mo (HR = 0.46) [n = 331]
Target PFS effect	C vs. P: HR = 0.50 V vs. P: TBD/not reported
Observed OS effect	C vs. P: 26.6 vs. 21.1 mo (HR = 0.85) [n = 330] V vs. P: 28.0 vs. 16.4 mo (HR = 0.99)
Subgroups	Yes, Biomarker RET +ve showed improvements in PFS and OS
Target OS effect	C vs. P: HR = 0.67 V vs. P: NR
PPS	Not identified
Utility [ERG utility]	FACT-G mapped to EQ-5D, no utility recorded in trial Pre-progression: 0.84 [0.8] Post-progression: 0.64 [0.54] Decrements of –0.11 for adverse events
Incremental cost	C vs. P: £72,734 V vs. P: £79,745
Incremental QALY	C vs. P: 0.48 V vs. P: 0.23

(Continued)

TABLE 6.5 (CONTINUED)

Comparison of Cost-Effectiveness Considerations from 2 Licensed Drugs

Detail of HTA	Cabozanitib + vandetanib TA516
HRQoL	No overall improvement in HRQoL based on a condition-specific measure (FACT-G)
ICER[a]	C vs. P: £150,874 V vs. P: £352,508
Other ICER	Range from £66,779 to £195,593, depending on data set
Mean survival time	The mean survival time and its standard error were underestimated because the largest observation was censored and the estimation was restricted to the largest event time
ERG main concerns	
Subsequent therapy confounding/ crossover	Confounding of OS due to subsequent treatments occurred; vandetanib was not compared to placebo but some other treatment including vandetanib itself Patients in the placebo arm who discontinued randomized treatment were unblinded and given the option to take open label vandetanib Rank-preserving structural failure time (RPSFT) approach reported to be unsuccessful in disentangling crossover effect
Modeling	Partitioned survival approach based on a partitioned survival structure implemented using the discretely integrated condition event (DICE) approach
Extrapolation	it was not possible to fit a parametric regression model to the observed KM data; due to relatively sparse data in the restricted population as producing KM curves with long steps would lead to inaccurate estimates of the median survival function when extrapolated for the economic model
Evidence synthesis	Currently, there is one Phase III trial supporting the use of vandetanib according to the EU label. Therefore, it is not possible to undertake a meta-analysis at this time. No direct comparison of V vs. C NICE has identified cabozantinib as a comparator in this appraisal, as part of this submission, however Sanofi Genzyme have not undertaken any indirect or mixed treatment comparisons for this treatment for two main reasons. Mixed treatment comparison uncertain due to differences in populations
Overall	No improvement in OS Improvement in PFS No improvement in HRQoL Time-to-pain worsening improved OS confounded by subsequent therapy Cost-effective

[a] *Notes:* ICER based on modeling; V: vandetanib; C: cabozantinib.

6.6 Exercises for Chapter 6

1. Compare and contrast the different types of adaptive trial designs and their implications for cost-effectiveness analyses.
2. Design a clinical trial for cost-effectiveness in any cancer trial. What important issues should you consider?
3. What is the difference between a retrospective and prospective economic evaluation?
4. Distinguish between a multicenter trial and a trial conducted in several countries. What are the challenges one might encounter in an economic evaluation from such trials?

7

Models for Economic Evaluation of Cancer

7.1 Types of Health Economic Models

Economic evaluation of cancer drugs is often conducted using special modeling techniques that are of two kinds: mathematical simulation or statistical (or stochastic, which refers to analyzing patient-level data). A health economic model can take on several forms. Table 7.1 shows the common models that have been used for HTAs of in the UK. We shall introduce some of these models in brief and discuss the more ubiquitous ones at some length. What is noticeable from Table 7.1 is that a type of statistical model called a 'partitioned survival model' is more common for the economic evaluation of cancer drugs. This chapter is more about understanding the key concepts around these models rather than expecting the reader to 'build' models, although it should provide some direction on how to approach the problem. Interested readers on building such models may consult references such as Drummond et al. (2015), Khan (2015), and Gray (2011) others.

7.2 Decision Tree Models

Decision trees are adequate for a decision at one specific point in time and are mathematical constructs. Although less useful for economic evaluation of cancer treatments for deriving cost per QALY from survival outcomes, they have been used for management of cancer; for example, to determine whether the use of 2-fluoro-2-deoxyglucose positron emission tomography (FDG-PET) in addition (Kenneth et al., 2001) to computed (axial) tomography (CT) is helpful in managing recurrent colorectal cancer (CRC). A decision tree set-up is described in Figure 7.1.

The objective of the decision tree model in Figure 7.1 was to compare the cost-effectiveness of FDG-PET (experimental) with CT alone (standard of care) in the management of patients with recurrent CRC. The squares are decision nodes; circles are chance nodes; and triangles terminal nodes.

TABLE 7.1

Health Economic Models used in Non-Small-Cell Lung Cancer

HTA body	Indication	Status	Comparator	Analysis Type	Model Design	No. of States	Disease Progression Criteria	Time Horizon	Cycle	Survival Analysis	Drug
pCODR 2013 (pCODR, 2013a)	1L EGFRm+	Accepted	Pemetrexed/ cisplatin Gefitinib Erlotinib	CEM (QALY and life-years)	Partitioned survival model	3 states: PFS; PD; death	RECIST	10 years	Not reported	Kaplan-Meier data used up to month 16 Extrapolation of the data not detailed	Afatinib
TA310 (NICE, 2014b)	1L EGFRm+ (TKI-naïve)	Accepted	Gefitinib Erlotinib	CUA (ERG have later recommended CMA)	Partitioned survival model	3 states: PFS; PD; death	RECIST	Lifetime (10 years)	1 month (half cycle)	Kaplan-Meier data used up to month 16 Extrapolated using standard parametric survival models	Afatinib
920/13 (SMC, 2014)	1L EGFRm+ (TKI-naïve)	Accepted	Erlotinib	CMA	–	–	RECIST	1 year	Per day	–	Afatinib
07-2013 (PBAC, 2013)	1L EGFRm+	Accepted	Gefitinib Erlotinib Cisplatin/ gemcitabine	CMA and CUA	Partitioned survival model	3 states: PFS; PD; death	RECIST	5 years	–	Kaplan-Meier data for 22 months extrapolated to 10 years	Afatinib
TA296 (NICE, 2013)	2L ALK+	Rejected	BSC Docetaxel (pooled chemotherapy)	CUA	Semi-Markov (using AUC)	3 state: PFS, PD, death	RECIST	Life time (15 years)	30 days (half cycle)	OS and PFS extrapolated from the clinical trials using standard parametric survival analysis and using hazard ratios	Crizotinib

(*Continued*)

TABLE 7.1 (CONTINUED)

Health Economic Models used in Non-Small-Cell Lung Cancer

HTA body	Indication	Status	Comparator	Analysis Type	Model Design	No. of States	Disease Progression Criteria	Time Horizon	Cycle	Survival Analysis	Drug
865/13 (SMC, 2013)	2L ALK+	Accepted	BSC Docetaxel (pooled chemotherapy)	CUA	Markov	3 state: PFS, PD, death	RECIST	Life time (15 years)	–	Standard parametric survival analysis used to extrapolate beyond trial data (including one single arm trial)	Crizotinib
pCODR 2013 (pCODR, 2013b)	2L ALK+	Accepted (resubmission)	Crizotinib/ pemetrexed/ docetaxel vs. gemcitabine/ platinum agent/ pemetrexed/ erlotinib	CEM (QALY and life-years)	–	–	RECIST	Lifetime (5 years)	–	Standard parametric survival analysis used to extrapolate beyond trial data	Crizotinib
TA258 (NICE, 2012)	1L EGFRm+	Accepted	Gefitinib	CUA	Semi-Markov model (partitioned survival model [PFS])	3 state: PFS, PD, death	RECIST	10 years	Per month	Kaplan-Meier data used up to month 16. Standard parametric survival analysis used to extrapolate beyond trial data	Erlotinib
TA162 (NICE, 2008)	2L	Accepted with restriction (revision of TA162 + TA175 is under development [ID620])	Docetaxel	CUA	Markov (Partitioned survival model)	3 state: PFS, PD, death	RECIST	2 years	Per month	No extrapolation	Erlotinib

(Continued)

TABLE 7.1 (CONTINUED)

Health Economic Models used in Non-Small-Cell Lung Cancer

HTA body	Indication	Status	Comparator	Analysis Type	Model Design	No. of States	Disease Progression Criteria	Time Horizon	Cycle	Survival Analysis	Drug
TA227 (NICE, 2011)	MTx (platinum-based first-line chemotherapy)	Rejected	BSC (ITT; stable disease) Pemetrexed (non-squamous)	CUA	Partitioned survival model	3 state: PFS; PD; death Subgroups defined by response	RECIST	Lifetime (5 years)	1 month (half cycle)	Standard parametric survival analysis used to extrapolate beyond trial data	Erlotinib
749/11 (SMC, 2012)	1L EGFRm+	Accepted	Pemetrexed/ cisplatin	CUA	Semi-Markov model	3 state: PFS, PD, death	–	–	–	Standard parametric survival analysis used to extrapolate beyond trial data	Erlotinib
220/05 (SMC, 2006)	2L	Rejected	Docetaxel	CUA	–	–	–	–	–	–	Erlotinib
	2L	Accepted (resubmission 2006)	Docetaxel	CUA	–	–	–	–	–	–	Erlotinib
S0037 (CADTH, 2005)	2L, EGFRm+ or unknown	Accepted	Docetaxel	CEM (cost per life-year)	–	–	–	–	–	–	Erlotinib
1066/2005 (TLV, 2008)	EGFR+	Accepted	Docetaxel	–	–	–	–	–	–	–	Erlotinib
07-2013 (PBAC, 2013)	1L EGFRm+	Accepted (resubmission)	Cisplatin and gemcitabine Gefitinib	CUA	Markov	3 state: PFS, PD, death	RECIST	5 years	Month	Constant hazard from months 1–3 and then from month 3 onward	Erlotinib
TA192 (NICE, 2010b)	1L EGFRm+	Accepted	Gemcitabine/ carboplatin Paclitaxel/ carboplatin Vinorelbine/ cisplatin Gemcitabine/ cisplatin	CUA	Markov (partitioned survival model)	4 states: TR, SD, PD, death	RECIST	Lifetime (5 years)	21 days	Standard parametric survival analysis was used to extrapolate beyond trial data	Gefitinib

(Continued)

TABLE 7.1 (CONTINUED)

Health Economic Models used in Non-Small-Cell Lung Cancer

HTA body	Indication	Status	Comparator	Analysis Type	Model Design	No. of States	Disease Progression Criteria	Time Horizon	Cycle	Survival Analysis	Drug
615/10 (SMC, 2010b)	1L	Rejected	Gemcitabine/carboplatin Gemcitabine/cisplatin Paclitaxel/carboplatin Vinorelbine/cisplatin Pemetrexed/cisplatin	CUA	Markov (using survival models)	4 states: TR, SD, PD, death	–	5 years	21 days	Standard parametric survival analysis was used to extrapolate beyond trial data	Gefitinib
07-2013 (PBAC, 2013)	1L	Accepted	Gemcitabine/carboplatin	CUA	–	–	–	5 years	–	Extrapolated (17 months median in trial)	Gefitinib
S0003 (CADTH, 2004)	2L	Accepted	Gemcitabine/cisplatin Paclitaxel/carboplatin	–	–	–	–	–	–	–	Gefitinib
TA181 (NICE, 2009)	1L	Accepted	Gemcitabine/cisplatin	CUA	Markov (treatment sequencing)	4 states: response, stable, PD, death	RECIST	Lifetime (6 years)	21 days (half cycle)	30-month trial data converted to constant probabilities	Pemetrexed
TA124 (NICE, 2007)	2L	Rejected	BSC	CUA	Markov (treatment sequencing)	4 states (plus AE sub-states): response; stable; PD; death	–	Lifetime (3 years)	21 days	Constant transition probabilities	Pemetrexed

(Continued)

TABLE 7.1 (CONTINUED)

Health Economic Models used in Non-Small-Cell Lung Cancer

HTA body	Indication	Status	Comparator	Analysis Type	Model Design	No. of States	Disease Progression Criteria	Time Horizon	Cycle	Survival Analysis	Drug
TA190 (NICE, 2010a)	MTx (following other treatment)	Accepted	BSC	CUA	Trial based + survival model (OS AUC)	4 states: pre-progression (based on treatment cycles); PD; terminal; death (OS)	RECIST	Lifetime (6 years)	21 days (half cycle)	Empirical data for 29 months; extrapolated using exponential and Weibull remainder 43 months	Pemetrexed
TA309 (NICE, 2014a)	MTx (following the same treatment)	Rejected	BSC	CUA	Markov (based on PFS and OS AUC)	3 states: pre-progression; post-progression; death	RECIST	Lifetime (15.99 years)	21 days (half cycle)	A survival hazard model to extrapolate beyond the trial (exponential, Weibull, log-logistic, log-normal, Gompertz and gamma)	Pemetrexed
531/09 (SMC 2010a)	1L	Rejected	Gemcitabine/ cisplatin	CUA	Markov	3 states: TR, SD, PD	–	Lifetime (6 years)	–	–	Pemetrexed
	1L	Rejected (resubmission 2009)	Gemcitabine/ cisplatin Gemcitabine/ carboplatin Docetaxel/ cisplatin	CUA	Markov	3 states: TR, SD, PD	–	Lifetime	–	–	Pemetrexed
	1L	Accepted (resubmission 2010)	Gemcitabine/ carboplatin Gemcitabine/ cisplatin.	CUA	–	3 states: TR, SD, PD	RECIST	Lifetime (6 years)	–	A survival hazard model to extrapolate beyond the 29-month trial	Pemetrexed

(Continued)

TABLE 7.1 (CONTINUED)

Health Economic Models used in Non-Small-Cell Lung Cancer

HTA body	Indication	Status	Comparator	Analysis Type	Model Design	No. of States	Disease Progression Criteria	Time Horizon	Cycle	Survival Analysis	Drug
342/07 (SMC 2008)	2L	Rejected	Docetaxel	CUA	Markov	–	–	3 years	21 days	–	Pemetrexed
	2L	Rejected (resubmission 2008)	BSC	CUA	Markov	–	–	–	–	–	Pemetrexed
	2L	Accepted (resubmission 2008)	Docetaxel	CUA	Markov	4 states: TR, SD, PD, death	–	3 years	21 days	–	Pemetrexed
PBAC 2010 03-2010 (PBAC, 2010)	1L	Rejected	Gemcitabine/ cisplatin	CUA	–	–	–	–	–	–	Pemetrexed
pCODR 2013 (pCODR, 2013c)	2L	Accepted	BSC or placebo	CUA	–	–	–	9 years	21 days	–	Pemetrexed

Notes: AUC: area under the curve; BSC: best supportive care, CEM: cost-effectiveness analysis, CMA: cost-minimization analysis, CUA: cost-utility analysis;

DSA: deterministic sensitivity analysis; SA: sensitivity analysis; PSA: probabilistic sensitivity analysis;

NICE: National Institute for Health and Care Excellence; SMC: Scottish Medicines Consortium; PBAC: Pharmaceutical Benefits Advisory Committee; pCODR: pan-Canadian Oncology Drug Review; TLV: Dental and Pharmaceutical Benefits Agency; CADTH: Canadian Agency for Drugs and Technologies in Health;

MTx: maintenance treatment; OS: overall survival; PD: progressive disease; QALY: Quality-adjusted life-year; RECIST: Response Evaluation Criteria in Solid Tumors; SD: stable disease; TR: treatment response;

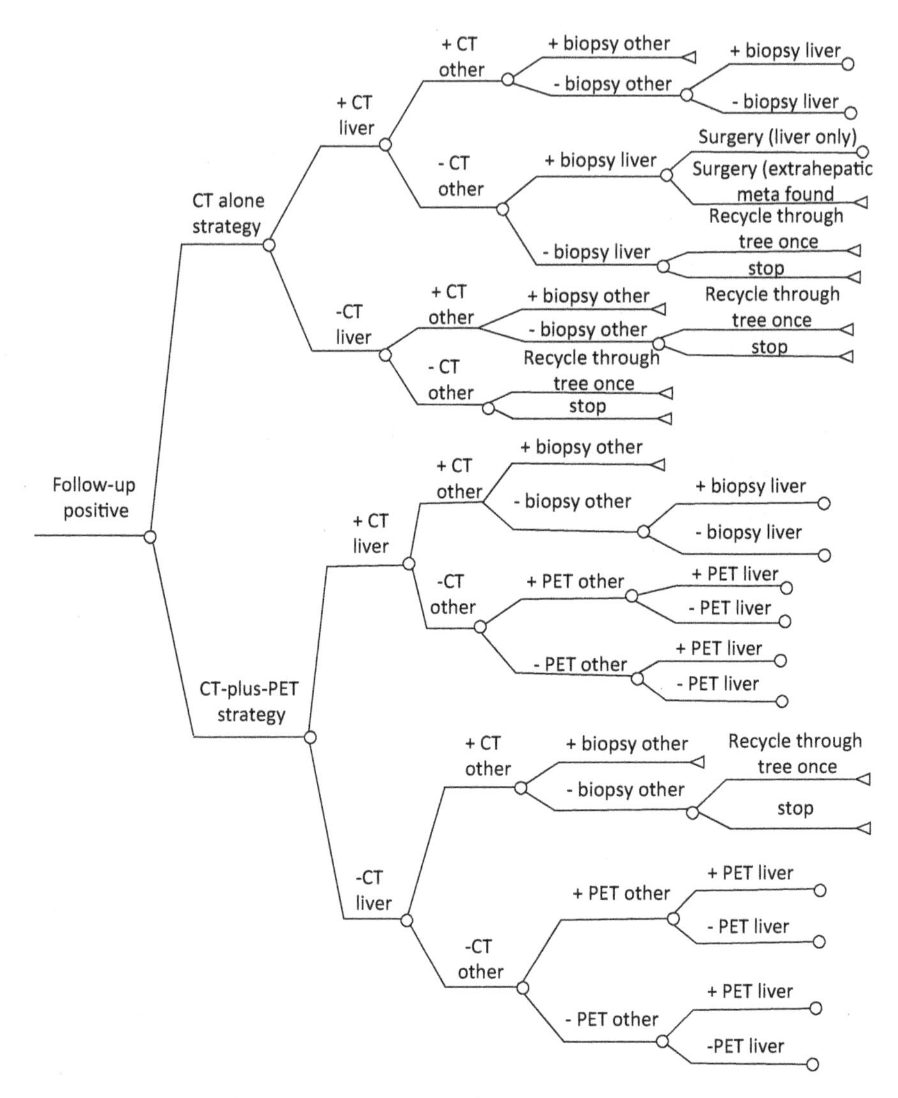

FIGURE 7.1
Example of a decision tree.

Source: Kenneth et al., 2001.

At each branch, the chance of patients in each subsequent 'group' ('recurrent in liver,' 'other part of the body,' and 'no recurrence') is determined from literature. Costs and effects (life expectancy, surgery) are also determined from literature. These are then used to determine the incremental costs and effects of FDG-PET versus CT alone. In this example, all inputs were from literature. However, one may also build a decision tree model using data from a clinical trial as inputs, to determine the expected costs and effects (determined by multiplying the probabilities at each branch with the costs associated with each branch). The expected life expectancy and the expected cost of care associated with each strategy are determined by multiplying the probabilities of certain events (e.g. recurrence) by the life expectancy and costs. For example, if the mean cost of surgery is £3,000 and the probability of recurrence is 0.20, then the expected cost is £600.

Example 7.1: Costs and Effects of Treating Side Effects of Chemotherapy

Take as another example the need to treat a patient for a single infectious episode with a given antibiotic. If one is concerned about the possibility of, say, permanent hearing loss (a rare side effect of chemotherapy), this simple decision can be decomposed into its constituent parts:

- The treatment alternatives (aminoglycoside vs. another antibiotic)
- The consequences (permanent hearing loss or no hearing loss)
- The probability of hearing loss

The percentage of patients with permanent hearing loss as a side effect is estimated to be between 20% and 60% with an average of 40% (Table 7.2). There are only two possible outcomes (health states): it is either present (hearing loss is valued as 1) or not (no hearing loss valued as 0). Based on this simple example we will introduce some further basic concepts.

All patients are in the same initial health state (no hearing loss) and can move (transit) only to permanent hearing loss or stay in their initial health state. The average possibility of a transition is expressed as a probability (between 0 and 1). Each outcome has been assigned a value (a pay-off). To formally choose between the two alternatives we then calculate the expectation (in its mathematical sense) of each outcome. That is the value of the outcome in question multiplied by its probability of occurrence (its incidence in this case) and we then sum these for all outcomes. So the expected pay-off of aminoglycoside treatment is equal to $(1 \times 0.40) + (0 \times 0.60) = 0.40$ and otherwise equals $(1 \times 0.10) + (0 \times 0.90) = 0.10$. We then choose the option with the minimum expected loss as a basis for deciding the antibiotic.

TABLE 7.2

Decision Table for Example 7.1

	Outcome Probability		Outcome Valuation		Expected Pay-Off
Decision	Permanent hearing loss	No hearing loss	Permanent hearing loss	No hearing loss	
Aminoglycoside	0.40	0.60	1	0	0.40
Alternative antibiotic	0.10	0.90	1	0	0.10

7.2.1 Further Possible Improvements to the Decision Model

- Valuation of the Outcomes

Instead of using a 0 or 1 (absence/presence) we could have given a score for the hearing loss state say (0 and 100) (the higher the score the worse the hearing loss). We could also give the hearing loss a subjective HRQoL value either as a score or as a utility loss, in this case by interviewing patients with existing hearing loss or those who lost their hearing after the treatment. Assume that no hearing loss is anchored at 0 and hearing loss is evaluated at a mean of 0.50 utilities (on a utility scale of 0 to 1). If we had chosen to value the outcomes as utility gains we could simply change the sign of the utility score (0 gain if no loss, –0.50 if loss) and choose the option with the highest expected outcome; or also give a score of 1 to no loss and a score of (1 – 0.50) = 0.50 to hearing loss. This is what is commonly done in cost-effectiveness analysis where patients are in some health state at the time of the decision with some (average) utility value attached to it (either 1 or some lower value depending on their starting health state). For example, cancer patients who have been diagnosed shortly before starting treatment would have a utility score below that of the general population of the same age and gender because of the psychological impact of the diagnosis; for some other patients it may be due to the presence of symptoms.

- Introducing More Health States

We now assume that hearing loss can be either complete or only partial, so we have three health states: 'partial loss,' 'complete loss,' 'no loss.' For each of these we will have corresponding probabilities. To even further refine the model, we could also introduce a difference between temporary hearing loss and permanent hearing loss. By now we are realizing that by adding more and more states, the decision tree will start to yield more branches and get more complex. If we were now to introduce another adverse side effect of the treatment like diarrhea (none, mild, severe) we would end up with 6 × 3 = 18 outcome states in each arm. This is sometimes called the 'outcomes curse' as it rapidly leads to an exponential explosion of health states to account for and is typical of all 'state transition' models.

- Probability Distributions

Instead of using a single fixed (average) probability of some event, one could use values from a distribution of probabilities. For example, if the hearing loss probability is between 0.20 and 0.60 (depending on the published literature) we could use a uniform distribution (a distribution that assumes an equal probability across possible values, as for example in the roll of a dice where the chance is 1/6 for each possible outcome) of all possible values between 0.20 and 0.60 instead. The mean of a uniform distribution for some range (a, b)

is $(a + b)/2$, which in this case is 0.40 (0.6 + 0.2/2). Alternatively, one could simulate from some given values (e.g. simulate from a distribution with a probability of 0.40). Inevitably, for each simulated probability, we would need to compute our expected costs and effects repeatedly. However, this has now replaced a fixed value with a random element and introduced uncertainty (rather than assuming a fixed value). It would be rare to believe the true probability of hearing loss can only be 0.40. There are likely to be several ways to introduce uncertainty by using different assumptions around the probability of distributions (see also Chapter 9 on uncertainty). The same is true about other estimates (mean costs, mean life-years). A caveat is that care should be taken when simulating or using probabilities such that their values sum to 1.

- Extending the Time Horizon of the Consequences (Outcomes)

In a decision tree, events unfold over time in some implicit way, from the initial decision node to the outcomes of interest. The period (of time) over which events happen and the way consequences are assessed are not explicitly defined in such models. For example, in the above scenario, we could use a 7-day antibiotic therapy period (the model used just states antibiotic use, but usually such drugs are taken as a course of treatment). Similarly, the outcome duration is undefined, i.e. hearing loss is permanent over a patient's remaining lifetime. It is up to the analyst to specify the time frame. For example, extending the duration of antibiotic therapy to 10 days instead of 7 would likely impact the cost of therapy, but also the adverse event probabilities and possibly their severity. If we were to define the outcome in QALYs then we would also need to specify the time horizon over which these are calculated (for the next 5 years, 10 years, lifelong).

- Time-Dependent Parameters

Once we consider longer time periods, i.e. extend the time horizon, most clinical and HRQoL parameters and costs will vary over time. For example, the incidence of post-surgery complications is highest in the first few days, or first weeks, after surgery, and then wanes over time. The same can be said about other treatments such as radiotherapy or chemotherapy. A decision tree approach accumulates these incidences over its implicit time horizon. For example, if we observe a scar infection incidence or wound dehiscence of 5% in the first month and this falls to 2% in month 2, and 1% in month 3, we could use a 3-month time horizon and consider using an adverse event probability of 8%. However, we would need to adjust all parameters and rerun the model for different periods if we change the time horizon. Hence, it would be better to construct a model that takes into account the time component.

- Repeating Treatments/Events

Many clinical situations involve several repeating episodes like those typically observed in migraine attacks, asthma, and other conditions. These are treated in a sequential (step-up or step-down) fashion with a mix of different interventions. This is typically the case in oncology where patients are usually treated many times (therapy cycles) with the same treatment combination and go through different combinations of treatments (surgery, radiotherapy, chemo- or immunotherapy, and combinations of these) over several different lines of therapy (generally from 1 to 7 and sometimes more) and over time. This therefore calls for a modeling approach where time is explicitly modeled.

7.3 Markov Models

A Markov model is an alternative approach to using decision tree models in tackling some of the above problems (more states, time dependency, etc.). It can be thought of as a recurrent number of decision trees over time. In Markov models, time is divided into separate, fixed, discrete time periods (weeks, months, years). In each time period, patients can 'move' or transit from varying health states. There can be a large number of health states. In oncology, there are usually three health states: alive and progression-free, progressive disease, and death. Patients enter the model in the alive and progression-free health state. Figure 7.2 shows such a model. Once death has been reached (an absorption state), the patients remain there. Patients may 'transit' between the other two states.

All patients are considered to start in a similar health state (alive and progression-free). Patients can move between health states over time, at discrete

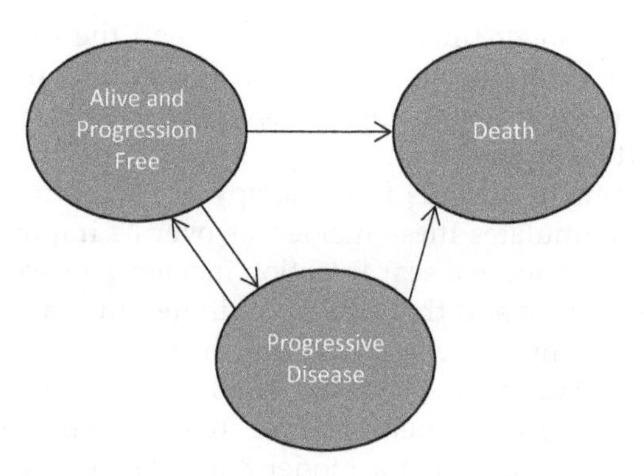

FIGURE 7.2
A 3 state Markov model for cancer.

time points (e.g. by week, month, year). The transition matrix is essentially a table of probabilities describing the chance of moving from one health state to another at a given time point. An elementary example of a transition matrix (see Chapter 4) would in fact be a survival curve where only two transitions are allowed: from 'alive to alive' and from 'alive to death' – two health states. In cancer trials, movements between health states is described by a transition matrix similar to that shown in Table 7.3.

In Table 7.4, all patients start in the same health state and are considered similar (homogeneity assumption) in time period zero (t_0). In the next period t_1 they could have progressed (e.g. after month-1 follow-up) or have died without progression. Each time period, t_i, corresponds to a new state of the system, i.e. a new distribution of the patients across the different health states.

At the first time point 1 (t_1), we see that 25 patients have progressed and 5 died (t_1 could be days, months, years, or any sensible discrete division of time). Using days for time increments would require more calculations for patients living years; using time increments of years for patients who live only a few months would be not be sensible either. All the deaths originated from the alive state in that period. The patients at risk in time 1 number

TABLE 7.3

Example of Probability Transition Matrix

From/to	Alive PF	Progression	Death
Alive PF	0.70	0.25	0.05
Progression	0	0.85	0.15
Death	0	0	1

TABLE 7.4

Example of Markov Chain Calculation for a Given Treatment Group (e.g. Control Arm)

Time (t_i)	Alive Stable	Progression	Death	Total Deaths	Total Probability
0.00	100.00	0.00	0.00	0.00	100.00
1.00	70.00	25.00	5.00	5.00	100.00
2.00	49.00	38.75	7.25	12.25	100.00
3.00	34.30	45.19	8.26	20.51	100.00
4.00	24.01	46.98	8.49	29.01	100.00
5.00	16.81	45.94	8.25	37.25	100.00
6.00	11.76	43.25	7.73	44.99	100.00
7.00	8.24	39.70	7.08	52.06	100.00
8.00	5.76	35.81	6.37	58.43	100.00
9.00	4.04	31.88	5.66	64.09	100.00
10.00	2.82	28.10	4.98	69.07	100.00

70 alive with stable disease and 25 in progression. At the start of period 2, from these 70, 49 (70 × 0.7) were still in stable condition, but 17.5 (70 × 0.25) had progressed and 3.5 (70 × 0.05) had died. Of those in progression 21.25 (25*0.85) were still in progression and 3.75 (25*0.15) had died after progression. We therefore end up in that period with 49 stable, 38.75 (21.25 + 17.5) in progression and 7.25 (3.5 + 3.75) dead patients, to which we have to add the previous deaths (5) to account for all the 100 patients, and so on.

- Different Starting Health States

To improve the above, where we assume all patients start in the same health state, we could assume that some patients enter the model in differing health states (any other state, except death), so long as we assume that their transitions are similar. We could therefore start with a mix of stable and progressed patients for example, with the progressed patients following their own transition trajectory from time 0 onward. We leave this as an exercise for the diligent reader (Table 7.5).

- Time Varying Transition Probabilities

The above are examples of Markov chains because:

(a) The transition probabilities do not vary over time but are fixed (constant) for all periods.
(b) The distribution between the different states at time period t depends only on the number present at the previous time period, t–1. So, the process has no memory.

TABLE 7.5

Markov Chain for Patients with Different Starting States

Time (t_i)	Alive Stable	Progression	Death	Total Deaths	Control All
0.00	80.00	20.00	0.00	0.00	100.00
1.00	56.00	37.00	7.00	7.00	100.00
2.00	39.20	45.45	8.35	15.35	100.00
3.00	27.44	48.43	8.78	24.13	100.00
4.00	19.21	48.03	8.64	32.76	100.00
5.00	13.45	45.63	8.16	40.93	100.00
6.00	9.41	42.14	7.52	48.45	100.00
7.00	6.59	38.17	6.79	55.24	100.00
8.00	4.61	34.10	6.06	61.29	100.00
9.00	3.23	30.13	5.34	66.64	100.00
10.00	2.26	26.42	4.68	71.32	100.00

One can allow probabilities to vary with time either by creating a set of transition matrices for different periods or by introducing a time-related equation for all or some probabilities, linking probabilities and the period. Care should be taken again to satisfy the summation of the probabilities to 1.

- Relaxing the 'No Memory' Assumption

Often in cancer treatments there appears to be a relation to past events. For example, an occurrence of febrile neutropenia in earlier cycles is likely to result in occurrence(s) at later cycles. The same can be said for many other treatment-related adverse events (AE). Resistance or progression observed in previous chemotherapy treatments may decrease the efficacy of subsequent treatment lines, including the same drug or drug family. Cross-resistance of drug A that induces resistance to drug B should also be acknowledged. A well-known effect is also the increased probability of AEs in relation to the number of chemotherapy cycles or increasing cumulative radiotherapy dose. This means that most toxicity-related probabilities will not only increase with average dosage, but also increase over time (or over cycles of treatment).

These therapeutic aspects can be dealt with, at least partially, by making the probabilities dependent on, for example, the total previous number of time periods or treatment cycles; or, as an alternative, dependent on the time spent in a given state following the cumulative dose received, by tracking these during the model simulation process and adjusting the transition probabilities accordingly. These models are sometimes called semi-Markov models.

- Reducing the Time Interval and Using Different Time Intervals in the Same Model

In reality, time is continuous; the shorter the discrete time intervals, the more closely they resemble continuous time. To reduce the approximation error with large intervals, one needs to apply a half-cycle correction (HCCor) or another type of continuity correction in state transition models. The standard HCCor consists of adding half a cycle of the state membership at the beginning of the first cycle and subtracting half a cycle of the membership at the end of the last cycle. There is some debate about the accuracy of the HCCor, leading to the recommendation to use the cycle-tree HCCor, which calculates state membership as the average of state membership at the beginning and end of each cycle (for further details see Mahony (2015); Elbasha (2016). It is also possible to construct a Markov chain with different time intervals, for example, a short one for the treatment phase (say monthly or weekly) and a longer one post-therapy (Chattwal, 2016). In the next section we can observe the impact of discrete cycle times on the expected survival time. More on the different simulation modeling approaches can be found in Petrou and Gray (2011a).

7.4 Continuous Time Markov Models

Reducing the time interval in a discrete Markov chain leads to a continuous Markov chain model. That is, the time interval t, t+1 (e.g. month 1, month 2) can become smaller (week 1, week 2, or day 1, day 2). As the interval gets smaller, the discrete Markov model with the time to a transition (e.g. from progressive disease to death) follows a (continuous) exponential distribution with rate $\lambda(t)$. This approach might be used for modeling disease transmission through infections because the health state of another person might change at any time due to infection. In cancer, however, health states are likely to be reported at discrete intervals. Although death can occur at any continuous time, the transition from progression until death will not be continuous because progressive disease is determined through scans at discrete time intervals (e.g. every three months). Time, therefore, progresses at fixed intervals (e.g. yearly or monthly cycles) whereas in continuous models, transitions do not have to occur at say the beginning or end of a cycle. Cost-effectiveness is therefore not influenced by the cycle length (and so applying corrections, such as the half-cycle correction as noted above, is not required). We can demonstrate the difference between a continuous and discrete Markov model in Example 7.2

Example 7.2: Discrete and Continuous Markov Models

Let us assume there are only two health states, alive and dead. Alive is the starting position of the Markov chain (obviously!). The transition to death is assumed to occur at a constant rate λ. This means that the time to the event of death follows an exponential distribution $\exp(-\lambda t)$. The average time to death is $1/\lambda$.

Let $\lambda = 0.1$, $t = 1$ year, and the cycle length varies according to the form $1/2k$ (k takes on discrete values from 0 to 6). Hence, the transition probability (transition from alive to dead) is: $P_{10} = 1 - \exp(-0.1 \times 1) = 0.0952$ (here 1 is the cycle length, or $k = 0$ in the expression $1/2k$). The expected mean time to death based on the continuous distribution is $1/\lambda = 1/0.1 = 10$. Based on a discrete form, the expected time to death is determined as $1/P_{10} \times (1/2k)$. Hence for $k = 1$, this is $1/0.0952 = 10.51$. The expected mean time to death is biased upward. As the cycle length becomes smaller, say $k = 6$ (the larger the value of k, the smaller the cycle length and the more it appears to be continuous), such that $1/2k = 0.015625$, $P_{10} = 1 - \exp(-0.1 \times 0.015625) = 0.9984$. Hence, the expected time to death in a much smaller cycle length is: $1/(1 - 0.9984)*0.015625$, which approximates to 10 (in fact 10.01), and has a much smaller bias.

Few continuous semi-Markov models have been applied in cancer treatment, although some have been applied in cancer-screening applications (Graham et al., 2014; Hettle et al., 2015; Rivera et al., 2017; Anderson, D.F., & Kurtz, T. 2015). For this reason, we turn to the most common models used in economic evaluation, specifically, using Markov modeling with individual patient data from clinical trials.

7.5 The Partitioned Survival Model

A common question is what would be the use of building a mathematical simulation model (like those above) if we have already conducted a trial and have access to the individual patient level data? This situation is the most common, where an RCT has been conducted, and a cost-effectiveness analysis is required using the available patient-level data. In contrast to using data from a reported trial where summary statistics (mean costs, mean effects, or proportions), available patient-level data eliminates the need to simulate. However, simulation for assessment of uncertainty is still required.

Using patient-level (Markov-type) micro-simulation also allows for greater patient heterogeneity, reflecting the original trial data better (having statistical summaries such as mean values does not tell us the relationship between these statistics and factors such as age, gender, etc.). This could lead to a better understanding of the uncertainty in specific subgroups (e.g. older patients might have larger effects, or where there are only a few patients in this subgroup).

Despite the advantages of using patient-level data, evidence from a single trial is seldom enough (except in rare or 'ultra-orphan' indications). Hence, for health policy purposes it is usually preferable (and requested by reimbursement agencies) to include all available evidence beyond a single trial. Here a 'de novo' model construction would probably be warranted where patient-level trial data and published reported data might be synthesized to provide inputs for the economic model.

7.5.1 Developing an Economic Model Using Patient-Level Data Using a Partitioned Survival Model Approach

An economic model using data from a cancer trials consist of two parts:

(a) Modeling the efficacy data (survival data)
(b) Modeling the cost and utility data

7.5.1.1 Modeling the efficacy data (survival data)

The total survival experience is divided into progression-free survival (PFS) and post-progression survival (PPS). PFS is computed from the time from randomization (or first dose received) until progression or death (whichever occurs first). Overall survival (OS) is computed from the time from randomization (or first dose of treatment) until death. In clinical trials, patients are not always followed until death (it might be impractical or too expensive to do so). Consequently, the PFS is modeled along with OS and future (extrapolated) survival proportions for each of PFS and OS are estimated. Survival proportions over time are typically represented as a Kaplan-Meier curve that plots the proportion of patients alive, died, or progressed (depending on the outcome) over time. In general, the mean survival time is represented as:

$$\mathbf{OS} = \mathbf{PFS} + \mathbf{PPS} \tag{7.1}$$

In general, the approach to modeling is as follows:

(i) Plot the KM curve for each treatment group for each of OS and PFS.
(ii) Extrapolate these survival times to generate mean OS and PFS. Hence, derive PPS by subtraction (OS minus PFS). This requires modeling survival beyond the trial follow-up. That is, 'estimating' the survival trajectory once the trial follow-up period is complete. This will require choosing a parametric survival model (Chapter 4). If all patients have died in the trial, extrapolation is not required. A judgment should be made whether extrapolating in the case of just one or two patients who are censored (alive at the end of the trial) is required (or useful).
(iii) If covariates are included that might influence the predicted survival times, then these could be included as part of the model.

Modeling the Cost and Utility Data

(i) Generate the mean utility for each treatment group.
(ii) Generate the mean costs for each treatment group, taking into account any censoring. For both costs and utility, model-based estimates using covariates should be used. For estimation of future costs (for patients left alive), these could be estimated by multiplying the predicted survival by the predicted cost (or using methods such as those of Lin (2861997; 2872000) mentioned in Chapter 5).
(iii) Derive the mean QALY for the PFS and PPS, that is, generate a mean PFS QALY and a mean PPS QALY for each treatment group.
(iv) Compute the incremental (mean) cost and QALY and derive the ICER

We now present a step-by-step example of a partitioned survival model introduced earlier in Chapter 3 applied in the context of an economic evaluation using a case study from a UK NICE HTA.

7.5.2 Case Study of an Economic Model Using Patient-Level Data: A Partitioned Survival Model

We use the example of the multiple technology appraisal, NICE TA516 case study: cabozantinib and vandetanib for treating unresectable locally advanced or metastatic medullary thyroid cancer. Full details are found on the NICE website (NICE HTA516, 2018).

(i) The indication: medullary thyroid cancer. This is a rare cancer (<1% cases in the UK). About 71% of patients survive 10 years if they have Stage III and 21% survive 10 years if they are diagnosed as Stage IV. Table 7.6 provides a summary of the trial design and results.
(ii) Cabozanitib and vandetanib (CV) are the only disease-modifying drugs licensed for this indication.
(iii) Comparators and existing treatments: surgery is the preferred (curative) treatment if the disease is locally resectable. Otherwise, depending on the prognosis either of:
   (a) Vandetanib + best supportive care (BSC).
   (b) Cabozantinib + BSC.
   (c) Vandetanib (300 mg once daily (QD)) or cabozantinib (140 mg QD) + BSC (treatment continued until disease progression).
   (d) BSC (palliative care – symptom relief).
(iv) Clinical trials: in this evaluation, data from one Phase III trial was submitted (ZETA trial) for economic evaluation. A further Phase III trial (EXAM trial) was included for comparing the efficacy but cost-effectiveness analyses were not provided. The two trials were not considered to be directly comparable. The differences in the trial population, impact of prior and post-progression therapies, and presence of crossover in the ZETA trial (not allowed in the EXAM trial) made it inappropriate to formally compare the two treatments, in the absence of head-to-head trials comparing vandetanib with cabozantinib. The results presented here are for the restricted population of patients (those with symptomatic and progressive medullary thyroid cancer plus a biomarker status).
   (a) EXAM trial: a Phase III double blind of cabozantinib versus placebo (BSC), sample size of 330 (219 on cabozantinib, 111 on placebo).
   (b) ZETA trial: a Phase III double blind of vandetanib versus placebo (BSC).
(v) Sample size of 331 (231 on vandetanib, 100 on placebo).
(vi) A summary of the ZETA trial and cost-effectiveness parameters are shown in Table 7.6.

Summary of the Methods, Results and Conclusions

(i) Trial Results

Both vandetanib and cabozanitib showed statistically improved PFS (primary endpoint). Vandetanib does not appear to show improvement in OS after 50% of the death events (HR = 0.99). However, the lack of statistical difference in

TABLE 7.6

Trial Design and Cost-Effectiveness Features of the ZETA Trial

Trial Design	Design	EXAM Phase III double blind	ZETA Phase III double blind
	Sample size	330 (219 vs. 111) 80% power, HR = 0.67 for OS	331 (231 vs. 100) 80% power, HR < 0.5
	Treatment	Cabozantinib vs. placebo until PD	Vandetanib vs. placebo until PD
	Trial follow-up	Median 13.9 months	Median 24 months
	Primary endpoint	PFS	PFS
	Secondary endpoints	OS, response, DoR, safety	OS, response, DoR, HRQoL, safety
Trial results	PFS[a]	11.2 mo vs. 4.0 mo (median) HR = 0.28 [CI: 0.19, 0.40; p < 0.001]	30.5 mo vs. 19.3 mo (median) HR = 0.46 [CI: 0.31, 0.69; p < 0.0001]
	OS	26.6 vs. 21.1 mo (median) HR = 0.85 [CI: 0.64, 1.12; p = 0.241] Death events: about 30% died (70% still alive by the end of the trial, hence extrapolation of OS will be needed)	Not reported/not reached[b] HR = 0.99 [CI: 0.72, 1.38; p = 0.975] death events about 50% (50% still alive at end of trial, hence extrapolation of OS will be needed)
	Crossover present	Yes – crossover from BSC to cabozanitib; hence adjustment for treatment switching needed	Yes – crossover from BSC to vandetanib; hence adjustment for treatment switching needed
Health economics	Horizon		20-year horizon (life time)
	Discounting		Yes, 3.5% for costs and QALYs
	Cycle length		Monthly
	Perspective		UK NHS
	Comparator		Placebo/BSC
Costs	Drug costs		£5,000 per 30 × 300 mg and £2,500 per 30 × 100 mg tablets[f]
	Adverse event costs		Varied depending on the type of AE
	BSC costs		£788 if in PFS state, £7,195 if in PD[c]
	Palliative care		£189.75[d] per day
	Palliative chemotherapy		£827
	Monitoring costs[f]		£400 in year 1 (per patient) and about £200/year in subsequent years
Utility	EQ-5D		None collected. Utility determined from FACT-G using Dobrez et al. algorithm (see below for details) PFS utility 0.84 PD utility: 0.64
Efficacy	PFS		Modeled using Weibull, log-normal, log-logistic

(Continued)

TABLE 7.6 (CONTINUED)

Trial Design and Cost-Effectiveness Features of the ZETA Trial

	Design	EXAM	ZETA
Trial Design		**Phase III double blind**	**Phase III double blind**
	OS		Modeled using Weibull, log-normal, log-logistic[g]
	Crossover handling	Crossover to cabozantinib not allowed, but other treatments allowed (including vandetanib)	Crossover at any time Extensive crossover could not be adjusted for statistically (see below) 10% of those on vandetanib crossed over and 28%[k]
Uncertainty		Not provided	PSA using CEAC Deterministic by varying parameters[i] Incremental QALY Scenario analyses[j]
Results	ICER		Incremental QALY: 1.34 Incremental costs: £42,215 ICER: £31,546[h]
	Probability of CE		88% at a WTP of £50,000/QALY

[a] *Notes:* Both central review- and investigator-based assessment of progression were reported. We only report the independent assessments for simplicity. Other results could be included as part of sensitivity analyses.

[b] For the ZETA trial, for the vandetanib group, the median could not be estimated, although for placebo it was estimable. However, reporting a median for one group and not the other is of little comparative benefit.

[c] These were estimated by multiplying the unit costs for items such as scans (£148/scan) by the frequency in either a PFS state or a PD disease state. mo: months; CI: 95% confidence intervals.

[d] These were estimated as the mean of different types of palliative care such as inpatient, specialist, or outpatient.

[e] Prior to applying discounts.

[f] Once a patient starts treatment, they are monitored (e.g. for ECG, biochemistry, etc.) – for vandetanib this was 8 times during the first year.

[g] This included extrapolated survival.

[h] This is based on the manufacturer's model. The ICER based on the NICE assessor's analysis was £66,000/QALY.

[i] Parameters varied included cost of monitoring, cost of care, AE costs, utilities in PFS and PPS states, and crossover rates (i.e. the proportion that crossed over).

[j] An example of one scenario was setting discount rates at 0% and 5%, removing post-progression costs, alternative methods of utility adjustment, setting the time horizon to 5 and 10 years and assuming a crossover vandetanib dose of 300 mg (patients could have taken either 100 mg or 300 g, but in this scenario only 300 mg is assumed).

[k] What this means is that some patients on both arms received alternative treatments. Since progression is determined by central review (experts who look at scans to determine progression), some patients took alternative treatment before the final date of progression was known (it takes time to get all the information across to determine PD status). Hence, the PFS was also confounded (that is some of the PFS could have been due to alternative therapy). One approach is to censor the patient at the date the crossover treatment was taken.

OS does not imply that a positive cost-effectiveness conclusion is not possible. OS was a secondary endpoint and the benefit is likely to be driven by the PFS endpoint. In addition, part of the reason for a lack of OS benefit is largely due to patients on the BSC switching over to vandetanib, which makes the treatments appear more similar. This is discussed further below.

(ii) Cost-Effectiveness Model

A partitioned survival model was used by the HTA assessor group using three health states: progression-free, post-progression (i.e. PD), and dead. The available patient-level data were used to estimate transitions (survival rates). Since there was censoring, parametric survival models were used including covariates for the presence of symptomatic disease and biomarker status. The empirical Kaplan-Meier for both PFS and OS were generated and then Weibull functions were selected to model both OS and PFS, assuming independent (non-proportional) hazards between treatment groups. Once a model was fitted, for uncertainty (PSA) the parameter estimates from these models were simulated to generate thousands of QALYs (and compute incremental QALYs). The mean survival times were computed, but it was noted that these could be underestimated because the longest survival time was censored. An example of a model fit is shown in Figure 7.3.

7.5.3 Crossover

An attempt was made to adjust the treatment effect for crossover. Methods introduced earlier such as rank-preserving structural failure time (RPSFT) models

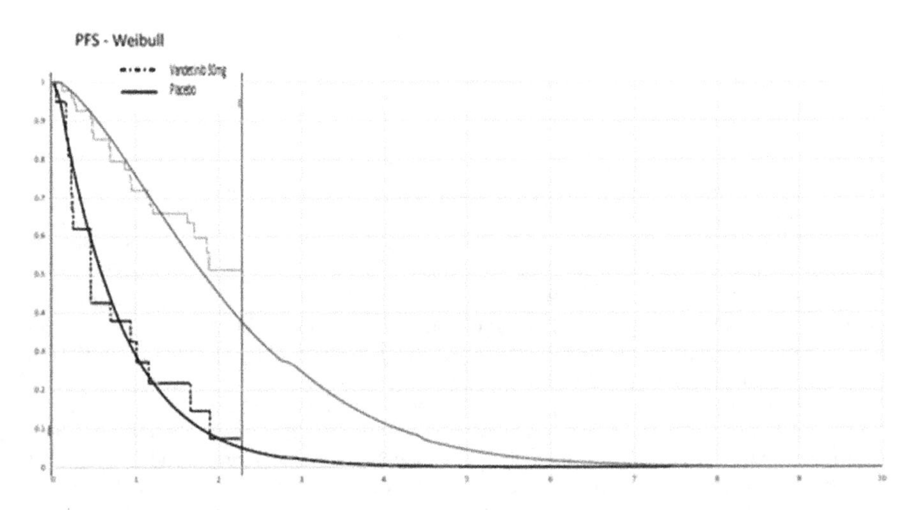

FIGURE 7.3
Source page 118 of HTA TA516: empirical PFS with modeled PFS beyond trial follow-up using a parametric survival model.

and inverse probability-of-censoring weights (IPCW) method were used. These methods failed to provide an estimate of treatment effect unconfounded by the crossover (from placebo to vandetanib). This resulted in an analysis that restricted the label to patients who were progressive and with symptomatic medullary thyroid cancer with rapid biomarker doubling (hence the consequences of crossover can be severe). RPSFT has been attempted in several previous NICE HTAs.

Since adjustment for crossover could not properly be carried out, the treatment benefit of vandetanib over placebo is likely to be underestimated. If vandetanib is indeed effective and prolongs survival, crossover is likely to result in rapid attenuation of any differences in OS. Hence, a traditional ITT analysis, will underestimate vandetanib's effect on OS. This also relates to the theme of estimands raised in Chapter 4.

(iii) Utilities

No EQ-5D utilities were collected during the trial. HRQoL data using a condition-specific FACT-G were collected. An algorithm to convert FACT-G responses to time trade-off (TTO) utilities was published by Dobrez et al. (Dobrez, 2004). The algorithm is based on directly elicited TTO utilities provided by a large sample of patients ($n = 1{,}433$) with cancer for their health state at the time as well as the patients' responses to the FACT-G. The algorithm gave an equation for utility –interested readers can consult the HTA report.

In addition, utility in the progressed state was determined from a few patients who completed FACT-G while in the PD state. These were not considered representative and a utility decrement was applied to the utility measured for the progression-free state (0.84). This decrement was obtained from an external study Beusterien et al. (2009).

(iv) Costs

Several cost items are shown in Table 7.6 and described in the footnotes of the table. The model structure states: "At each apportioning, values (in terms of quality of life and costs) are applied to each state and the resulting accruals are accumulated as outputs. This happens cyclically until the end of the time horizon." In other words, the proportions from each of the PFS and PD states are multiplied and summed over the time horizon. Little was mentioned by way of missing data, although its presence was noted.

(v) Results, Conclusion and Issues

The conclusions of the results were:

- Vandetanib was considered to be cost-effective with an ICER of around £66,000. This was almost twice that of the manufacturer's ICER of around £32,000.

- Some reasons for the discrepancy are due to:
    - The manufacturer included a single (first) progression event that corresponds to the partition between the PFS and PD health states. Patients receiving vandetanib after this in either arm are assumed to continue to do so until death, whereas in practice these patients are likely to have a second progression before death. This would likely mean that vandetanib would be discontinued. The manufacturer/company model failed to reflect this. Although adjustment for crossover was unsuccessful, including these costs of the drug in both groups would usually be reasonable, but assuming that all treatment post-progression continues until death will overestimate the costs of vandetanib in both groups. This bias strongly favors the intervention group because a higher proportion of patients receive vandetanib post-progression within the BSC group (proportion of patients on treatment post-progression). Therefore, removing the costs of vandetanib received post-progression in both groups will increase the ICER from around £32,000 per QALY gained to around £60,000 per QALY gained.
- Failure to adjust for treatment switching resulting in estimates of treatment effect that are potentially confounded by the use of open label vandetanib. The impact of open label vandetanib could not be addressed. The company's model included the estimated costs of post-progression vandetanib used within both the intervention and comparator treatment groups. The economic comparison made by the company's model is therefore vandetanib including continued use in some patients post-progression versus BSC with vandetanib use in most patients post-progression. The assessment group noted that this may not have been useful for decision-making. The manufacturer used a mapping model to estimate the EQ-5D utilities from the FACT-G whereas the assessor used estimates using a published algorithm.
- The duration over which QALY losses due to AEs are applied and differences in the inputs relating to the proportion of patients who discontinued vandetanib prior to PD.

The above example shows the complexity and detail with which HTAs are undertaken, and the care needed to evaluate all possible uncertainties. In the above case the drug was recommended, despite a high estimate of the ICER. However in other cases, drugs are not recommended after the biases have been addressed.

7.6 Summary of Cost-Effectiveness Models for Cancer Used in HTA Submissions

Table 7.1 presented the common economic evaluation models reported in the economic evaluation of (lung) cancer drugs from a UK NICE HTA perspective. Many of these models used individual patient-level data from clinical trials and then simulation to describe the uncertainty around the ICER. Table 7.7 shows a summary of health economic models in cancer. The sources for the model inputs – health resource use and utilities (not always from trial data) are shown. For example, for afatinib (NICE TA310, 2014), patient-level data were taken from two different trials (the LUX-Lung 3 and LUX-Lung 6 trials). Several parametric survival models were fitted to estimate future (extrapolated) survival rates (exponential, Weibull and Gompertz models); treatment costs were obtained from BNF 2011; and NHS reference costs were obtained (NHS reference costs for a given year are on the website, seehttps://improvement.nhs.uk). Utilities were taken from the clinical trials and all these data were fed into a model to derive the ICERs. Note that while combining trial data and historical data might be more informative, it could also introduce greater uncertainty because populations and experimental conditions from historical data may be different.

In Table 7.6, we have highlighted where survival models were used, often for extrapolation for estimating QALYs. Most submissions extrapolated the time-to-event survival data to cover a lifetime horizon, either through survival model fitting or by using Markov assumptions, using observed hazard ratios for the comparators. In addition, the key cost and utility inputs are provided for the model. The information in Table 7.7 can be summarized as:

- NICE in the UK have, to a large extent, recommended cancer drugs for first-line treatment and generally recommended against drugs for second-line and maintenance treatment. The SMC have also rejected, or approved with limitations, a number of drugs for first- and second-line treatment. Outside the UK, there has been a higher rate of success in terms of approval for use, with only two treatments (crizotinib first-line in Canada and afatanib second-line in Australia) being rejected.
- The main sources of efficacy data for the models were from the clinical trials: LUX-Lung 3, LUX-Lung 6, INTEREST, BR21, EURTAC, OPTIMAL, IPASS, PARAMOUNT, JMDB, PROFILE 1005, PROFILE 1007 (see references to HTA).
- Survival data were often modeled to generate QALYs using partitioned survival models.
- Costs were determined from literature and established sources such as National Health Service (NHS) reference costs, British

TABLE 7.7

Cost-Effectiveness Models Used in Lung Cancer

Treatment	Submission	Clinical Data	Resource Use/Costs	Utilities
Afatinib	TA310 1L (NICE, 2014b)	Estimates of OS and PFS based on data from LUX-Lung 3 (28% maturity) and LUX-Lung 6 (43% maturity), corresponding parametric survival models Exponential, Weibull and Gompertz explored as proportional hazard models; log-logistic and log-normal included for sensitivity analysis (goodness-of-fit provided) Second-line (docetaxel) PFS data from INTEREST trial Relative efficacy data retrieved from MTC	Treatment costs from BNF 2011 NHS reference costs (2010–11) and HRG data used for hospitalization (currency codes are provided); and PFS 2011 used for outpatient visits Other costs sourced from literature reviews such as (Billingham, 2002; Lees, 2002) Costs of AEs only applied in first year (no separate health states) – frequencies and duration from MTC, LUX-Lung 1, and LUX-Lung 3 EGFR mutation test from SMC 2012 (only in the first cycle)	Health state utilities derived from LUX-Lung and LUCEOR trials (Chouaid, 2012) in base case and assumed to be the same across treatment arms (not between 1L and 2L); other sources used in sensitivity analysis (Doyle, 2008; Lewis, 2010; Nafees, 2008) Disutilities sourced from LUX-Lung 1, LUX-Lung 3, and (Nafees, 2008)
	07-2013 1L (PBAC, 2013a)	Non-inferiority against gefitinib and erlotinib from MTC – submitted a cost minimization analysis (CMA). Outcomes were extrapolated from data at maximum follow-up of 22 months observed in LUX-Lung 3		Utility from LUX-Lung 3 and LUCEOR 2 trials. Utility decrements from studies conducted in patients receiving second- or third-line therapy (LUX-Lung 1 and Tabberer et al.)
Crizotinib	TA296 2L (NICE, 2013)	Extrapolation of OS based on the PROFILE 1005 trial, and PFS based on the PROFILE 1007 trial. Trial 1005 was single arm but more mature. Trial 1007 was assumed to have the same trends but included comparators. Both proportional hazard models (Weibull, exponential, and Gompertz) and accelerated failure time models (log-logistic and log-normal). Crossover accounted for using RPSFT, IPTCW (base case)	Administration and routine medical management from NHS reference costs and PSSRU, acquisition cost from BNF 63 (2012), and resource use from clinical experts. Treatment cost until disease progression ALK testing costs were applied to the crizotinib arm of the model – assumed as the cost of one test multiplied by the number of patients needed to be tested to identify one ALK+ patient (all patients identified eventually) Treatment for AEs related to crizotinib and chemotherapy. Cost of AEs occurred the first out of the 30 treatment days (only included neutropenia)	Utility collected in PROFILE 1007 using the EQ-5D Calculated EQ-5D in PFS by weighting the value at each time point by the number of patients at each time point A weighted average utility at the end of treatment was extrapolated to post-progression health states No utility decrement was applied to AE occurrences
	865/13 2L (SMC, 2013)	Taken from clinical trial, including Phase II (single arm) study to increase sample size and extrapolate the data	Costs included cost of medicine and administration, cost of ALK-testing (FISH test), routine care before and after progression Price with PAS was proposed by SMC	Utility data was derived using EQ-5D from the clinical trials. Values for BSC were assigned using assumptions
	pCODR 2013 2L (pCODR, 2013b)	Extrapolation of the PROFILE 1007 clinical trial using information from Phase II trials	All costs relevant for the publicly funded healthcare.	Utility data was derived using EQ-5D from the clinical trials.

(Continued)

TABLE 7.7 (CONTINUED)

Cost-Effectiveness Models Used in Lung Cancer

Treatment	Submission	Clinical Data	Resource Use/Costs	Utilities
Erlotinib	TA258 1L (NICE, 2012)	EURTAC clinical trial	Cost data sourced from previous NICE technology appraisals in a NSCLC, specifically: TA227, TA181, and TA192	Utilities were taken from (Nafees, 2008); a study commissioned for second-line NSCLC, with 100 members of the general population, using SG and VAS techniques
	TA162 2L (NICE, 2008)	BR21 clinical trial for erlotinib (Holmes, 2004) for docetaxel	Cost data sourced primarily from published sources Docetaxel drug administration based on data from expert panel	
	749/11 1L (SMC, 2012)	EURTAC clinical trial	Cost data sourced from NICE appraisal of 1L pemetrexed/cisplatin	Primary study derived from a survey that used the standard gamble technique with 100 members of the UK public
	220/05 2L (SMC, 2006)	Indirect comparison from 2 trials (erlotinib vs. placebo; docetaxel vs. pemetrexed	Cost data sourced primarily from published sources Resource use and AEs were estimated from an expert panel	Primary study from a sample of the UK general population using appropriate methods (not specified)
	07-2013 1L (PBAC, 2013b)	Main clinical trial was EURTAC, supplemented by OPTIMAL trial compared to chemotherapy. Also used IPASS, NEJGSG, Study 0054, and WJTOG3405 to compare to gefitinib.		Utilities for patients with stable disease and progressive disease directly from (Nafees, 2008)
Gefitinib	TA192 1L (NICE, 2010b)	IPASS study (gefitinib vs. paclitaxel/carboplatin) Odds ratios for treatment response for the indirect comparators were sourced from an MTC	Various sources including: BNF, NHS reference costs,	Most utilities were sourced from (Nafees, 2008) Progression-free and therapy were sourced from an ERG report (2006) Disutility for anemia was sourced from Eli Lilly (2009)
	615/10 1L (SMC, 2010b)	Effectiveness of gefitinib and paclitaxel/carboplatin: from the pivotal gefitinib trial results Effectiveness of the other double chemotherapy: from an MTC, within which paclitaxel/carboplatin provided the link to the results of the pivotal gefitinib trial	Adverse events costs: from industry submissions to NICE	Sourced from literature (not specified)
	07-2013 1L (PBAC, 2013c)	IPASS study (gefitinib vs. paclitaxel/carboplatin)		Utilities were adapted from HRQoL data reported in the trial

(*Continued*)

TABLE 7.7 (CONTINUED)

Cost-Effectiveness Models Used in Lung Cancer

Treatment	Submission	Clinical Data	Resource Use/Costs	Utilities
Pemetrexed	TA181 1L (NICE, 2009)	Transition probabilities calculated based on response rates and PFS from JMDB trial data (pemetrexed/cisplatin and gemcitabine/cisplatin) by estimations of the median time. Death derived from median time of OS and PFS, converted to transition probability. This assumes an exponential form. No direct comparison of gemcitabine/carboplatin or docetaxel/cisplatin was available. Indirect analysis conducted to adjust the data to the JMDB population	Acquisition costs and administration doses taken from the trial and the treatments' SPCs UK unit cost sourced from the BNF Administration costs estimated using national HRGs Resource use associated with adverse events informed by a survey of clinician experts commissioned by the manufacturer (Lilly) Unit costs were sourced from the UK NHS reference costs 2008	Utilities were taken from (Nafees, 2008); a study commissioned for second-line NSCLC, with 100 members of the general population, using SG and VAS techniques
	TA309 MTx (NICE, 2014a)	Curve fitting and extrapolation of OS and PFS KM curves were undertaken (maturity up to 80%) using exponential, Weibull, log-logistic, log-normal, Gompertz and gamma (goodness-of-fit, curves, and values are presented)	NHS reference costs and HRG used for hospitalization and monitoring (currency codes provided) Treatment costs from BNF 2012 Resource uses (including AEs) taken from the PARAMOUNT trial Monitoring use from (Beckett, 2012)	EQ-5D data from a mixed regression model of the PARAMOUNT trial. No significant different in AEs between maintenance treatments in trial
	531/09 1L (SMC, 2010a)	Data was sourced from the 29-month pivotal Phase III trial of pemetrexed/cisplatin vs. gemcitabine/cisplatin and extrapolated using standard survival model fitting	Acquisition costs of pemetrexed/cisplatin and gemcitabine/cisplatin were based on doses used in the trial The dose for gemcitabine/carboplatin was based on that applied in the NICE appraisal of pemetrexed for first -line treatment of NSCLC Other resources and costs were taken from literature, guidelines, or using expert opinion	Sourced from a utility valuation survey using SG in 100 members of the general population in the UK
	342/07 2st line (SMC, 2008)	Median survival rates were taken from a retrospective subgroup analysis of the results of the clinical study of pemetrexed and docetaxel (randomized, open label Phase III study)	Most resource use associated with adverse events was based on clinical expert opinion NHS reference costs were used Data for febrile neutropenia was taken from literature	Sourced from a study of 100 members of the general population using SG to value 18 states and adverse events)

Notes: AE: adverse events; ALK: anaplastic lymphoma kinase; BNF: British National Formulary; BSC: best supportive care; CI: confidence interval; CMA: cost-minimization analysis; EGFR: epidermal growth factor receptor; EQ-5D: EuroQoL five dimension; ERG: evidence review group; FISH: fluorescence in situ hybridization; HRG: healthcare Resource Group; HRQoL: Health-related quality of life; IPTCW: Inverse probability of treatment and censoring weighted; KM: Kaplan Meier; MTC: Mixed-treatment comparison; MTx: maintenance treatment; NICE: National Institute for Health and Care Excellence; NHS: National Health Services; NSCLC: non-small-cell lung cancer; OS: overall survival; PAS: patient-access schemes; PBAC: Pharmaceutical Benefits Advisory Committee; pCODR: pan-Canadian Oncology Drug Review; PFS: progression-free survival; PSSRU: Personal Social Services Research Unit; RPSFT: rank-preserved structural failure time; SG: standard gamble; SMC: Scottish Medicines Consortium; SPC: summary of product characteristics; TA: technology appraisal; VAS: visual analogue scale.

National Formulary (BNF), and Personal Social Services Research Unit (PSSRU). Some resource use has also been sourced from clinical experts and systematic reviews of the literature, especially for adverse events.

- Health state utilities have commonly been sourced from a study by Nafees et al., 2008 and where available from the clinical trial.
- MTC has been used frequently but some submissions use direct comparisons.

Criticisms of Health Economic Models: Examples from Lung Cancer

Criticisms of some cost-effectiveness models used in lung cancer are shown in Table 7.8. Many of these models used patient-level data. For example, in the case of afatinib, there were issues with model fit, mix of the patient population (EGFR + ve and EGFR –ve), generalizability, and inadequate survival projection.

7.7 Summary

We have discussed at some length the types of cost-effectiveness models used for cancer. A common approach is the partitioned survival model. We have also seen the common criticisms from HTA assessors in the context of lung cancer, but these criticisms can be generalized. We have not discussed some other types of models such as discrete event simulation (DES) models. A DES model consists of entities (patients) that enter the system, get serviced (by a resource unit) one or more times, and then exit, or make a delay and then exit the system. Resource units can be physical agents (doctors, nurses, other hospital personnel) and/or equipment or materials, or a mix of these, as is usual in healthcare. DES has not yet gained wide acceptance in the cancer field. A search in PubMed with search terms 'discrete event' AND 'model' OR 'simulation' AND 'cancer' yielded only 34 hits (as of June 2018). Most of those before 2011 mostly concerned cancer-screening policies. A complete introduction with practical applications of DES models in healthcare can be found in Caro et al. (2015).

7.8 Exercises for Chapter 7

1. Distinguish between a decision tree, Markov model, and patient-level model in the context of cancer.

TABLE 7.8

Key criticisms of HTA Submissions: Lung Cancer

Treatment	Area	Critiques	Submission
Afatinib	Clinical data	The results of an MTC carried out using the currently available trial evidence comparing erlotinib and gefitinib were unreliable, especially as they included both EGFR-positive and EGFR-unknown/mixed patient populations in the networks Eliminating these studies results in predominantly studies with Asian patients that may not be generalizable to all patients	NICE, 2014b (TA310) 1L SMC, 2014 (920/13) 1L PBAC, 2013a (07-2013) 1L
		The MTC relied on proportional hazards, but the ERG suggested that the assumptions supporting this were not valid	NICE, 2014 (TA310) 1L
		Despite a statistically significant improvement in PFS, there did not appear to be a corresponding gain in OS for TKIs vs. chemotherapy, based on similar information from previous erlotinib and gefitinib submissions, after adjusting for crossover	NICE, 2014 (TA310) 1L
	Survival analysis	The modeled PFS survival projection for afatinib did not reflect the LUX-Lung 3 trial afatinib data from which it was derived	NICE, 2014 (TA310) 1L
		The OS data was not yet mature at the time of submission	NICE, 2014 (TA310) 1L SMC, 2014 (920/13) 1L PBAC, 2013 1L
		Recommended to use RPSFT to account for crossover data. The SMC tested this and it gave a higher ICER than in the original model	SMC, 2013 (865/13) 2L
	Comparator	Erlotinib and gefitinib were appropriate comparators in first-line, but data were derived from an MTC that had methodological limitations The data in the MTC was only in first-line use. As such, relative benefits in the second-line setting are unclear	NICE, 2014 (TA310) 1L SMC, 2014 (920/13) 1L
		Chemotherapies from LUX-Lung 3 and LUX-Lung 6 were not appropriate comparators for the stated decision problem	NICE, 2014 (TA310) 1L
		Proposed comparators should be (a) first-line that includes EGFR testing compared to TKI for positive tests and chemotherapy for negative tests, and (b) compared to chemotherapy treatment without EGFR testing	PBAC, 2013 1L
	Utilities	The generated QALYs were not supported by clinical data The utility decrement between stable and progressive disease was not supported	PBAC, 2013 1L
	Costs	Maintenance treatment with pemetrexed before disease progression would only incur costs and no additional efficacy	PBAC, 2013 1L
	Others	The submission did not present clinical- or cost-effectiveness evidence to support the use of afatinib for TKI-naïve patients in a second- or third-line setting	NICE, 2014 (TA310) 1L
		Since the clinical data was not appropriate to calculate reliable ICERs, the ERG proposed a CMA exercise	NICE, 2014 (TA310) 1L SMC, 2014 (920/13) 1L PBAC, 2013 1L
		The assumption that all patients receiving first-line chemotherapy who progress will receive a second-line treatment was inconsistent with clinical practice	PBAC, 2013 1L
		Assumption that EGFR mutation negative patients in the comparator arm will receive erlotinib in second-line may not be reasonable	PBAC, 2013 1L
		A significant limitation is that the model failed to account for false positives in the EGFR testing, as this would probably not be 100% and therefore lower the efficacy of afatinib	PBAC, 2013 1L

(*Continued*)

TABLE 7.8 (CONTINUED)

Key criticisms of HTA Submissions: Lung Cancer

Treatment	Area	Critiques	Submission
Crizotinib	Clinical data	Limitations of the MTC include the small number of studies included	SMC, 2013 (865/13) 2L NICE, 2013 (TA296) 2L
		Probabilities for progression and mortality were updated in this resubmission from the PROFILE 1001 study in the first submissions as these were inappropriate	pCODR, 2013 2L
	Survival analysis	No significant difference in OS data as it was immature and subject to high crossover. Extrapolation of the trial data using single arm studies may introduce bias	SMC, 2013 (865/13) 2L NICE, 2013 (TA296) 2L
		The survival data did not focus on ALK+ patients	NICE, 2013 (TA296) 2L
		The extra trials used to estimate the survival (PROFILE 1005, GFPC 05-06, JMEI, and TAX 317) were not comparable to the main clinical trial (PROFILE 1007)	NICE, 2013 (TA296) 2L
	Comparator	The primary relevant comparator is docetaxel	NICE, 2013 (TA296) 2L
	Utilities	The utilities from PROFILE 1007 were overestimated – particularly the assumption that treatment effect was maintained, to some extent, post-progression	pCODR, 2013 2L NICE, 2013 (TA296) 2L
	Costs	Testing for ALK mutation was included but assumed the same in both arms – the ERG raised concerns that this underestimated the costs	pCODR, 2013 2L
		Removing the cost of ALK-testing reduced ICER by £1,000 – this scenario may be likely in the future	SMC, 2013 (865/13) 2L
		Treatment duration was assumed to last until progression but in some instances within the trials treatment continued longer. Using trial duration increased the QALY Discontinuation rule for crizotinib was inappropriate	SMC, 2013 (865/13) 2L NICE, 2013 (TA296) 2L
	Other	The screening of ALK patients contained three issues: validity of the approach where the model did not use the same test that was used by NHS), cost of the test, and prevalence rate of ALK+	NICE, 2013 (TA296) 2L
		The ERG proposed a 2-year time horizon as opposed to 5 years	pCODR, 2013 2L
		The base case ICER was estimated to be overly optimistic toward crizotinib for several reasons (as mentioned above)	NICE, 2013 (TA296) 2L
Erlotinib	Clinical data	Questioned the strength of the indirect comparison/mixed treatment comparison due to the comparability of the studies included	NICE, 2L SMC, 2011 (749/11) 1L SMC, 2006 (220/05) 2L
	Survival analysis	Extrapolation method utilized did not appropriately fit the trial data for both the intervention and comparator; the method utilized overestimated benefit for the intervention and underestimated benefit for the comparator	NICE, 2006 (TA162) 2L
		The model solely relied on PFS data since no significant difference was identified for OS, and assumed that PFS gains automatically convert to OS gains, which was unreliable	NICE, 2012 (TA258) 1L
	Comparator	Comparators included in the model were not comprehensive of clinical practice. Efficacy of pemetrexed as a first-line treatment for patients with EGFRm+ did not exist and therefore was inappropriate as comparator	NICE, 2012 (TA258) 1L
		Pemetrexed should not be included as maintenance only in the comparator arm	PBAC, 2013 1L

(Continued)

TABLE 7.8 (CONTINUED)

Key criticisms of HTA Submissions: Lung Cancer

Treatment	Area	Critiques	Submission
	Utilities	Assumption that utilities are independent of time is not reflective of real-world circumstances	NICE, 2006 (TA162) 2L
		Utility estimates were not based on the full EQ-5D questionnaire	NICE, 2006 (TA162) 2L
		All utilities should preferably have been derived from trial rather than the use of vignettes	PBAC, 2013 1L
		Different utility values for first-line progression-free treatment and second-line progression-free treatment were not supported by the evidence	PBAC, 2013 1L
	Costs	Assumption that costs are independent of time is not reflective of clinical practice	NICE, 2006 (TA162) 2L
		Assumption that there is no drug wastage is not reflective of clinical practice	NICE, 2006 (TA162) 2L
		Assumption that there is no vial sharing is not reflective of clinical practice	NICE, 2006 (TA162) 2L
		Cost and resource use data extracted from expert opinion was not validated against any observational datasets	NICE, 2006 (TA162) 2L
		The duration of therapy was uncertain, especially if treatment would continue beyond disease progression in real-world practice	PBAC, 2013 1L
		The model was not comprehensive of the costs included in clinical practice. Specifically, transportation costs associated with treatment delivery were omitted	NICE, 2006 (TA162) 2L
	Others	The detection of all EGFR mutations using a standard test was considered too optimistic and that false positives should have lower efficacy. PBAC had identified a number of studies showing inferior results of TKI in patients with no EGFR mutation (TORCH, DELTA, TAILOR, TITAN, IPASS) – lowering the prevalence of EGFR increased the ICER	PBAC, 2013 1L
		Assumption that patients cannot suffer from multiple adverse events is not reflective of clinical practice	NICE, 2006 (TA162) 2L
Gefitinib	Clinical data	The trial data (IPASS) did not focus on EGFRm+ and was not powered to evaluate this	NICE, 2010 (TA192) 1L
		The trial data (IPASS) may not have been generalizable to England and Wales	NICE, 2010 (TA192) 1L
		ERG believed that the first SIGNAL trial should have been included in the submission	
	Survival analysis	Concern was expressed over whether using the Cox proportionate hazards method to calculate hazards ratios was appropriate (only valid if the hazard ratio for the two groups remains constant over time)	NICE, 2010 (TA192) 1L
		Concern was expressed about the immaturity of the survival data as relatively few deaths had occurred	NICE, 2010 (TA192) 1L
		Concern was expressed about the poor fit of the parametric model to the data	NICE, 2010 (TA192) 1L SMC, 2010 (615/10) 1L

(Continued)

TABLE 7.8 (CONTINUED)

Key criticisms of HTA Submissions: Lung Cancer

Treatment	Area	Critiques	Submission
	Comparator	Comparators included in the model were not a comprehensive reflection of clinical practice	NICE, 2010 (TA192) 1L
		The handling of second-line treatments may be inappropriate	SMC, 2010 (615/10) 1L
	Costs	Comparator costs included in the model were inaccurate	NICE, 2010 (TA192) 1L
	Others	Concern that resource utilization was not reflective of clinical guidelines	NICE, 2010 (TA192) 1L
		Cost for the management of adverse events was considered inaccurate	PBAC, 2013 1L
		The model assumes 100% specificity of the EGFR test, which likely overestimates the benefit of the treatment (since treatment effect on false positives would be lower than on true positives)	PBAC, 2013 1L NICE, 2010 (TA192) 1L
		Other cost data were considered to be inaccurate	PBAC, 2013 1L
		Uncertain prevalence of EGFR, which affects the ICER	SMC, 2010 (615/10) 1L
		Time horizon (5 years) was not considered to be reflective of the approximated length of life for the patient group, where the longest possible time horizon should have been used (6 years)	NICE, 2010 (TA192) 1L
Pemetrexed	Clinical data	Clinical trial population differed from clinical practice	NICE, 2013 (TA310) MTx
		Unlimited maintenance treatment cycles not reflective of clinical practice	NICE, 2013 (TA310) MTx
		The ERG believed the approach to evidence synthesis (pooling of absolute median) adopted by the company was not meaningful; as a consequence, indirect comparisons provided in the submission were not considered to be appropriate	NICE, 2007 (TA124) 2L
		Re-analysis of clinical trial data indicates that there is no additional benefit provided to patients by pemetrexed once disease progression is confirmed	NICE, 2013 (TA310) MTx NICE, 2007 (TA124) 2L
	Survival analysis	The ERG questioned whether the estimated survival from the economic model was consistent with the mean and median clinical outcomes in the trial	NICE, 2009 (TA181) 1L SMC, 2010 (342/07) 2L
		The survival estimates are inaccurate in the long term	NICE, 2009 (TA181) 1L
	Comparator	Comparators included in the model were not comprehensive of clinical practice	NICE, 2009 (TA181) 1L PBAC, (2010) 1L
		The validity of the indirect comparisons was questioned	NICE, 2009 (TA181) 1L
	Utilities	The QALY weights used were considered inappropriate as they were not treatment-specific	PBAC, 2010 1L
		Some of the utility values were not justified	PBAC, 2010 1L
	Others	The chosen model design was not obviously suitable for modeling the disease and treatments	NICE, 2009 (TA181) 1L
		The ERG questioned whether the model structure accurately replicates the trial data	NICE, 2009 (TA181) 1L
		The ERG highlighted several flaws in the economic model making it impossible to estimate robust ICERs	NICE, 2009 (TA181) 1L
		The ERGs corrected errors in economic model and it resulted in substantially less favorable results than in the submission	NICE, 2013 (TA310) MTx

Notes: ALK: anaplastic lymphoma kinase; BSC: best supportive care; CMA: cost-minimization analysis; EGFR: epidermal growth factor receptor; ERG: evidence review group; EQ-5D: EuroQoL five dimension; ICER: incremental cost-effectiveness ratio; MTC: mixed treatment comparison; MTx: maintenance treatment; NICE: National Institute for Health and Care Excellence; NSCLC: non-small-cell lung cancer; OS: overall survival; PBAC: Pharmaceutical Benefits Advisory Committee; pCODR: pan-Canadian Oncology Drug Review; PFS: progression-free survival; QALY: quality-adjusted life-year; RPSFT: rank-preserved structural failure time; SMC: Scottish Medicines Consortium; TA: technology appraisal; TKI: tyrosine kinase inhibitors.

2. Discuss the main criticisms of cost-effectiveness models submitted to reimbursement authorities. How can these criticisms be addressed?
3. Conduct and appraise an HTA submission (find a published one from a relevant website). Provide a summary of your findings and compare them with those of a colleague. Do you agree?
4. Explain in detail how a partition survival model works including how uncertainty (PSA and deterministic) could be undertaken.

8

Real-World Data in Cost-Effectiveness Studies on Cancer

8.1 Introduction to Real-World Data

Real-world data (RWD) is a relatively recent term that refers to data generated outside an experimental setting (often a clinical trial). It is the fact that these data are collected outside experimental conditions, that is, under real clinical practice conditions, that properly defines it as 'real-world data'. The conclusions derived from the use of RWD are sometimes termed as 'real-world evidence' (RWE). The strength of RWE must be subject to many of the principles of statistical inference and methodological rigor.

RWE offers a means of evaluating the natural history of disease development and understanding important factors that influence clinical outcomes outside of controlled settings. Generalizability of treatment effects, regional equity, under studied populations and access to cancer care, cannot be properly addressed using data collected in a multicenter RCT of say 5 or 20 centers all located in a confined geographical area. Some questions about treatment and outcomes are also more appropriately addressed in observational or other types of trials and not RCTs. For example, whether some NSCLC patients live shorter lives because of lack of access to treatment due to age, ethnicity, or social demographics cannot be adequately (or easily) answered from data generated in a clinical trial. Moreover, in clinical trials, patients may receive treatment at specialist center; however, the target population may actually be treated in a community setting or general hospitals where the quality of care given can be quite different. Hence, treatment effects from patients treated at specialist centers may be different compared to those treated in real-world community settings.

Although the terms RWD and RWE are new, collecting RWD is not so new. Its scope, however, has increased in recent years. In many clinical trials, the use of adverse events (adverse events monitoring well beyond the trial is completed) continues through the use of pharmacovigilance databases. This practice has been ongoing for many years but is often subject to underreporting. Their use has often been limited to adverse event signal detection for public safety reasons. RWD is now seen in some ways as an enhancement and extension of such data collection to include outcomes beyond safety.

RWD are generated through designing studies, collecting data from electronic health records (EHR) such as pharmacy claims data sets, disease registries, and other data sources for which:

(a) The medicinal product is prescribed in the usual way in line with marketing authorization approval; and, in some cases, through off-label use.
(b) The assignment to treatment is not determined on the basis of a pre-specified protocol but is given according to current treatment guidelines or practices.
(c) No further additional diagnostic or monitoring procedures are used to gather data, outside routine practice.

Table 8.1 shows the differences in objectives between an RCT and a study using RWD.

For the purposes of economic evaluation, RWD can provide valuable information on actual health resource use involved in delivering a cancer intervention, rather than protocol-defined healthcare. These aspects have been discussed in Chapters 2–5.

TABLE 8.1

Key Features that Differentiate RWD and Clinical Trials

Key Feature	RCT	RWD
Objective	Efficacy	Effectiveness and safety Where does treatment fit in the current pathway
Setting	Usually small sample sizes	Larger, possibly millions of records
Design	prospective	Retrospective or prospective
Time to get the results	Longer	Relatively quick, especially retrospective designs
Costs	High	Generally high[a] for prospective (observational type), mid for retrospective case control type studies and low for registry data studies
Statistical methodology	Usually less complex	More complex
Economic evaluation	ICER based on trial follow-up; relatively simpler approaches	ICER based on external factors, model uses complex simulation to quantify uncertainty
Implications	Drug registration	Clinical, economic, policy evaluation

[a] *Note:* The costs are lower in relation to comparable RCTs.

8.2 Using RWD to Support Cost-Effectiveness Analysis

In Chapter 6 we introduced observational studies as one of several methods for collecting data when an RCT is not feasible. Such data might provide insights on, for example, real-world drug utilization (e.g. compliance or preference) and treatment regimens (e.g. which doses are more common, dose per body weight in the wider community), patient characteristics, longer-term safety clinical outcomes, additional treatments, or, indeed, additional care. The longer-term side-effect data of oncology drugs are often limited in clinical trial databases. Moreover, once the drug is prescribed in a wider community setting, the treatment and management of the consequences of cancer treatments becomes apparent in hospitals or visits to GPs. For example, for a new drug with a novel mechanism of action such as palbociclib (Kish, 2018), an observational study was set up to examine the real-world occurrence of neutropenia and how providers monitored and managed these events (e.g. through dose modifications or other interventions or care). In a clinical trial, if neutropenia is severe enough, patients come off treatment and exit the trial if dose modifications fail. No further data is often collected when the patient leaves the trial. During the first year post-licensing, such types of data might be particularly important for economic evaluation.

The main reasons for generating RWE are:

(i) To enhance the external validity and generalizability of clinical trial evidence. Clinical trials may involve highly selected patients with limited follow-up.
(ii) It is sometimes impractical to conduct research in wider populations (not used in the main clinical trials because of heterogeneity introduced in the data and also the costs of running the trial). The recruitment challenges and costs associated with RCTs can be significant. Access to readily available data can be a much cheaper option. In any case, some form of data collection in trials might be considered burdensome (patients already have many other assessments) and intrusive.
(iii) To bridge the gap between the experimental and real-world setting by adding in the knowledge that RCTs are unable provide. In addition, longer-term prediction of event rates or outcomes can be made beyond the (limited) RCT follow-up. This is especially important for populating transition probability matrices used for Markov modeling.
(iv) Technology and computing power have increased substantially so that the generation of RWE is more feasible (large amounts of data on patients are readily available, yet nothing is being done with it to improve patient healthcare). The opportunity cost for not using the data is greater than for using it.

(v) To support claims or challenge claims such as: "response rates for drug A appear to be higher than drug B." The hope is that such claims (whether factual or embellished) will influence the prescribers or other groups, depending on the strength of evidence. A market access department has an objective to increase market share and the use of RWD is one means to this objective. The methodology for such claims should be rigorous.

(vi) Some licensing authorities (e.g. FDA) endorse gathering further data to support clinical trials when, for example, survival data are not mature (i.e. many patients are censored at the end of the study). Further follow-up might be needed to ensure survival rates (i.e. the primary efficacy endpoint) are sustained over a longer period. This might be part of a conditional approval process – where, so long as the manufacturer provides additional data, a license or reimbursement may be awarded.

(vii) To document the interconnection between the different sequential lines of therapy in oncology patients, which are often poorly documented or not documented at all in cancer RCTs.

In single arm trials, where there is limited evidence of efficacy, but a high unmet need or rare tumor population, follow-up data from patient registries could be used to complement clinical trial evidence (see Examples 6.1 and 6.2); one way might be to compare outcomes from a group of similar (matched) patients using RWD to those from the single arm trial. This use of real-world data might provide useful comparative evidence of safety and effectiveness for decision-makers. Another useful context might be in the case of 'promising' cancer medicines through early access schemes (such as EAMs). Here, a license may be provided 'quickly' under a special EAMS protocol (a document that states the conditions under which the treatment may be given). Data collection from such patients under routine clinical care could be generated for understanding the economic value of the treatment.

(viii) Where enhanced anti-tumor activity is observed in patients with some specific genetic (bio)marker, the number of patients might be limited in such subgroups. The proportion with or without a biomarker depends on the prevalence of the biomarker in the target population The potential to provide more evidence when the drug is used in the wider community can be realized by collecting such data from patient registries. However, this does require each patient having recorded in the registry the biomarker (or test) outcome (e.g. EGFR +ve or –ve) along with clinical and demographic data; or, at the very least, the ability to link the biomarker data with registry data that holds other clinical data merged (linked) through a common unique identifier (e.g. NHS number or health insurance number), or in some cases through probabilistic matching.

(ix) For generating evidence for cost-effectiveness and hence the value of the new treatment in real-world clinical practice. Real-world data sources can contain a variety of data not collected or not possible in clinical trials – such as elective and non-elective surgery, outpatient visits, GP visits – all of which might be related to the cost-effectiveness of the drug. Even where this is collected in an RCT using health resource CRFs, the data is limited to the trial follow-up and, as we noted earlier in Chapter 5, the data depends on retrospective recall.

Table 8.2 shows possible ways RWD could be used during pharmaceutical development.

8.3 Strengths and Limitations of Using RWD to Support Cost-Effectiveness Analysis

The strengths and limitations will depend on where the RWD are generated from (e.g. case control study, observational study, registry, administrative data). Camm and Fox (2018) provide a useful summary of the strengths and limitations of using RWD from various sources. The main strengths of RWD are: the wider populations studied; the ability to evaluate real-world effectiveness; a limited need, if any, for scheduled assessments; more treatments able to be compared, rather than just the comparators in the trial; and data captured at the point of care (or in real time). In particular, some larger databases have massive amounts of data that allow detailed interrogation of the relationship between multiple factors like treatment, outcomes, compliance, dosing, ethnicity, geography, social class, and so forth. Such large databases allow for the investigation of treatment benefit in some rare populations. The access to data can be relatively cheap and quick (in contrast to large expensive RCTs). Where healthcare resource use is available, the unit costs are also readily available (e.g. NHS reference costs in the UK, or from claims databases) and complement this, so that comprehensive economic evaluations can be performed.

RWE is also increasingly accepted by regulators and other bodies to support disease management and decision-making. It has been argued (Khoizin et al., 2017) that current FDA regulations support the use of evidence from emerging sources as evidence for making regulatory decisions. In 2008, the FDA launched the Sentinel Initiative in response to the FDA Amendments Act (FDAAA) calling for monitoring the safety of approved drugs and

TABLE 8.2

Possible Real-World Data Use During Drug Development

	Phase I	Phase II	Phase IIb/III	Launch Phase IV
Epidemiology and treatment patterns	Incidence of myeloma in population Incidence of biomarker mutation status		Source data sources and registries	Compare Phase III observed data with that expected in the general population
Trial design	Scoping of secondary source data for the target product profile	Feasibility of inclusion/exclusion	Feasibility of inclusion/exclusion	Real-world findings that have implications for altering or modifying the trial design in future/expanded indications
Health economics	Identify appropriate HRQoL measures HRQoL features that impact symptom and function		Burden to health system? Cost-efficiency and budget impact of new drug	
Post-marketing clinical evidence (therapeutic utilization, effectiveness)			How is the treatment used compared to alternatives?	How is the treatment used compared to alternatives? Real-world survival? Optimal duration of therapy? Subgroups
Post-marketing drug safety				Incidence of specific SAEs in usual care compared to RCT Comparative OS? e.g. at 1 year
Comparative effectiveness vs. usual care				Real-world benefit in a different tumor type; market size of new indication; potential long-term safety concerns to be evaluated using long-term studies or real-world data

medical products. In collaboration with insurers, universities, and hospitals, several surveillance reports have been generated using data contained in Sentinel's (FDA, 2017) network of claims and electronic health record- (EHR) related content.

In oncology, the Information Exchange and Data Transformation (INFORMED) initiative (FDA, 2018) is a multidisciplinary group focusing on building technical and organizational infrastructure in several key areas of 'big data' analytics to investigate how data from EHRs and digital health solutions can be used in making regulatory decisions. The 21st Century Cures Act in 2016 in the US also allowed for the potential use of RWD to support new product indications and post-approval requirements. In other words, whereas a post-approval clinical trial might have been conducted previously to gather evidence of longer-term efficacy and safety post-marketing, EHRs may be used as an alternative. However, a caveat in using RWE of this type is that it must still subscribe to scientific rigor in terms of study design and data collection (e.g. minimizing bias). Before discussing designing studies for gathering RWE, it is useful to determine where RWD will be collected from.

In Europe, the European Medicines Agency (EMA) does not dismiss the use of RWD out of hand. While it is acknowledged that such data cannot be used primarily as a basis for providing evidence of efficacy, they may be used to contextualize the evidence provided in a clinical trial. For example, if a single arm trial is conducted and reference to historical data is made, it may not be acceptable to compare a historical control arm using RWD of, say, several thousand patients with an experimental arm of 150 patients. For cost-effectiveness, however, because the decision-making framework is not always inferential (p-values do not matter), providing the biases were addressed as best as possible, expected net benefits could be generated to provide a direction of cost-effectiveness. As a caveat, just because the problem is not inferential, this does not mean that biased estimates of treatment effects should be used to justify cost-effectiveness.

8.3.1 Limitations

The main limitations of RWD are issues such as recall bias, loss to follow-up (censoring and missing data), selection, and other biases due to lack of randomization (for example, there may be limited data on some treatment due to clinical preference for one treatment over another). There can also be restrictions on the amount of data that may be extracted, and it can cost more, for example, to access 20 million records compared to 5,000. There is also a lot of additional programming time that may be needed, because data are not often collected at fixed time intervals, but as and when care is needed, and may also need complex extraction and linkage procedures.

A key issue in the use of EHRs is the quality of the data. This relates to the systematic and non-systematic bias (see Section 8.4) in the way the data have been collected (e.g. outcomes on only those who might attend a hospital). Registry data often have, for example, incoherent dates (e.g. date of death before a date of progression) and incoherent data collected – often left to be collected by untrained staff – whose main reason for collection is part of their administrative role, rather than with a research objective in mind. The coding of the data may also be erroneous (see 8.4.4) and therefore unreliable for inferential purposes.

In clinical trial data, rigorous data management and monitoring efforts are used to be able to verify the data source. Where EHRs are used, the fundamental principles of Good Clinical Practice – to be able to reconstruct the trial results may not be possible. The governance issues in 'source data verification' (i.e. making sure that the data in the records corresponds with patients'/doctors' notes) might require access to patients' personal records. In Europe, given the new GDPR directive, this will be difficult. Acceptance of data that does not conform to the basic principles of GCP may not be acceptable to regulatory agencies for establishing efficacy, but may be acceptable for reimbursement depending on what safeguards are in place to ensure an acceptable degree of data quality (e.g. more than 70% missing data is likely to be unacceptable).

However, if these biases can be limited and/or managed, use of RWD has potential for providing very valuable data on the longer term cost-effectiveness of many (expensive) cancer drugs.

8.3.2 Internal Validity versus Generalizability

The usual RCT framework provides strong internal validity of clinical findings (efficacy). The ideal conditions and assumptions in which trials are executed attempt to limit the plausibility of external factors influencing observed treatment benefit – in other words, yielding unbiased estimates of treatment effects. In reality, not all biases are quantified, and sometimes if a bias is there it may not even be known.

Although, strong internal validity is needed for experimental settings, the restrictive eligibility criteria can exacerbate differences in outcomes between patients in real practice and ideal settings, and consequently limit external validity. Hence, external validity needs to be strengthened so that results from experimental settings can be readily applied for the health of the general public (Steckler & McLeroy, 2008). This may also explain the reason why some reimbursement agencies treat the estimates of treatment effects from experimental trial conditions as being uncertain when there is a desire to generalize these effects to a wider population.

It is argued that a "balanced approach based on prospective collection of RWD can protect against common threats to internal validity" while at the same time augmenting the external validity of clinical research (Khozin et al., 2017). It would be misleading to believe, however, the impact of evidence from RCTs alone does not apply to a real-world setting. For example, an early phase RCT demonstrating the presence of a food effect, suggests treatment should be taken with food. If, in a real-world setting, patients do not take food, whether this is a limitation of the external validity of the trial or because patients simply don't follow clinical advice, is something that should be distinguished. A lack of treatment effect may be due to poorer drug absorption when taken with/without food. The adage 'read the label on the tin' applies to many products and services, and a treatment should not be penalized because elementary instructions for taking treatment have not been followed. This type of criticism of external validity is different to testing treatments in trials with specific populations (e.g. Caucasians) and then extrapolating to others (ethnic minorities).

A separate question is whether a trial should be designed for external validity alone. Let us take the above example on the food effect. If, in the real-world, patients are unlikely to take treatment with food, the question is whether regulatory agencies, such as the FDA and EMEA, should mandate food effect studies, because (after all) they don't reflect the real world. During Phase III, if patients are not going to follow the protocol, some patients who take food with the drug may have poorer clinical effects compared to those who do not take food (e.g. worse effects because the drug might be less well absorbed); one scenario (taking food) is reflective of the real world and one is not (take it according to the label). However, both situations (taking the drug with or without food) are reflective of the real-world setting. There will be patients who take drug according to the label and those who do not. Therefore, it may be very difficult to design trials that cover this type of internal and external validity. A related question is whether real-world studies themselves have credible internal validity and whether statistical methods can account for all the biases involved in estimating treatment effects to strengthen such internal validity.

8.4 Sources for RWD Generation

RWD can be determined from several sources including electronic health records, disease registries, and other sources of administrative data. RWD is sometimes used synonymously with electronic health records (EHR). Ultimately, all or most data is found in some form or another of an EHR. It is perhaps the way that it is populated in the EHR that is important: A definition focused on the original intent of data collected at the point of care can distinguish RWD from conventional clinical trial data. Where the purpose of collecting data is 'research,' then data can be gathered from a clinical trial or similar experimental design (with or without an intervention). A summary of the data sources for RWE generation is shown in Table 8.3.

TABLE 8.3

Sources of Real-World Data

Source	Example	Advantages	Disadvantages
National registries including primary care	Cancer registry SACT	Can be linked	Biases and confounding
	CPRD	Protocol required	Government regulations
	HES	Relevant records	Limited/no HRQoL data
	THIN	Natural disease history	Data quality issues
		Cheaper than a clinical trial	Missing data
		Large sample size	Costs more to extract large amounts
		Real time	Limited inference
		Useful for rare outcomes	Biased estimates
		Useful for economics	No randomization
		Quick access/studies	Switching between treatments
		Interrogate multiple associations	
Audit data/HER	Hospital consultants collect data	Cheaper than a clinical trial	Smaller sample sizes
		Based at hospital/point of care	Maybe single arm data
		Useful for economics	Data quality issues
		Real time outcomes	No randomization
		Useful if rare outcome is studied at site	Missing data
		Private/commercial companies	Private companies charge more
		Can pool across hospitals	
		prospective	
Observational studies	Prospectively designed	Prospective	No randomization
Retrospective		Defined outcomes	Loss to follow up

(*Continued*)

TABLE 8.3 (CONTINUED)

Sources of Real-World Data

Source	Example	Advantages	Disadvantages
		Cheaper than RCTs	Sample, observational and recall bias
		Useful for economics	Can require long follow-up for rare outcomes
Social media, internet logs	Twitter, blogs, internet, meta data	Cheap, easy access	Complicated/large amount to make sense
			Little HRQoL data
Administrative/claims database	Medicare/Medicaid	Longitudinal	Missing data
		Large database	Errors in coding/data quality
		Useful for economics	Confounding and bias
		Useful for rare tumors	Switching between treatments
		Quick studies – easy to access	
		Multiple associations	

8.4.1 Registries

Registries are national or public electronic health records (EHRs). These are essentially large repositories of data collected at the patient level. Examples of these in the UK include the National Cancer Registry (NCR), (see Section 8.5), Hospital Episodes Statistics (HES), systemic anti-cancer therapy (SACT) data. The HES data is an administrative source of data collected for commissioning purposes. In other countries, such as France or the US however, no comprehensive national cancer registry exists. Local registries do however exist (see for example: http://invs.santepubliquefrance.fr/surveillance/cancers/acteurs.htm.

In these registries/sources, patient-level data recording each episode of an event (e.g. death, hospitalization, adverse event) may be available. To use the data, a data dictionary might be needed because conditions are often coded using the international classification of diseases (ICD) or ICD-O (for oncology). It is also possible to link some registries (data) at the patient level. In the UK, the National Health Service number is a unique variable that allows merging across data sets such as HES, cancer registry data, cancer treatment data (SACT), and general practice (primary care) data. Particularly useful are linkages between cancer registries and official death records to assess cancer incidence and long-term survival. The registries may have restricted commercial use and, where used, a protocol (prior to authorization for data access) is often required. Moreover, charges for data extraction may also be levied and in many cases only aggregate data are made available because of national confidentiality regulations.

Some cancer registries increasingly collect important prognostic factors of survival useful for oncologists, policymakers, and others in order to make decisions on expected survival rates for subgroups of patients. For example, calculating the survival probability for an individual (or group of individuals) who is female, aged 50 (on average), with Stage III cancer, is a particularly useful statistic for policymakers and planners, especially for future costing of cancer treatments. However, in many countries, such as Belgium or France, survival data are not routinely collected/calculated in the cancer registries. In Section 8.5, cancer registries will be discussed in more detail.

Example 8.1: Real-World Data on Metastatic NSCLC from Canadian Cancer Registries

An example of an RWD study with cost-effectiveness implications was reported by Scherer et al. (2015). This study was undertaken to better understand the consequences of real-world chemotherapy patterns in NSCLC. Registries were identified in Canada (using the Ontario Cancer Registry) and were linked (merged) together. Patients were tracked using existing cancer registry data over several years (retrospectively). The data from each patient record included:

- Diagnosis date
- Institution and region of diagnosis
- Stage
- Pathology
- Age
- Sex
- Date of death

Treatment records included:

- The chemotherapy regimen
- Dose
- Treatment dates
- Treating hospital
- Line of therapy
- Radiotherapy treatment dates and doses

Oral agents, performance status, and comorbidities were not systematically included in these databases. After linking databases, and performing statistical analyses, the researchers concluded the following:

- Most patients with (metastatic) NSCLC in the general Canadian population did not receive systemic therapy.
- Patients selected for first- and second-line systemic treatment, had survival outcomes comparable to clinical trial results.
- Older patients and patients with squamous histology are less likely to receive chemotherapy.

The policy implications were:

- *To ensure all patients with newly diagnosed advanced NSCLC receive timely consultation with a trained oncologist.*
- *The gap between the diagnosis and the initial oncology consultation in this study was 30 days. In a disease such as metastatic NSCLC, with often short survival and where patients deteriorate clinically, 30 days should be reduced; this might improve the number of patients who are candidates for systemic therapy.*
- *An increased use of screening methods for NSCLC in at-risk populations might be needed.*
- *To further investigate other unknown factors contributing to low treatment rates – and consequently to improve treatment access and outcomes in this population.*

8.4.2 Audits

Many researchers collect data on cancer patients at secondary care sites (hospitals). These data are often used for auditing, or assessing the quality or performance of, for example, cancer treatment delivery at specific hospitals. Although data from hospital registries tends to be rich, and often contain key cancer outcomes, unfortunately some audit data sets are limited to small sample sizes, limiting their generalizability. To strengthen generalizability, similar data sets would need to be merged together to address a study question. Wilson (1999) differentiates audit and research: "research is finding out what you ought to be doing; audit is whether you are doing what you ought to be doing."

The primary aim of research is to derive knowledge that is new and generalizable, with clearly defined questions, aims, and objectives for which there is often a well-written protocol detailing the methodology. An audit, on the other hand, is a way of understanding whether cancer treatment or care is reaching a defined standard. The treatment itself is defined (unlike in research where it could be randomized). Hence, when a new treatment is licensed and is considered to be the standard of care, data from a clinical audit might be useful to determine whether the standard of care is being reached. Outcomes such as survival may also be collected.

Example 8.2: Lenalidomide Alternative Dose Proposal for Treating Multiple Myeloma

As an example, the lenalidomide alternative dose proposal (Popat et al., 2015) used audit data to gather evidence in 39 patients on whether alternate dosing was a potentially a more cost-effective dosing regimen compared to daily dosing, without impacting survival benefit. This example was discussed earlier in the context of modeling (Chapter 4, Example 4.5). Its relevance in the context of RWD shows how it may be possible for non-trial data to be used to propose a more cost-effective dosing regimen with the view that efficacy is not compromised.

8.4.3 Primary Care Databases: CPRD, THIN, QResearch

The Clinical Practice Research Datalink (CPRD) database was established in 1987 in the UK.. It operates as part of the UK Department of Health. It covers more than 644 general practice databases, exceeding 13 million patient records and covering about 7% of the general UK population. It offers the ability to extract anything adequately recorded in primary care.

The Health Improvement Network (THIN) database was established in around 2003. The database consists of data from over 560 practices exceeding 11 million patients or about 6% of the UK populations. There is some overlap with the CPRD, although there may be more efficient patient matching for sociodemographic characteristics.

QResearch is a collaboration with the University of Nottingham containing data from over 754 practices consisting of over 13 million patients (about 7% of the UK population).

In all the above primary care databases, patient-level data is available on clinical and demographic characteristics, disease status, and other treatment details in primary care settings. Typical examples might include data on diabetes management. The CPRD can also be linked with cancer registries.

8.4.4 Insurance Claims Databases

In the US, there are claims databases, or databases that consist of EHRs of millions of transactions between patients and healthcare providers, including hospitals, nursing homes, and pharmacies (Ferver, 2009). In general they tend to be used by health insurance companies to decide the risks associated with groups of patients and whether cover should be offered. Ferver et al. (2009) have provided a very useful summary of how claims data are used, outlining their strengths (anonymous, cheap, plentiful, widely available in an electronic format, and useful for identifying rare subgroups) and limitations (the databases were not designed for research, non-essential data for billing is often excluded, there is missing information from some claims, health resource use is incorrectly classified, chronic diseases are underreported because only one diagnosis is enough for a reimbursement). The databases nevertheless contain much information on healthcare resource use, covering many disease areas including cancer, however, as in the case of any registry, the potential for confounding and bias exists and robust methodology should be used in the analysis of this type of data (Ferver et al., 2009).

8.4.5 Digital Data Sources, Social Media and Applications

In recent years, phenomenal growth in information technology solutions has offered a means to develop an integrated approach for generating RWE from EHRs and other data sources, such as mobile applications and internet search logs. Because of the dynamic way in which data processing works, using digital applications (apps) with web-based analytical tools may enable earlier detection of adverse events or disease progression, than can be obtained in clinical trials. Since clinical trials collect data at specified discrete time points, coinciding with scheduled visits, the opportunity for identifying the consequences of such events is delayed. The type of data available could include patients taking medication for treating adverse reactions, taking subsequent therapy, delaying subsequent therapy, missing a potential tumor progression, or reporting worsening HRQoL (perhaps an indication of disease progression). These data may have implications for cost-effectiveness. RCTs that use web-based tools showed potential for several health benefits including close monitoring of symptoms (Basch et al., 2017; Denis et al., 2017).

Example 8.3: Example of Digital Real-World Web-Mediated Follow-Up Compared with Routine Surveillance in NSCLC Patients

This example is taken from Denis et al. (2017). Patients with NSCLC were randomly assigned to web-mediated follow-up (experimental) or usual follow-up while taking their usual maintenance chemotherapy, or TKI, or no treatment. Patients were followed-up in both arms every three months. CT scans were more frequent in the control group compared to web-mediated follow-up because the web-based application was found to be reliable in detecting patient relapse as a result of self-evaluated symptoms assessed weekly. The trial results reported in Denis et al. (2017) showed improved survival in patients using the web-based follow-up (called e-FAP) compared to patients in the control group. The e-FAP also reported a decrease in the number of imaging tests (which would lead to a reduction in health resource costs).

8.4.6 Commercial Data Sources

More recently, private initiatives and collaborations with health researchers have developed and enabled wider access to real-world data. However, there are often strict governance issues on the commercialization of what is in effect data that belong to the public. Audit data may effectively be used as research where there is an agreed partnership with local investigators (e.g. offering small grants), and strong methodology is used to ensure factors such as bias has been adequately assessed. Some national charities, non-profit organizations, and patient society networks also collect data. In some larger national registries, an absence of HRQoL makes their use for an economic evaluation limited. National charities and patient networks may have the potential to offer or collect this type of data.

Access to patients and their records for nonclinical purposes has been and will continue to remain under scrutiny. Although research ethics committees (REC) safeguard access to patient data for research purposes, audits are often below the radar, unless the database is available on a larger scale. Guidelines published by the UK Royal College of Physicians recommend submission to a research ethics committee if doubt exists about whether a project is audit or research.

8.4.7 Pragmatic Clinical Trials

Another source of real-world type data is through the conduct of a pragmatic RCT. In such a trial, observation and follow-up of patients is carried out under a routine clinical setting. For example, rather than stipulating in the trial protocol that scans will occur every two months, scans occur according to routine practice. Additional tests specified in a trial protocol may not be undertaken in routine practice. In short, the main difference between a pragmatic RCT and a highly controlled RCT is the degree of experimental control involved in conducting the trial. Patients in a pragmatic RCT (PRCT) may have less restrictive inclusion/exclusion criteria. PRCTs are designed to produce results that uniquely support clinical decision-making at the point of care (Kish, 2018; Khozin, 2017). Since PRCTs are conducted in the real world, data collected may form part of the usual administrative process for recording and entry. A trial conducted in this setting, providing that the technology is available, and data security and integrity are preserved, is likely to yield rich data, including HRQoL (e.g. through the use of mobile phone applications), and data on health resource use. HRQoL are rarely available in cancer registries. A well design PRCT using EHRs can "bring the real-world evidence base to drug development while driving the focus on improving quality, patient safety, and value in cancer care delivery" although their cost may be high (Khozin et al., 2017).

8.4.8 Prospective Observational Research Studies

Observational studies were discussed in Chapter 6. New hypotheses can be generated from observational studies as supportive evidence for reimbursement agencies (in some cases this is specifically requested by agencies who might wish to have more data on longer-term outcomes. Longer-term assessment of safety, effectiveness, patients excluded in conventional cancer trials, patients with poor performance status, history of prior malignancies, organ dysfunction, or other metastases (e.g. brain) can be evaluated. Evidence also suggests that well-designed and well-conducted observational studies can yield results similar to those in RCTs. This might be an opportunity for building capability and methods in using EHR-based observational research to enhance generalizability (Anglemyer et al., 2014; Konnerup et al., 2012; Vázquez et al., 2015). In Section 8.4, an example of how data from a real-world observational study is analyzed and reported is given.

8.4.9 Case Control Studies

Case control studies make use of EHRs because of their retrospective nature. Even if a group of patients with the outcome (e.g. disease progression) in question are followed up for other data, they can be matched uniquely (1:1 matching) to a patient control (another patient without the disease or outcome, but who is otherwise 'identical' in terms of age, gender, and other characteristics). A single patient in the group with the disease or outcome of interest (case) can be matched with several (*m*:1, many-to-one matching) historical cases. Alternatively, several cases can be matched to several controls (m:n many-to-many matching). These studies are less expensive to conduct and more efficient especially for rare diseases or outcomes, and where time to an outcome is long (e.g. long-term death or toxicity). Clearly, the data will be subject to selection bias, and information on outcomes and treatments is likely to be subject to observation bias. In addition, incidence (new events or outcomes) cannot be computed. Special statistical methods for analyzing such data are needed.

8.5 Using Cancer Registries

Cancer registries have their own unique history. The first-known systematic collection of cancer data was the general census of cancer in London in 1728 (Hutchinson et al., 2004). Since then registries have developed further (e.g.

TABLE 8.4
Cancer Registries in Several Countries

Country	Years	Details	Coverage	Sample for NSCLC	Coding
Denmark	From 1943	Inpatient/outpatient oncology	Nationwide	>23,000	ICD-10
France	From 1997	All tumors	Regional	>900,000	ICD-O-3
Germany	From 1998	General population	Bavaria	>12 million	ICD-10
Italy	From 2012	NSCLC	General	>2,500	ICD-10
Norway	From 1973	General population	General	>317,000	ICD-10

1842 in Verona, 1913 in Chicago), such that in the early 1900s cancer registries were used to systematically track the etiology and survival of cancer patients. Their ubiquitous capabilities led them to being developed in several Western European countries. Table 8.4 gives examples of several cancer registries in several countries (there can be multiple registries in each country).

Merging data is likely to be highly complex. However, the data could be analyzed locally to furnish evidence across countries. It is often the case that economic evidence is required at the local level and hence local registries used. However, it is possible that evidence from a registry in one country might be admissible in another, especially where the target population is similar. However, the differences in health systems will make the quantification of health resources more challenging.

How Registries Work in Brief

For a national cancer registry, each cancer and its subtype are coded using ICD low-level codes, of which there are several thousands (updates to these codes are made yearly). The 2018 ICD-10 codes for cancer, termed 'neoplasms' are coded as C00-D49. For example, a code of C00-C14 in the registry will have information on malignant neoplasms of lip, oral cavity, and pharynx, which are then further divided into other subtypes.

- C00 Malignant neoplasm of lip
- C01 Malignant neoplasm of base of tongue
- C02 Malignant neoplasm of other and unspecified ...
- C03 Malignant neoplasm of gum
- C04 Malignant neoplasm of floor of mouth
- C05 Malignant neoplasm of palate
- C06 Malignant neoplasm of other and unspecified ...

- C07 Malignant neoplasm of parotid gland
- C08 Malignant neoplasm of other and unspecified
- C09 Malignant neoplasm of tonsil
- C10 Malignant neoplasm of oropharynx
- C11 Malignant neoplasm of nasopharynx
- C12 Malignant neoplasm of pyriform sinus
- C13 Malignant neoplasm of hypopharynx

The potentially rich patient-level of data in cancer registries covers a wide spectrum of tumor types. So, for example, if someone wanted to determine the incidence of a given cancer, the number of occurrences of a given code between two consecutive years divided by the population might be extracted.

8.5.1 Examples of Registries in the UK for RWE

In the UK there is a unified healthcare system with multiple sources of rich data across primary and secondary care settings. There are also strong academic registries supported politically through 'big data' in health philosophy. EHRs are used extensively in primary care and there is an impetus to use these extensively in secondary care. The challenges revolve around private access to public healthcare data, lack of a consistent and clear method of access, inability to link databases together, and a complicated governance structure with a cautious attitude toward RWE by regulators or payers. For example, lung cancer data can be obtained from the National Cancer Registration Service (NCRS). Different files exist that contain patient-level data on:

- Radiotherapy
- Chemotherapy
- Imaging (scans)
- Primary care
- Hospital episodes (resource use)
- Specific cancer data
- Genetic data (biobank)
- National Lung Cancer Audit Lung Cancer Data (e.g. previously held by University of Nottingham), which details chemotherapy
- SACT data set, which consists of five sections (demographics, clinical status, treatment regimen, number of cycles, details of drugs such as reductions, and outcomes such as death and disease progression)

In Europe, the commercial availability of RWD is limited. In oncology, most data is used for market research (e.g. number of prescription sales) and currently not very suitable for evidence generation. Companies are now creating strategic portals for accessing data to support market access groups. Some Nordic registries can be accessed through commercial companies, whereas access to some public cancer data sets require academic partnerships.

8.6 Statistical Analyses of RWD: Addressing Selection Bias

As noted above, RWD has potential for much confounding and bias. Selection bias might occur when the chance of receiving treatment differs between patients; and, moreover, the characteristics (e.g. age, gender) are also related (confounded) with outcomes. Selection bias is likely to lead to incorrect conclusions that treatment effects are generalizable. Confounding occurs where an outcome (death) might be associated with an independent factor (treatment) and consequently thought to be causal (treatment effects from good quality RCTs are considered to be causal), but if the measure of treatment effect is influenced by a third factor (ECOG), a valid estimate of treatment effect cannot be determined, unless we know about ECOG status. In this case, ECOG status is said to be a confounder. As an example, suppose it was observed in a cohort of people that many of those who drank alcohol died from lung cancer. One might think that alcohol is more likely to be related to liver cancer. However, there is a confounder – a third factor, smoking. Since those who drink more alcohol also tend to smoke, smoking is the confounding factor leading one to incorrectly conclude that alcohol 'causes' lung cancer. Therefore, some specific statistical methods and designs are used for the analyses of data from registries and observational studies to control for selection bias, mainly:

(i) Propensity score modeling
(ii) Instrumental variable methods

A general overview of methods for selection bias correction can be found in Keeble et al. (2015).

8.6.1 Propensity Score Modeling

Comparing treatment differences in RWD studies will be influenced by differences in baseline characteristics. The propensity score approach allows one way of adjusting treatment differences to take into account the (known) baseline differences. Without delving into the technicality of these models (see bibliography and references therein), propensity score models (PSM) involve modeling the treatment received in terms of the baseline characteristics (Pan & Bai, 2015; Guo & Fraser, 2014).

In the case of two treatments, patients that receive treatment (exposed to treatment) may be coded as 1 and those that do not (controls) are coded as 0. These outcomes are then modeled using a multivariate logistic model (for more than one treatment, a multinomial approach can be used). We are in fact modeling the chance of receiving treatment given (conditional on) what we know about baseline characteristics. In an RCT (1:1 allocation), the chance of receiving treatment is expected to be equal (regardless of patient characteristic).

In RWD, it is not uncommon to find unequal numbers of patients in a cancer registry taking either the experimental treatment (once approved) or the standard of care. The systematic nature of the unequal numbers receiving treatment may be related to some baseline characteristic (e.g. Stage III, poor performance status) – thereby violating the idea that patients have an equal chance of receiving treatment. It may well be possible that 80% of males receive treatment A and 90% of females receive treatment B, which complicates a comparison between treatment A and B.

Example 8.3: Propensity Score Modeling Using Data from a Cancer Registry

The following data (Table 8.5) are reported from a cancer registry. There are two types of treatment: chemotherapy (C) alone and chemotherapy in combination radiotherapy (C+R). Five-year survival rates from lung cancer patients are of interest. Several baseline/clinical characteristics (age, gender, ECOG, stage) are included in this fictitious example. The objective is to compare nonrandomized C with C+R in terms of 5-year survival rates using data from linked registries.

Selection bias is first addressed by a straightforward comparison of the data in the registry. Some imbalance in the baseline characteristics is observed (Table 8.5).

As can be observed in Table 8.5, there are statistically significant imbalances in the baseline clinical characteristics that may lead to confounding and potentially misleading conclusions when comparing survival rates between C versus C+R. It is also important to note that with such large sample sizes, the p-value will be small. Hence, attention should be paid to the magnitude of any differences. A propensity score (PS) analysis will be performed that allows for differences between groups.

The first step is to derive the propensity score. Hence, we model the treatment group (C or C+R) in terms of the covariates using a logistic regression model. In this case:

$$\textbf{Treatment Group}(\textbf{C}/\textbf{C}+\textbf{R}) = \textbf{Age, Gender, ECOG, Stage}$$

From this model, a propensity score is computed for each patient. We compare the baseline characteristics and the 5-year survival rates,

TABLE 8.5

Comparison of Clinical Characteristics Using Cancer Registry Data

	C (N = 4,217)	C+R (N = 2,687)	*p*-Value
Age (years)	68.7	74.6	$p < 0.0001$
Gender:			
Male	2,911 (69%)	1,564 (58%)	$p < 0.0001$
Female	1,306 (31%)	1,123 (42%)	
ECOG			
0	2,145 (51%)	1,852 (69%)	$p < 0.0001$
1	1,347 (32%)	575 (21%)	
2	725 (17%)	260 (10%)	
Stage			
I	1,441 (34%)	1,021 (38%)	$p = 0.0345$
II	2,542 (60%)	1,575 (59%)	
III–IV	234 (6%)	91 (3%)	
5-year survival rates	25%	39%	$p < 0.001$ Odds ratio = 1.91

adjusting for the PS in the model. The propensity scores can be categorized (e.g. using quantiles) or included as a continuous covariate when adjusting for the difference between C versus C+R. The results in Table 8.6 show what happens when the propensity scores are included in a statistical model when comparing 5-year survival rates. The model is of the form:

$$\textbf{Survival (yes / no)} = \textbf{Treatment, PS, Age, Gender, ECOG, Stage}$$

As can be seen from Table 8.6, without adjusting for differences in baseline characteristics, the 5-year survival rates appear to be 91% higher with C+R versus C (OR = 1.91). After adjusting for PS as a continuous outcome, this difference is no longer statistically significant and falls to 54% higher for C+R versus C. The differences in baseline characteristics may well have contributed toward a higher favorable treatment for C+R.

Example 8.4: Performing a Propensity Score Model Using Matching to Compare Health Resource Determined from a Cancer Registry

A researcher wishes to understand how various factors and health resource use differ between patients treated with existing standard chemotherapies in multiple myeloma patients. Data from linked registries were used. A sample of 937,182 patients who received the current standard of care (control) and 44,215 patients who received an alternative treatment (CAP: chemotherapy for advanced prostate cancer) were extracted from the linked Hospital Episodes (HES) database and linked with cancer registry data. The registry also contained many potential confounding variables including age, gender, ECOG, and hospital site.

TABLE 8.6

Comparison of Clinical Characteristics Using Cancer Registry Data Adjusting for PS

	Odds ratio	95% CI	*p*-Value
Unadjusted	1.91	1.06, 3.58	0.028
Adjusted for PS (continuous)	1.54	0.95, 3.12	0.078
Adjusted for PS (categorical)	1.58	0.97, 3.22	0.069

TABLE 8.7

Data Structure for Example 8.3 Prior to Matching

Patient	Age	Gender	ECOG	Site	Comorbidity	Treatment
1	65	Male	2	1	Yes	Control
2	59	Female	3	2	Yes	Control
3	44	Male	3	3	No	Control
937,182	..	..	..	..	..	Control
1	45	Male	3	1	Yes	CAP
2	55	Male	2	2	No	CAP
3	65	Female	1	3	Yes	CAP
..	..	..	..	..	..	..
44,215	..	..	..	..	..	..

An important question to answer from the data is how hospital admissions and other health resources (e.g. elective admissions, nonelective admissions, etc.) differ between CAP and control groups. An example of the data structure prior to matching is shown in Table 8.7.

In this example, 36,386 CAP patients randomly selected from 44,215 were matched to the same number of controls of which there were 937,182 (Table 8.8).

Step 1: Matching:

In order to perform the matching, several options are available:

(i) 1:1 matching. We could take a sample of patients from the 937,182 controls available in the registry who are identical in every respect to those that were treated. For each patient who was treated, say aged 50, with ECOG of 2, and male, we will seek to match an identical patient who takes the control treatment. The more factors there are to match, the harder it may be to get a matched patient.

(ii) Many-to-1 matching. Here there may be several control patients who are similar to the ones treated. Hence, we could have two patients taking the control treatment for each treated (with a different treatment) patient.

(iii) m:n matching, A third type of matching is called many-to-many (m:n) matching). Where there is an abundance of those taking treatment and control (as is the case in some large national registries), this might be used.

TABLE 8.8

Summary of Baseline Characteristics

	Prior to Matching			Post-Matching			
	CAP (N = 44,215)	Control (N = 937,182)	*p*-Value	CAP (N = 36,386)	Control (N = 36,386)	*p*-Value	Standardized Difference
Age (years)	70.7	78.6	$p < 0.0001$	79.1	79.5	0.0327	0.0215
Gender:							
Male	23,911 (54%)	525,514 (56%)	$p < 0.0001$	17,432 (48.2%)	17,524 (48%)	0.631	0.0051
Female	20,304 (46%)	411,668 (44%)		18,862 (51.8%)	18,954 (52.1%)	0.622	0.0051
ECOG							
0	523 (1%)	12,852 (1%)	$p < 0.0001$	456 (1.3%)	444 (1.2%)	0.689	0.0030
1	1,347 (3%)	37,520 (4%)		969 (2.7%)	1,167 (3.2%)	<0.001	0.0322
2	40,206 (91%)	813,570 (87%)		33,210 (91.3%)	33,128 (91%)	0.750	0.0079
3	90 (<1%)	2,733 (<1%)		79 (<1%)	68 (<1%)	0.364	0.0067
>3	2,049 (5%)	70,507 (7%)		1,672 (4.5%)	1,579 (4.3%)	0.128	0.0054
Comorbidity Yes	14,222 (32%)	234,327 (25%)	$p < 0.0001$	11,779 (32.4%)	11,849 (32.6%)	0.648	0.0041

Once the matched data sets are formed, the success of matching needs to be determined, and then followed by estimates of treatment effects using propensity score methods shown in Example 8.3.

Step 2: Evaluate the successfulness of matching:

Table 8.6 shows the summary statistics for all patients before and after matching. For such large sample sizes, the p-value is small, even after matching, where the mean matched age is 79.1 versus 79.5 years (p = 0.0327). Therefore, the standardized difference (SDiff) should be used, which should be <0.10 for a conclusion of no difference in baseline characteristics between groups as evidence for successfulness of matching. In this case the SDiff is 0.0215, suggesting patients are matched on age between CAP versus control groups.

Table 8.8 shows the following:

(a) Prior to matching, the baseline factors were imbalanced showing strong statistical differences (even when the differences were small, such as gender). There were more comorbidities in the treated group ($p < 0.001$).
(b) After taking a matched control group so that we have 36,386 patients in each group who are as similar as possible, the baseline characteristics are now somewhat balanced. The propensity scores (Figure 8.1) confirm this. In Figure 8.1b the propensity scores are practically superimposed between CAP and control after matching.

This propensity scores in Figure 8.1 are determined by modeling the treatment group assignment related to covariates as before in Example 8.3. The model generates a propensity score (PS) for each patient. This score will be used to adjust the differences in outcomes such as survival at 5 years and health resource use between treatment groups.

Step 3: Use the matched samples to compare groups and draw inferences.

Under the assumption that matching has been successful so that valid comparisons from nonrandomized samples can be made, we model the

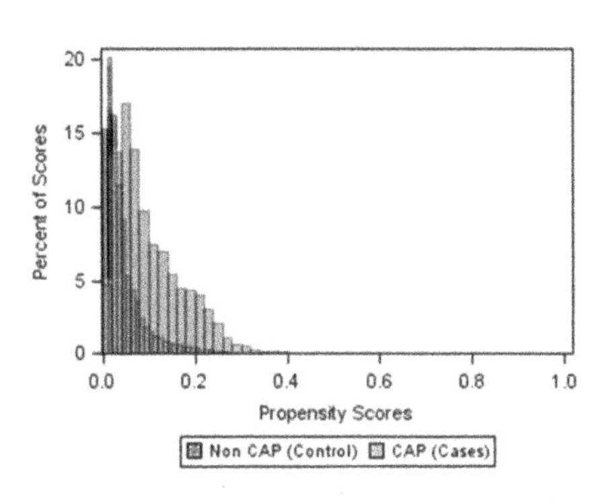

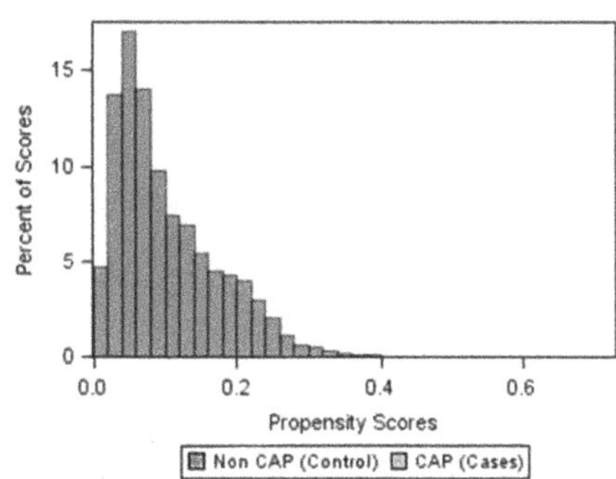

FIGURE 8.1
(a) Prior to matching, and (b) post-matching propensity scores.

response or outcome of interest in the usual way and adjust for the propensity scores.

Hence, we would use the treatment group (matched samples of 36,386 per group) for our usual statistical analysis. There are several health resource items of interest: elective admissions, nonelective admissions, bed stays, outpatient appointments, and emergency attendance. Since we are modeling the frequency of these occurrences, we will be interested in either the mean count or incidence of using a given health resource. That is, we might be interested in the mean number of elective admissions or an incidence rate ratio. If the incidence rate ratio (the ratio of the mean counts) is, for example, 1.19, this is interpreted as a 19% increase in the rate of usage of that particular health resource item.

Table 8.9 shows the results using two types of models: a two-part hurdle model and a negative binomial model (NBM). The main difference between the hurdle model and a model such as the NBM is that for count models (i.e. NBM) values equal to zero and greater than zero are assumed to come from the same data-generating process. For a hurdle model, these two processes are not considered to be the same. The hurdle approach models (as a mixture of two distributions): first whether a health resource value is zero or not, and second, whether the 'hurdle' is crossed, the conditional distribution (conditional on crossing zero) is modeled. However, if it is the case that data have been collected from hospital records, then it may be unrealistic to assume that zero health resource use is a plausible value. Consequently, if zeros are not plausible values, an alternative model, such as a generalized linear model (GLM), assuming a Gamma distribution could be used (Khan, 2015). Further details of hurdle models and negative binomial models can be found in Khan (2015) and Agresti (2013).

The mean number of elective admissions determined from the hurdle model for those taking treatment was 4.78 elective admissions compared to about 3.58 elective admissions ($p < 0.0001$) for the control (Table 8.9). Hence, the incidence of elective admissions was 19% higher for those treated compared to those not treated with the chemotherapy of interest. When using a negative binomial model, the conclusion was the same but with a slightly higher incidence. Note how the mean (count) number of elective admissions differs between the models, but the ratio is similar. This is reflected in the way the models compute effects.

Note also that the propensity score is included as part of the adjustment into the model. The uncertainty of the incidence of elective admissions was expressed in terms of the 95% CI: the true increase in the number of elective admissions for those with treatment compared to untreated range somewhere between 16% to 21% for the hurdle model and 19% to 32% for the negative binomial model. The hurdle model appears to model the within and between subject variability better, resulting in lower standard errors.

8.6.2 Instrumental Variable Methods

In addition to the various types of propensity score modeling methods for handling selection bias, another technique called the instrumental variable

TABLE 8.9

Statistical Modeling of Treatment vs. Standard of Care Health Resource Use (Hurdle and Negative Binomial Models) on Matched Data

	Hurdle Model				Negative Binomial Model			
Health Resource Item	**Treated Mean (SE)**	**Control Mean (SE)**	**Incidence Rate Ratio (95% CI)**	***p*-Value[a]**	**Treated Mean (SE))**	**Control Mean (SE)**	**Incidence Rate Ratio (95% CI)**	***p*-Value[b]**
Elective Admissions	4.34 (0.024)	3.58 (0.022)	1.19 (1.16, 1.21)	<.0001	2.57 (0.121)	2.13 (0.097)	1.25 (1.19, 1.32)	<.0001
Nonelective admissions	2.55 (0.002)	2.04 (0.002)	1.24 (1.22, 1.27)	<.0001	1.28 (0.018)	1.21 (0.014)	1.27 (1.24, 1.30)	<.0001
Bed stays	24.99 (0.023)	17.06 (0.015)	1.46 (1.45, 1.47)	<.0001	3.47 (0.151)	2.10 (0.090)	1.67 (1.61, 1.74)	<.0001
Outpatient appointments	8.97 (0.011)	8.10 (0.010)	1.09 (1.09, 1.10)	<.0001	4.40 (0.092)	3.71 (0.082)	1.13 (1.11, 1.15)	<.0001
A&E attendances	2.71 (0.003)	2.20 (0.000)	1.23 (1.20, 1.25)	<.0001	1.28 (0.018)	1.22 (0.015)	1.25 (1.23, 1.28)	<.0001

[a] *Notes:* Using a hurdle model adjusted for covariates without adjustment for multiplicity.
[b] Using a negative binomial model adjusted for covariates.

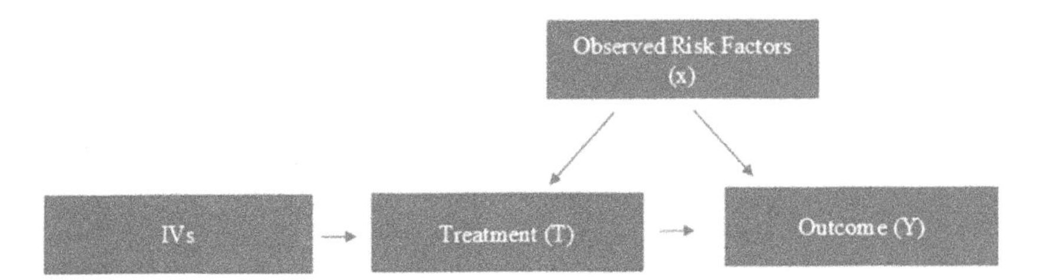

FIGURE 8.2
Description of instrumental variables methods.

(IV) method can be used. Methods such as those described above (e.g. propensity models) use observed variables (age, gender, etc.) to adjust for selection bias. IV methods assume that there is a set of unobserved factors that influence treatment received and confounding. Figure 8.2 shows how IVs are represented.

Observed factors (X) may influence both treatment received and outcome. Usual methods (regression or propensity score models) can deal with confounding for observed factors, but not unobserved factors. IV methods aim to find instruments correlated with treatment selection but not directly with outcome. An example is summarized from Faries et al. (2010).

Example 8.4: Example of IV: Comparison of Compliance Rates

This example is adapted from Faries et al. (2010) :

- A number of observed potential confounders (**X**) were collected (age, gender, number of previous drugs, number of complete cycles of treatment). These were different between the two drugs. Therefore, it was assumed that if differences existed between treatments A and B for observed variables, such differences could also exist for unobserved variables.
- The outcome was compliance rates (cycles of chemotherapy completed) (**Y**).
- Instrumental variable (**IV**) was the prescribing preference of clinicians. The most recent prescription (treatment A or B) was a dichotomous variable. Those who were newly prescribed to A or B were likely to be influenced by their cancer consultant/prescriber.
- Patients who had been recently prescribed were extracted from databases (N = 1,426 of which N = 611 took drug A and N = 815 drug B).
- Selection bias was likely to exist because the two treatments had different toxicity profiles. This would influence both patient and clinician choice.
- Traditional methods (regression) may not have estimated the treatment effect on the outcome properly.
- The objective was to compare compliance rates between two drugs (cancer drugs) over a 6-month period.

TABLE 8.10

Summary of Baseline Factors and Compliance

	A (N = 611)	B (N = 815)	
Age (years)	55.5	56.0	
Gender:			
Male	56%	54%	
Female	44%	46%	
No. of previous therapies	2.1	2.3	
No. completed all cycles (mean)[a] (Y)	66%	59%	P = 0.0071
Preference for drug (IV)	47%	53%	OR=3.44 (95% CI: 2.76, 4.29)

[a] *Note:* For each patient, the number of cycles received divided by the planned number of cycles expressed as a percentage.

Results

Table 8.10 summarizes the results of the IV method.

The unadjusted mean compliance (%) was statistically different. This could indicate better cancer management with A compared to B and how prescribing is done in practice. However, since we suspect that selection bias persists due to clinician bias in prescribing, an IV modeling approach is used to disentangle persisting bias.

In Table 8.10, the values of 53% and 47% suggest the IV is predictive of prescriber preference (A appears to be preferred more). The next thing is to check the relationship between the IV and the observed factors (X) – i.e. we check the independence assumption (e.g. if prescribers are giving more females drug A than drug B). The results of a comparison between the models (raw, adjusted using regression, and IV model are compared in Table 8.11). Compliance rates between drugs for the raw unadjusted values were: 66% versus 59%; after using standard regression techniques adjusted for observed confounders this was 67% versus 61%; using an IV model this was 73% versus 72% (Table 8.11). Clearly, compared to the unadjusted case where all patients were assumed to have used drug A, the IV model provided more comparative compliance rates. In some cases (Brookhart et al., 2006; Landrum & Ayani, 2001), differences can be much larger between unadjusted and IV models.

In summary, standard regression methods use observed factors to adjust for confounding. IV models make use of an IV variable that models both observed and unobserved factors. This can be very important because, despite propensity matching appearing successful, a question that often comes up is "have you controlled for the unobserved confounders?" An important challenge in using IV models is how an instrument is determined

TABLE 8.11

Comparison of Average Compliance for Each Model

Model	Treatment	Compliance (Mean) (%)	95% CI (%)	*p*-Value
Unadjusted (raw values)				
	A	66		
	B	59		
	Difference	7	(1.9, 12.1)	0.007
Regression	A	67		
	B	61		
	Difference	6	(0.9, 11.1)	0.0095
IV	A	73		
	B	72		
	Difference	1	(–3.6, 5.7)	0.0676

and validated. In the above example, it was assumed that the prescriber's last prescription preference affected the subsequent patient's prescription. The assumption that the previous patient's prescription is related to the next patient's choice of treatment is likely to be untenable.

Example 8.5: Cost-Effectiveness Analysis of Potentially Curative and Combination Treatments for Hepatocellular Carcinoma with Person-Level Data in a Canadian Setting (Thein et al., 2017; Cancer Medicine, 2017; 6(9):2017–2033).

In this example, the cost-effectiveness of various combination treatments for hepatocellular carcinoma (HCC) is evaluated using the Ontario Cancer Registry, using linked administrative data. The sample size used was 2,222, of which about 11% received radiofrequency ablation (RFA), 14% had surgical resection (SR), and 10% received liver transplantation (LT) monotherapy; a further 53% received no treatment (control). Hence the comparison was between RFA, SR, and LT alone (monotherapies), or in some combination, versus control.

The ICD-9 classification was used to identify patients with the code 155.0 along with other codes for histology (codes 8170–8175). The period of data extraction was between January 1, 2002 and December 31, 2010. Hence diagnosis of HCC should be on or after January 1, 2002. In brief, a summary of this analysis is:

- Health resource use: this was obtained from previously published sources. This included items such as outpatient visits, emergency department visits, acute inpatient hospitalizations, surgeries, medicines, home visits, and long-term care.
- Effectiveness data: the date between diagnosis and death – obtained from the registry. The utility data were based on a separate published sources.

- Estimation of effectiveness: the statistical methodology used propensity models to address selection bias and multiple imputation to address missing data.
- Cost-effectiveness: the cost-effectiveness was determined using a net benefit approach, using the derived QALYs, which were obtained by weighting survival time with utility (taking into account disease stage). Other issues such as multicollinearity (when independent variables are correlated) were also addressed.
- The results show that RFA in combination with transarterial chemoembolization (TACE) have a high chance of cost-effectiveness (probability of 100%) when compared to no treatment (cost/QALY of $2,465); while RFA alone versus no treatment gave a cost/QALY of $15,553.

The above example shows the possibility of using real-world data to reach an important cost-effectiveness conclusion that alternative treatment options for HCC, which offer good value for money, should be considered. The study was not free from limitations, such as limited long-term effectiveness beyond 9 years, and the impact of the stage of HCC. Hence when data are not available in a registry, the conclusions will be restricted.

8.7 Summary and Conclusion

The use of RWD has become increasingly common for conducting economic evaluations (Gansen, 2018). However, there exist a number of methodological limitations that require addressing, including how a study that uses routine data is designed, analyzed, and interpreted. The results from this review only found one cancer indication that used RWD, hence it is difficult to identify cancer-specific issues. However, the issues identified can be generalized across diseases, some of which are shown in Table 8.12, but should be considered along with other criteria for reporting economic evaluations, such as the Consolidated Health Economic Evaluation Reporting (CHEERS) checklist (Husereau et al., 2013). The most important consideration is to ensure wherever possible the myriads of different types of bias. These will need to be either designed out or adjusted for in the analyses:

- Selection bias: due to variation in access to care; or study population not representative of the true distributions in the overall population.
- Confounding bias: association between treatment and outcome being influenced by the presence of extraneous variables; due to patient characteristics and comorbidities; or EHR diagnostic and

TABLE 8.12

Considerations When Using RWD for an Economic Evaluation

Design	Considerations
Identify registry	Availability of target data, completeness of target data, is linkage possible? Insurance claims, national registries? Can the data be collected during an EAMS designation or other early promising medicine designation?
Identify outcome of interest	Is outcome related to health resource use? Mortality, complications, incidence, HRQoL, QALYs, biomarker data?
Cost category	Inpatient treatment, medication (drug), outpatient treatment, intervention, medical aids, social care, rehabilitation, sickness benefits
Comparators	Are comparators of interest in the registry – unlikely if the treatment has not been approved/marketed
Key measures of effectiveness	Can all of these be identified from the registry? Which are the efficacy/safety outcomes? Are these available at the times of interest?
Completeness of the data	How much missing data per variable is there?
Geographical variables	Is inequality an issue?
Time horizon	What is the reference point in time – how far back?
Inflation adjustment and discounting	Past costs to be estimated at current prices
Any HRQoL – preference-based outcomes	If not, where will these be found?
Sample size and matching	How will sample sizes be derived? Will there be any matching, and, if so, how? Will samples be taken at random?
Analysis	
Has selection bias been addressed	For example, using propensity score models. How is the matching determined? How much has been stated upfront? Is a statistical plan available?
Can an economic model be populated	Is there sufficient data in the registry to populate the model?
Assumptions	Assumptions around missing health resource use, or other assumptions on treatment delivery
Uncertainty	How uncertain are the estimates from the registry?
Unobserved confounders	How will these be addressed? How will instrumental variables be defined and validated?
Evidence	Does the analysis really answer the question of interest? What is the uncertainty in the conclusions? Has this been quantified (e.g. using confidence intervals). Any evidence that addresses a safety concern of a drug must be robust enough to defend not doing a long-term follow-up study (which is more expensive than using data registries)

therapeutic codes; regional variations in standards of care; or available therapies.

- Compliance bias: due to patient third-party formularies; nonadherence to treatment; or variations in patient adherence to planned treatment affecting study outcomes.
- Information bias: due to erroneous or inaccurate capture of patient variables in the EHRs.

8.8 Exercises for Chapter 8

1. Why are registries needed and what advantages do they have over performing a randomized trial? What are their disadvantages?
2. What is confounding and what could be done to avoid potential confounding when comparing treatments for cost-effectiveness?
3. Propensity matching is a replacement for randomization. Discuss.
4. Distinguish between a pragmatic trial, a randomized trial, a case control study, an observational study, and a registry study.

9

Reporting and Interpreting Results of Cost-Effectiveness Analyses from Cancer Trials

When looking at the cost-effectiveness of cancer trials there are several important results that need to be interpreted, both clinically and from a cost-effectiveness perspective. Some of these concepts were introduced earlier, and we will now interpret them with practical examples:

(i) Incremental costs
(ii) Incremental QALYs
(iii) Interpreting the ICER and the cost-effectiveness plane
(iv) Uncertainty analyses
(v) Value of information

9.1 Interpreting Incremental Costs and QALYs

For cost-effectiveness analyses we require the mean incremental costs. The mean incremental cost is computed as the difference in the mean costs between two groups. In RCTs, the mean of the cumulative costs over their observation period per patient in each group, is used for this purpose. In cases of imbalance (e.g. costs differ between groups in terms of their baseline characteristics), to compute the mean incremental cost the patient-level costs are often modeled using a statistical model. Many baseline factors can influence the mean incremental cost, such as age, gender, ECOG, disease stage (e.g. patients whose illness is more severe may also be associated with the larger costs). The observed distribution of the patient-level costs will also influence the type of regression method used (e.g. if the costs are heavily skewed, a different analysis technique might be needed). In Chapter 5, we observed patterns of costs that were very skewed and over-dispersed, and we assumed the costs followed a gamma type distribution (see Figure 5.4).

Usually, for cost-effectiveness, the primary analysis variable of interest in trials will be the cumulative (total) cost incurred by the patient up to the end of the trial. Alternatively, costs could be analyzed over a specified period (say during initial therapy) or a well-specified part of the treatment period (say staging, palliative care period, etc.) and broken down by type of cost items (drugs, radiotherapy, surgery, supportive care, etc.) to visualize the cost structure of the treatments.

Costs may also be incomplete (right censored) because at the end of the trial patients might still be alive, but no longer followed up, or because they are lost to follow-up during the trial period. Hence these costs are censored. Patients censored before the trial ends will typically have a lower cumulative cost than those who have not been censored, resulting in a biased estimate of the total mean cost (see example data generated in Figure 9.1). In such a case, one needs to apply some statistical method to correct for the bias.

9.1.1 Informative Censoring

A key issue present in most cost data is informative censoring due to the lack of a common rate of cost accrual over time among patients. Informative censoring means that the reason for censoring may well be related to treatment (e.g. because of toxicity or patients drop out more in one arm and incur lower costs) resulting in incomplete costs. To handle non-ignorable censoring, the popular approaches are either weighting-based (Bang & Tsiatis, 2000; Lin et al., 1997; Bang, H., & Zhao, H., 2014; Bang, H., & Zhao, H., 2016), or using Kaplan-Meier estimates as weights. The latter is less popular (Etzioni et al. 1999) demonstrated that standard survival techniques may yield biased estimates. Lin et al. (1997) proposed a nonparametric approach that splits the time period into small intervals and weights mean costs from each interval by survival probabilities estimated from the Kaplan-Meier curve. An example of this was shown in Chapter 5.

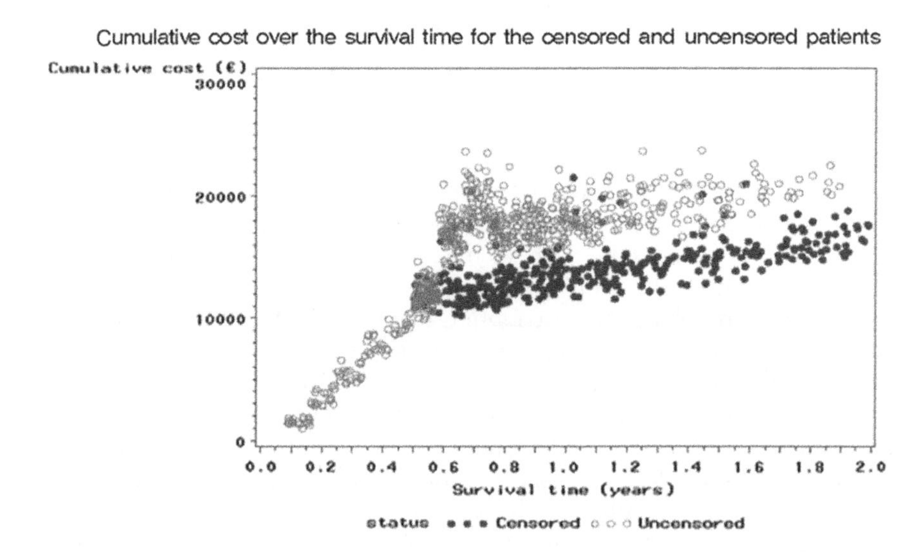

FIGURE 9.1
Simulated cumulative costs for uncensored patients compared to censored patients in a single arm.

Example 9.1: Modeling Costs from a Myeloma Cancer Trial

Table 9.1 shows the structure of (fictitious) data for 100 patients (50 randomized to treatment A and 50 to treatment B).

Since costs are positive, a skewed gamma distribution was assumed. To fit a gamma regression model, we added the value of 0.001 to (as in this example) patient 4 costs because the gamma is only defined for values >0. This creates a small bias in the estimate of the mean incremental costs but is of little practical significance. When many zero values are present, zero-inflated models would be preferable (see Dupuy 2018; Zuur et al. 2017).

Four covariates were used to estimate the mean cost: age, ECOG score, gender, number of previous chemotherapies, in addition to treatment arm. The results from the statistical output are shown in Table 9.2.

From the results in Table 9.2 we see that treatment and ECOG are the only statistically predictive factors ($p < 0.05$) of the incremental mean costs. Costs are increasing with all factors, particularly for treatment (A is more expensive) and ECOG (as patients worsen in the baseline status, the costs increase by a factor of £100.6 on average). The total costs for treatment A and B can be estimated as:

$$\text{Total Cost} = 3125 + 625.3 * \text{Treatment group}$$
$$+23.4 * \text{Gender} + 8.90 * \text{Age} + 100.6 * \text{ECOG}$$

TABLE 9.1

Example Data Structure for Modeling Costs in Terms of Other Factors

Patient	Cost	Age	ECOG	Gender	Previous Chemotherapy	Treatment
1	4,380	64	1	Male	2	A
2	6,290	49	2	Male	1	B
3	3,400	62	1	Male	3	A
4	0	75	2	Female	2	A
etc. …						
100	4,950	39	1	Female	2	B

TABLE 9.2

Results from Modeling Costs

Factor	Estimate	Standard Error	95% CI	*p*-Value
Intercept	3,125	233.45		
Treatment	625.30	195.52	(243, 1007)	<0.001
Gender	23.40	20.94	(−18, 64)	0.345
Age	8.90	8.11	(−7, 24)	0.551
ECOG	100.6	48.11	(6, 195)	0.021
		Difference		
LSmean A	4,275			
LSmean B	3,650	625	(243, 1007)	

Note that the model predicts the total cost for each patient. The mean of these predicted costs is called the adjusted mean (or least squares mean, LSmean for short). The lack of statistical significance of some terms (e.g. gender) does not imply that these should be dropped. They may still be used to predict the mean costs. Statistical significance is less of an issue than generating a reliable estimate of the mean incremental cost. If the treatment term was not statistically significant, for example, dropping it would not make sense because we still need a reliable estimate of mean costs for each treatment group.

Since treatment group takes the value of 1 for treatment A and 0 for treatment B, the cost of delivering treatment A to males aged 45 (mean age of the sample) and with an ECOG of 0 or 1 (coded as 1 if ECOG = 0 or 1, and coded as 2 if ECOG > 1) would be:

$$\text{Total Cost A} = 3125 + 625.3 + 23.4 + 8.9 * 45 + 100.6 = £4{,}275$$

One can compute the costs for treatment B in a similar way.

In practice, the adjusted mean costs are used to generate the mean incremental cost of £625. The corresponding 95% CI for this incremental cost is (£243, £1,007). These values are then used for estimating the numerator of the ICER:

$$ICER_{mean} = \frac{mean(C_1) - mean(C_2)}{mean(E_1) - mean(E_2)}$$

The wide 95% confidence interval for the cost difference between the two arms in Table 9.2 (£243 to £1,007), shows that there is considerable uncertainty in the mean cost difference (which is not unusual in cost data).

One alternative approach to computing the mean cost difference in case of a skewed distribution might be to compute a bootstrap estimate. Essentially, this involves executing the above analyses many times and from each analysis saving the mean incremental costs. This would give a distribution of mean cost differences from which we could use the 5th and 95th percentile to estimate the bootstrap confidence interval or use more technical ways (like bias corrected methods). When there are missing data (as distinct from zero costs) we can use a multiple imputation (MI) procedure. The validity of MI depends on the mechanism of missingness (see Chapter 4). Table 9.3 shows the table again with missing costs.

A statistical model using MI to predict the missing costs results in a model (e.g. a type of regression model with covariates) being repeatedly executed on the data (each bootstrap sample) where missing values are estimated. These are then essentially averaged over the number of times the model is executed (Van Buuren, 2018; Carpenter & Kenward, 2013). The mean costs and mean costs difference are then derived from each analysis and the uncertainty can be quantified (e.g. through use of confidence intervals). The next step is then to repeat the process for effectiveness measures.

TABLE 9.3

Data Example Showing Missing Costs for Multiple Imputation-Based Analyses

Patient	Cost	Age	ECOG	Gender	Previous Chemotherapy	Treatment
1	4380	64	1	Male	2	A
2	.	49	2	Male	1	B
3	.	62	1	Male	3	A
4	0	75	2	Female	2	A
etc.						
100	4,950	39	1	Female	2	B

9.2 Interpreting Incremental QALYs

The distribution of QALYs are the result of the patient's observed (whether censored or not) survival times and HRQoL (i.e. utility) score(s) over that period. The derivation and analysis of QALYs in cancer trials are not trivial. Each patient will have repeated measurements over time. The measures may be categorized as being observed in a progression-free (PF) period or post-progression (PP) period, so that we can be sure that utilities over time make sense (e.g. we expect mean PP utilities to be lower than PF utilities). Utilities can also be defined for other in-treatment or between-treatment periods and events (such as adverse events, partial response, or cure).

For each patient profile, we can estimate the QALY using estimates of the survival rates at each of the specified time points (to generate the QoL-adjusted survival curve). This was mentioned in Chapter 4 and we show a practical example below. For now, the QALY is derived over the entire overall survival time, ignoring the extrapolated survival period.

Example 9.2: Deriving the QALY Using the Kaplan-Meier Curve

We assume that the survival rates over time were observed as shown in Table 9.4 for one arm of a treatment, along with utilities at three-monthly time points. Note that utilities were not collected monthly whereas survival rates are reported monthly in Table 9.4 (this is arbitrary as they could be reported every two months, but it is useful to report them at time points where utilities are available). One way of computing the QALY is to derive, for each patient, the area under the HRQoL curve. So, for example, if a patient had measures of EQ-5D at 0, 3, 6, 12, and 18 months of 0.52, 0.58, 0.54, 0.43, 0.41, respectively, the QALY between time 0 and 18 months would be computed. The mean QALY across all patients can then be computed.

An important note is that the utilities used in Table 9.4 are derived from some external source (e.g. published data). If we have patient level HRQoL, then for each individual patient we could compute an individual $QALY_{AUC}$ and perform extrapolation (often drawing a straight line

TABLE 9.4

Survival Data with Corresponding Utilities for Example 9.2

Survival Time (Months) (t_i)	% Alive (S_i)	Mean Utility (Q_i)
0	100	0.54
1	85	
2	80	
3	75	0.52
4	71	
5	65	
6	60	0.53
7	48	
8	35	
9	25	0.42
10	20	
11	15	
12	10	0.39

not only between discrete time points but also between the last observed time point and some other arbitrary future time point).The assumption of constancy of utility between time points is strong but practical, as long as they are not too far apart in time.

To estimate the QALY we use the linear trapezoidal rule (which essentially divides the total area under a (continuous) curve into discrete intervals (trapeziums) and, using the formula for the area of the trapezium, we can compute the QALY) (Figure 9.2).

For the example, in Table 9.4, by 12 months, only 10% of the patients were alive (taking into account censoring). But the mean utility is only available at baseline (time 0), 3, 6, 9 and 12 months. Applying the trapezoidal rule, the mean QALY for all patients (for a given treatment group) is calculated as:

$$
\begin{aligned}
&\left[(0.54+0.52)/2*(1.00+0.75)/2*(3-0)\right] \\
&+\left[(0.52+0.53)/2*(0.75+0.60)/2*(6-3)\right] \\
&+\left[(0.53+0.42)/2*(0.60+0.25)/2*(9-6)\right] \\
&+\left[(0.42+0.39)/2*(0.25+0.10)/2*(12-9)\right] \\
&= (\text{left for the reader})
\end{aligned}
$$

When collected during the trial, mean utility estimates per time point for different health states can be estimated by statistical methods, such as a mixed effect (multilevel) regression model that accounts for the number of time points, possible treatment covariates, and any missing data that takes into account the intra-patient correlation. This is a separate and more efficient method to computing patient-level QALYs noted above,

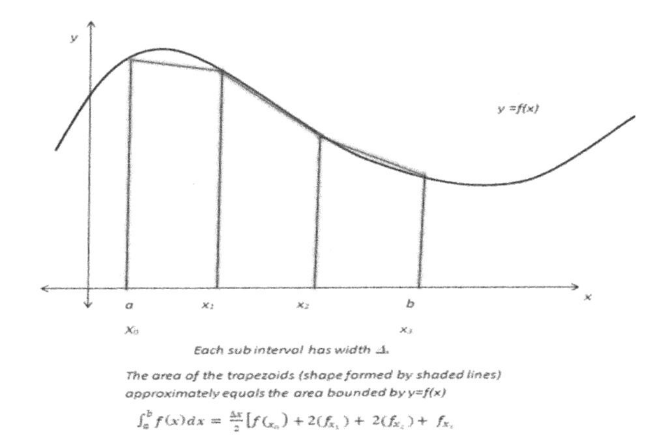

FIGURE 9.2
Using the trapezoidal rule.

because utilities at each of the time points are adjusted for possible confounders. In a similar approach to deriving mean incremental costs, non-parametric bootstrapping methods may be used to derive the confidence intervals for the QALYs per treatment arm and the incremental QALY.

The utility-adjusted survival will always be lower than the unadjusted survival (unless the HRQoL is 1 at each time point, in which case it will be the same as the overall survival curve). Depending on the relationship between survival length and HRQoL, the QALY value will vary with survival time (e.g. shorter or longer overall survival time) and possibly other factors (e.g. age, gender). It may also vary with other post-treatment factors – for example, non-responders may have a shorter survival time and a worse HRQoL than longer-term survivors (Figure 9.3).

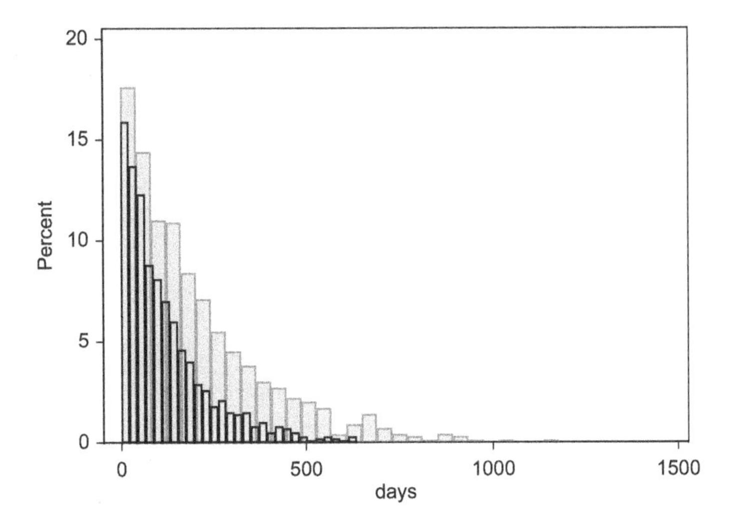

FIGURE 9.3
Comparison of simulated survival and quality-adjusted survival.

Example 9.4: Deriving a QALY with Extrapolated Survival Data

In Example 9.1, 10% of patients were still alive at the end of the trial at 12 months. In the following situation, extrapolation of survival rates beyond 12 months is estimated. However, utility data beyond 12 months needs to be estimated from published data or some assumptions have to be made about their behavior. For the purpose of this example, we shall assume a steady linear decline after 12 months. Table 9.5 shows extrapolated survival rates with estimated utilities after month 12. Note that after month 12 there is uncertainty in both survival rates and utilities. Using similar methods as used in Example 9.1, we can then estimate the QALY's.

The $QALY_{AUC}$ can be computed as follows using the trapezoidal rule:

$$QALY_{AUC} = [(0.632 + 0.588)/2 * (1.00 + 0.80)/2 * (3 - 0)]$$

$$+ [(0.63 + 0.80)/2 * (0.588 + 0.522)/2 * (6 - 3)]$$

$$+ [(0.43 + 0.36)/2 * (0.391 + 0.388)/2 * (13 - 12)]$$

$$+ [(0.17 + 0.15)/2 * (0 + 0.03)/2 * (24 - 23)]$$

Since the estimates of utility are assumed to fall at a constant rate after month 12, we can directly estimate the utilities at any time point beyond 12 without any need for interpolation. The fact that the utility at 24 months is estimated above zero should not be a surprise because of the use of a constant falling utility, which varies with time and not with the proportion alive – and, hence, is a limitation of assuming linear (constant) decline.

Another approach would be to estimate a fixed utility value for the last month(s) of life the patient was alive. In fact, estimating utility values beyond the trial observation horizon is fraught with difficulties and will need some scenario analysis with alternative utility assumptions related to the longer-term outcome of the still-surviving patients and their health state(s). For example, as shown in Chapter 3, utility may increase and then fall depending on whether other anti-cancer treatments have been given.

9.3 Relationship between Costs and QALYs

In many cases patient-level life-years and QALYs will be (positively) correlated with the patient's total costs. The longer patients survive, the more care and monitoring they will receive. In cancer trials it is only after an often long post-therapy period that the cancer-related costs might fall to zero, if at all. Even if considered cured, long-term survivors often have life-long sequelae that still need medical attention. Moreover, HRQoL may also improve over time as symptoms and treatment-related side effects wane. Generally, one

TABLE 9.5

Survival Data with Extrapolated Survival Rates for Example 9.3

Survival Time (months)	Alive (%)	Utility+
0	100	0.6323866
1	100	
2	89	
3	80	0.5885334
4	71	
5	69	
6	63	0.5227535
7	55	
8	55	
9	55	0.4569736
10	55	
11	49	
12	43	0.3911938
13*	36	0.3810000
14*	33	0.3600000
15*	32	0.3390000
16*	29	0.3180000
17*	29	0.2970000
18*	25	0.2760000
19*	23	0.2550000
20*	20	0.2340000
21*	18	0.2130000
22*	9	0.1920000
23*	3	0.1710000
24*	0	0.1500000

Notes: * Extrapolated survival rates and utilities.
+ Estimated as a linear (constant rate) decline beyond month 12.

would expect a U-shaped evolution of HRQoL over time for these patients. One might also expect the variance of costs to increase in relation to the length of (quality-adjusted) survival, resulting in a heteroscedastic relationship. Figure 9.4 shows such a typical (simulated) situation.

From Figure 9.4, at the patient level, the cost per QALY ratio or cost-effectiveness ratio (CER) is skewed. This is due to the skewed distribution of the individual survival times, even after the transformation of survival times to QALYs as shown in Figure 9.2. The highly right-skewed nature of the patient-level costs coupled with the similar skewed nature of the individual survival times can lead to very high cost per QALY ratios for some patients (those

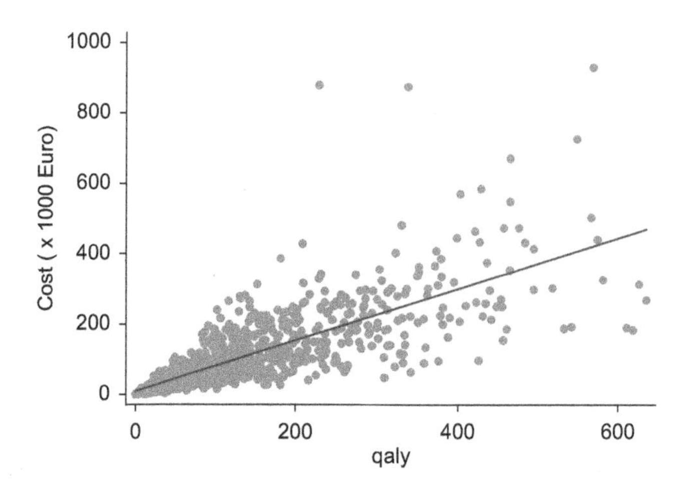

FIGURE 9.4
Relationship between patient-level costs and QALYs.

with large costs and relatively low survival or HRQoL). Plotting these per trial arm helps to yield some insights at the individual level between the treatments under study and may be worth investigating further (for example: Are the distributions overlapping? Similarly shaped? Any sub-groups? etc.).

9.4 Interpreting the ICER and the Cost-Effectiveness Plane

Once we have constructed the mean incremental cost and incremental effect, we need to construct the ICER and present the uncertainty around it. The 'base' or 'reference' case and (sometimes confusingly and wrongly called) the 'baseline' ICER are considered the key estimates of the mean ICER for which the uncertainty needs to be quantified. The ICER and its uncertainty, as presented on a cost-effectiveness plane divided into four quadrants, were introduced in Chapter 1. Table 9.6 shows the different ways of interpreting the ICER for two treatments (A and B) when the incremental costs and QALYs are positive or negative.

9.4.1 Uncertainty

Since the ICER is computed as a single value (given that it is based on the differences between two means), the uncertainty around its value is calculated by simulating several thousands of ICERs (in fact by simulating the initial

TABLE 9.6

Interpretation of the ICER for Two Treatments A and B

Incremental Costs (Cost Difference)	Incremental QALYs (Effect Difference)	ICER	ICER Interpretation
+ve (A > B)	+ve (A > B)	+ve	Cost are higher for A, A more effective
+ve (A > B)	–ve (A < B)	–ve	Cost are higher for A, A less effective
–ve (A < B)	+ve (A > B)	–ve	Cost are lower for A, A more effective
–ve (A < B)	–ve (A < B)	+ve	Cost are lower for A, A less effective

Notes: +ve = positive; –ve = negative.

trial by bootstrapping methods) to get a feel for their distribution and how many of these lie above or below the CE threshold.

Example 9.5: ICER and Cost-Effectiveness from a Lung Cancer Trial

Figure 9.5 shows 10,000 simulated incremental costs and effects for a NSCLC trial comparing erlotinib with BSC (Khan, 2015). The X-axis shows the mean incremental effectiveness (measured in QALYs) and the Y-axis the mean incremental costs. In addition, there is a vertical line at zero, which is presented to help interpret the graph (values to the right of 0 show the new treatment, erlotinib, is more effective and to the left of 0 show it is less effective). The Y-axis starts at £2,000, which shows that erlotinib is more costly. We could have started the Y-axis at zero, but since erlotinib is never cheaper than BSC, starting at £2,000 is fine for the purposes of this example. The other two reference lines (horizontal and vertical) show the observed mean incremental costs (horizontal) and the mean incremental effect (vertical). Where these two lines cross is where values of the ICER can be determined. In this case, the mean incremental cost is about £7,891 and the mean incremental effect is 0.139 QALYs, yielding an ICER of £7,891/0.139 = £56,777. A 95% confidence ellipse could be added to the graph to highlight the mean ICER of all bootstraps or the original trial ICER.

In Figure 9.5, there are some outlier incremental costs, which suggest that erlotinib could be very effective (e.g. incremental QALYs of >0.32) and in some cases erlotinib worse (incremental QALYs of <–0.03). This reflects the uncertainty around the true mean incremental costs and effects. There are also a few observations where the incremental effectiveness ≈ 0, in which case the ICER tends to infinity. However, what is less certain is that most ICERs are >£30,000. In Figure 9.9 we can visualize the uncertainty in a graph called the cost-effectiveness acceptability curve (CEAC).

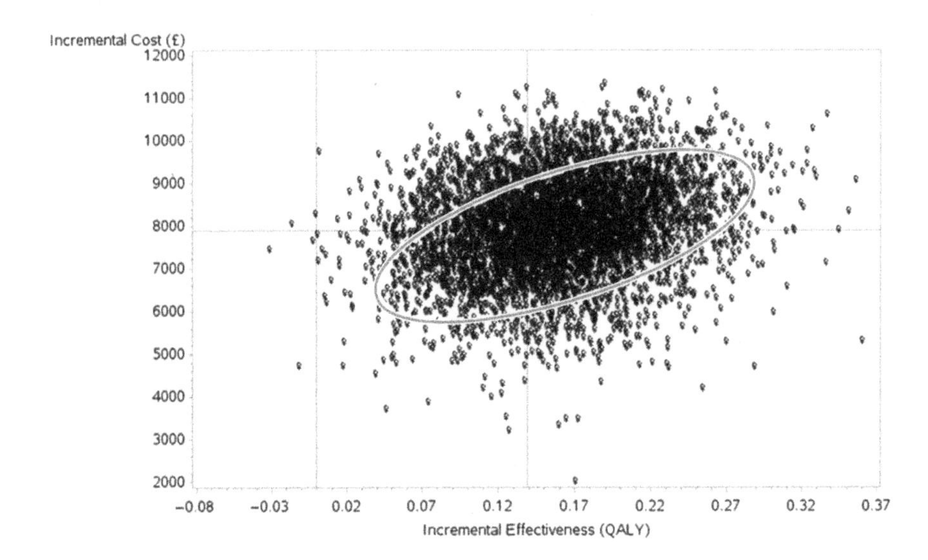

FIGURE 9.5
Cost-effectiveness of erlotinib versus BSC.

The more general form of the CE plane can be presented as shown in Figure 9.6 (reproduced from Chapter 1). We see that most of the simulated ICERs fall in the north eastern quadrant. Clockwise from Figure 9.6, we note these quadrants as NE (++), SE (−+), SW(−−) and NW(+−). The decision in case of the dominant SE quadrant is straightforward (accept new therapy), as is the decision in case of the NW quadrant (reject new therapy, Example 9.6). In the case of the SW quadrant, one has to make a value judgment about the new treatment: are we willing to forego some clinical efficiency for the sake of a (possibly much) lower cost of care? This could be a possible decision in very stretched health budgets whereby the health gain of one group of patients would be (hopefully slightly) decreased but would allow other patients get some care that would otherwise not be available to them.

For example, cancer patients would then lose some clinical benefit, but the money saved could be allocated to fund dialysis units for end-stage renal disease patients. This is then a policy decision across disease areas.

The most common situation when it comes to funding new treatments concerns patients with the same indication for which two (or possibly more) treatments are compared. Here also a value judgment has to be made: how much more are we willing to pay for an increased clinical benefit. That is, what is our (i.e. the decision-maker's) maximum willingness-to-pay (WTP) threshold for one unit increase in clinical benefit? In cancer, as in other fatal or deadly diseases, the clinical benefit would at least have to be expressed as a gain in life expectancy (i.e. life-years gained or LYG) or, even better, given the toxicity of most cancer therapies, as quality-adjusted life-years (QALY) gained. Another useful plot is to plot the LYG versus the QALYs, which shows the loss of life-years related to lower HRQoL. In fact, this is equivalent to an indirect estimation of

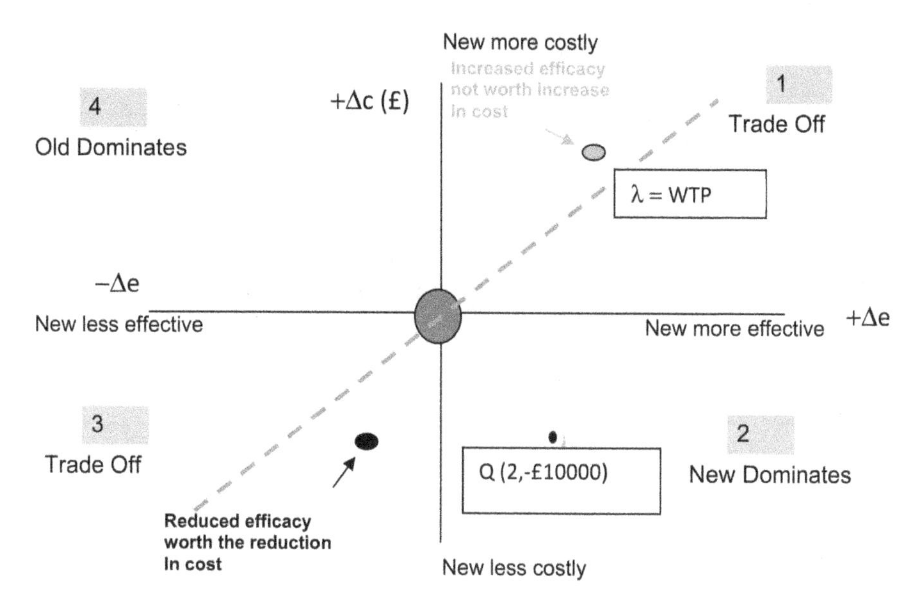

FIGURE 9.6
Cost-effectiveness plane.

years of life lost (YLL) from a decrease in quality of life (QoL) due to treatment toxicity and adverse events and sequelae.

The WTP may differ widely between stakeholder groups such as patients, physicians, and other health professionals, health economists, and decision makers (in reimbursement policy committees). This last group also includes clinicians and administrators at hospital level, when, for example, the hospital is funded by a fixed annual budget. In practice the WTP will also depend on other factors, such as the rarity of the disease, its health impact (morbidity and mortality), the demographic target group (children, women, the elderly, etc.), the existence of an alternative treatment or not (as in orphan or genetic diseases), and the overall wealth level of the country and healthcare system. We can readily plot this (or several) threshold(s) on the ICER plane once we have decided upon the WTP threshold(s). Often cited WTP thresholds in the UK are £15,000, £20,000–£30,000 and £50,000 per QALY gained (for end of life care). Finally, it should be noted that the ICER is expressed in an absolute value, i.e. for 1 QALY.

Example 9.6: Impact of Varying WTP Thresholds

In the following example we can readily see that if our WTP threshold is set at $100,000 per QALY then we would probably accept the new treatment, as most estimates fall below the threshold (a gain of 0.05 QALY = 2.6 weeks at a cost of $4,000 = $1,538 additional expenses per quality-adjusted week gained, or $80,000 per QALY in Figure 9.7).

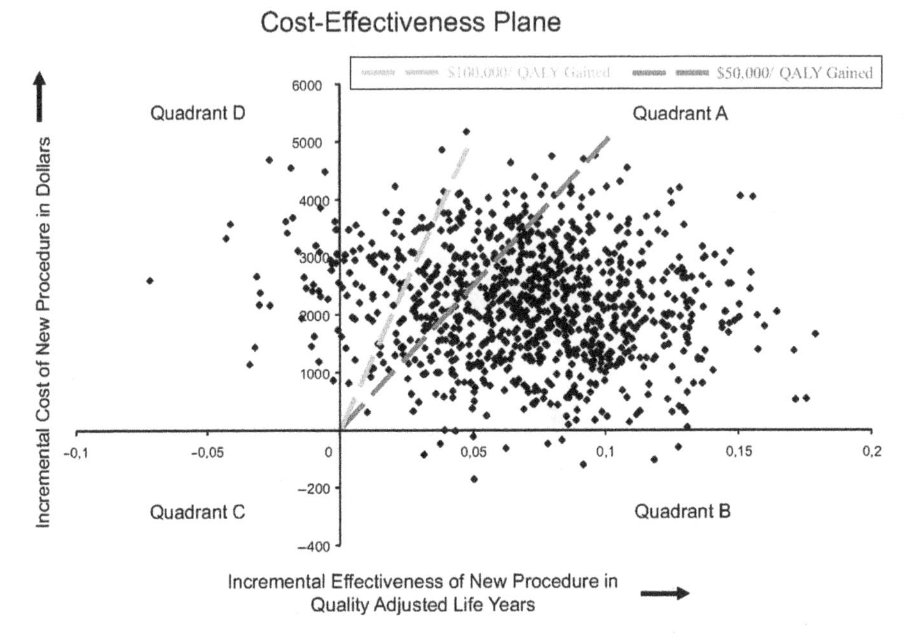

FIGURE 9.7
Impact of varying WTP (CE thresholds).

9.5 Presenting and Interpreting Results from Uncertainty Analysis

The purpose of sensitivity analysis in health economic evaluation is to assess the uncertainty of conclusions (such as those based on the ICER) by varying the model inputs. Data from a single clinical trial might be of limited value, especially if it is the only trial that has been carried out for the disease under investigation (or it is unlikely a similar trial will be conducted again in the near future). For example, assuming that the treatment-related adverse event rate is 5% for a particular treatment group, but the reliability of the rate is questionable (because, for example, the trial was unblinded and any assessment of treatment relatedness is biased; or the rate has wide confidence intervals), one might wish to assess the impact on the ICER if the adverse rate was larger or smaller than 5%.

In decision trees or Markov models and other simulation models used in HTA, uncertainty is assessed by techniques such as 'one-way sensitivity analysis,' 'two-way sensitivity analysis,' and 'probabilistic sensitivity analysis' (PSA). One-way sensitivity analysis is where single inputs (costs, or effects, or model parameters – e.g. estimates of key effects such as response rates) are varied by a certain amount. If there are multiple parameters, one factor is varied while the others are held fixed. For example, the cost of drugs, might be varied by ±10% and the impact on the reference ICER observed, while all other inputs are held constant. Second, the parameters are varied according to their lack of accuracy or uncertainty around their (mean) values. In this approach, different parameters may be varied by different amounts. For example, if it is not possible to have a response rate below 20%, then one could vary the parameter as far as 20% only.

Two-way sensitivity analysis is where two inputs are simultaneously varied. For example, the adverse event rate might increase by 10% and utilities reduce by 10% (at the same time). The effect on the ICER (i.e. how it has changed from the base case value) is then observed and plotted on a two-way graph. An alternative approach might be to work out the simultaneous percentage changes in one or two inputs (or sometimes three) simultaneously for a required ICER (i.e. working backward for a desired ICER), such as changing the price of new drug to attain an ICER threshold of £30,000 per QALY. With patient-level data, one can increment inputs (costs, effects) by a certain percentage (so multiplying each value on one arm by 1.10 would increase these by 10%).

In sensitivity analysis, the decision about the actual amounts to vary the inputs by is somewhat arbitrary. One could use 95% (or even 90%) confidence intervals to describe the uncertainty of some input variables. For example, one could calculate the 95% CI of the mean utility or mean QALYs for a given treatment group, and also report the 95% CI for the mean costs. The upper and lower confidence limits from these could then be used to assess the impact on the ICER in a further sensitivity analysis. The upper and lower 95% confidence intervals of inputs, although plausible, may result in some extreme but rare ICERs. An alternative approach is to simply present the 95% confidence interval for the mean ICER using a more complex statistical approach such as Fieller's theorem (O'Brien & Briggs, 2002) or some other CI estimation method.

The plausible range of values for the confidence interval of the observed (simulated) ICERs can lead to different interpretations, especially if the confidence interval covers two or more regions in the cost-effectiveness plane. It is therefore useful to count the proportion of ICERs in each region of the cost-effectiveness plane. For example, if the 95% CI for the ICER ranges from (–£456 to +£899) for a mean ICER of £678/QALY, there are two possible inferences: on the one hand, the new treatment is more expensive (£899) but also more effective; on the other hand, the new treatment is less effective but also cheaper (–£456). We need to know the position of incremental costs and effects (numerator and denominator) in the cost-effectiveness plane to interpret the results properly. In this example, if the cost effectiveness threshold was £1,000, both decisions could be implemented, although it would be doubtful if a decision-maker, health professional, or member of the public would accept funding a cheaper but less efficient treatment, certainly for cancer. This implies that only quadrants A and B are relevant for decision-making in practice.

We now provide examples and interpretations of each of the analyses:

(i) One-way sensitivity analysis
One way of displaying the impact on the ICER in a one-way sensitivity analysis is through the use of a type of plot called a 'tornado diagram.' These are essentially horizontal bar charts that attempt to show the influence of the factors (for both a positive and negative change per variable) that impact the ICER. An example of a tornado or influence plot is shown in Figure 9.8 for some simulated data for two treatments A and B (not the same as the above example). What is apparent from the plot is that varying treatment A costs by ±10% does not impact the ICER, whereas varying the costs of treating adverse events on treatment B by the same amount results in large changes in the ICER.

Example 9.6: One-Way Sensitivity Analysis

Assume the mean cumulative costs for treatments A and B are £3,000 and £4,000 respectively with mean utilities of 1.10 and 1.20. This gives a base case ICER of (£4,000 – £3,000)/(1.20 – 1.10) = £10,000/QALY for B versus A as our reference case ICER. This is the calculated mean ICER prior to any sensitivity analysis. We will now vary the mean cost and mean utility by + and – 10% one at a time. With all other factors (costs for treatment B, utilities for A and B) remaining the same. Reducing the cost of treatment B by 10% has the greatest impact on the ICER.

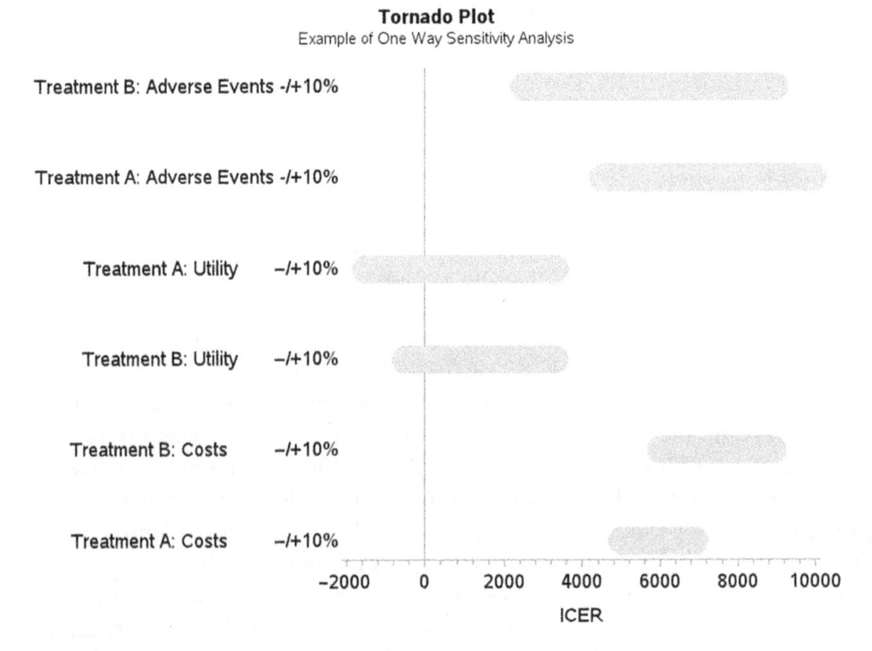

FIGURE 9.8
Tornado plot for one-way sensitivity analysis.

The impact on the ICER from one-way sensitivity analysis is shown in Table 9.7 below.

TABLE 9.7

One-Way Sensitivity Analysis for Example 9.4

	ICER
Base case	£10,000
Costs treatment A +10%	£7,000[a]
Costs treatment B –10%	£6,000[b]
Utility treatment A +10%	£9,090[c]

Notes: [a] A 10% increase of £3,000 = £3,300, so that the revised ICER = £4,000–£3,300/0.1 = £7,000.

[b] A 10% decrease of £4,000 = £3,600, so that the revised ICER = £3,600–£3,000/0.1 = £6,000.

[c] A 10% increase in utility of 1.1 = 1.21, so that the revised ICER = £4,000–£3,000/0.11 = £9,090.

(ii) Two-Way Sensitivity Analysis

Example 9.7: Two-Way Sensitivity Analysis

Following on from Example 9.6, we now show the impact on the ICER when two factors are varied simultaneously. In the first few rows of Table 9.9 we note that costs and utilities have been varied by a 10% increase for treatment A, while simultaneously we assume that costs and utilities for treatment B have decreases by 10%, resulting in a revised ICER of £2,307/QALY. In other words, if the costs of treatment A were to rise by 10% and HRQoL also improved by a similar amount, but treatment B costs were to fall along with the QALYs by 10%, treatment B would be cheaper but also less effective. In the second row, the contrary is assumed where treatment A costs and utilities are assumed to fall by 10%, whereas for treatment B they are assumed to increase. In this case the ICER rises to over £5,000/QALY. In Table 9.8 the ICER fell by 30% to 40% as a result of varying drug costs by ±10%.

(iii) Presenting Sensitivity Analysis

In TA299 (NICE TA299, 2013), the treatment for chronic myeloid leukemia with bosutinib was appraised and a one-way sensitivity analysis was not conducted:

Extensive one-way sensitivity analyses were not performed as Pfizer believed structural uncertainties were greater than parameter uncertainties. Scenario analyses were performed instead.

The resulting scenarios are shown in Table 9.10 using fictitious data but following a real situation.

TABLE 9.8

Two-Way Sensitivity for Example 9.2

			ICER
Treatment	Factor	Change	(Base case £10,000)
A	Costs	+10%	–£2, 307
A	Utility	+10%	
B	Costs	–10%	
B	Utility	–10%	
A	Costs	–10%	£5,151
A	Utility	–10%	
B	Costs	+10%	
B	Utility	+10%	

Example 9.8: Resulting Scenarios from Varying Inputs

What is noticeable from Table 9.9, is that real-world issues, such as taking additional treatments and higher dosing (e.g. in TA299, it was assumed the dosing could be increased from 200 mg used in the clinical trial to 500 mg in real-world practice) result in increased ICERs and can reverse the decision for a drug to be cost-effective.

TABLE 9.9

Scenario Analyses

Scenario	Revised ICER (£)	Impact of New Treatment vs. Comparator[a]
Base case	21,421	New treatment dominant
Reduce cohort age by 10%	23,662	New treatment dominant
Use the lower 95% CI for the hazard ratio	28,656	New treatment dominant
Use the upper 95% CI for the hazard ratio	18,332	New treatment dominant
Fitting exponential curve to both arms	22,843	New treatment dominant
Fitting Weibull model to both arms	24,982	New treatment dominant
Fitting exponential curve to one arm and Weibull to the other	25,333	New treatment dominant
Assuming mean OS increase by 20%	20,116	New treatment dominant
Time on treatment is increased by 6 months	29,155	New treatment dominant
Dosing in real life increase by 50%	33,213	New treatment dominated
Medical management costs increase by 20%	25,775	New treatment dominant
Additional treatment taken at a cost of £25 per month	25,999	New treatment dominant
Utilities 20% higher	18,994	New treatment dominant
Utilities 20% lower	31,669	New treatment dominant

[a] *Note:* Threshold is £30,000 per QALY.

(iv) Probabilistic Sensitivity Analysis

In probabilistic sensitivity analysis, the outcomes (mean costs, mean QALYs, mean OS) and/or inputs are considered to originate from a probability distribution. Hence, we need to simulate their uncertainty by drawing from a probability distribution (usually several thousand times). For example, if the trial size of the study was 300 per group, and we want to assess how a change in, say, the post-progression utility impacts the ICER, we could generate 5,000 samples, where each simulated sample consists of 300 values (e.g. utility, survival, costs). For each of the simulated trials we can then recalculate the mean utility, incremental utility, and ICER. We can then summarize all 5,000 ICERs and other values (incremental costs, QALYs).

An important feature of the data in an economic evaluation is that some variables are correlated and so the simulation will need to ensure that this correlation structure is preserved during the sampling so that the PSA gives sensible (and less biased) results. This can become complicated in practice though. If we wish to analyze the impact of increased dosing (as measured by the average dose received in one of the arms in the trial), we might expect an increase in drug costs and therefore the overall mean cost of the treatment. Furthermore, increased dosing would probably increase the occurrence of adverse events and possibly their severity (i.e. increase the arm's treatment toxicity), which in turn would increase the adverse events treatment costs in the arm. Higher toxicity will in turn impact post-treatment HRQoL. In some cases, it may even increase the toxicity-related deaths and therefore decrease the overall survival. These two latter effects will then decrease the mean QALYs. Hence, a change in one input (average drug dose) can have positive or negative consequences for other inputs, all of which would have to be considered. This is why, in practice, researchers often limit the sensitivity analysis to more aggregate variables.

The usual frequentist approach to PSA uses Monte-Carlo simulation to estimate the overall uncertainty of cost-effectiveness. In this respect it is like estimating a population parameter from a single trial as it considers that the observed trial values are a single realization of a large number of possible similar trials. This detailed approach is described as follows:

(i) Identify the inputs (variables) to vary (e.g. cost, utilities, survival, adverse events, etc.).
(ii) Identify the distributional parameters associated with the inputs (e.g. mean, standard deviation, rates).
(iii) Identify or estimate the correlation or covariance matrix of the set of variables from which to simulate, if required.
(iv) Determine whether the Monte-Carlo simulation will be from a univariate or multivariate distribution.
(v) Determine whether a multivariate simulation will take into account the 'mixed' nature of the distributions (i.e. will the simulation assume data are multivariate normal or a combination of normally and non-normally distributed data).
(vi) Write software code to simulate the pseudo-trials.
(vii) Compute the ICER for each simulation.

(viii) Plot the resulting ICERS on the CE plane and determine the proportion of ICERs above a certain CE threshold value (λ).
(ix) Plot the cost-effectiveness acceptability curve (CEAC).

Note that with two arms you have only one ICER and one CE plane, if there are more than two arms then one can overlay two or more comparisons on the same CE plane (arm A versus control; arm B versus control) or the same CEAC.

Example 9.9: Probabilistic Sensitivity Analysis

An example is taken from Lee (2012) for a lung cancer trial. The following costs and effects were simulated from a multivariate distribution for each arm (a joint distribution of several variables with each variable having his own distribution):

(a) Total costs – assumed to be normally distributed.
(b) Utilities – assumed to be beta binomial (pre- and post-progression utility separately).
(c) Overall survival and progression-free survival – assumed to be exponentially distributed.

Hence, four components of the ICER were to be simulated. The objective was to simulate from a multivariate distribution where variables (inputs) had different distributions. The mean and standard deviations for each cost component is shown in Table 9.10 below for the erlotinib treatment group.

As noted above, it would be incorrect to simulate these independently and then merge them together. What is needed is a correlation or covariance matrix. We assume that the five components have the correlation matrix shown in Table 9.11.

Simulating multivariate data from mixed distributions can be very complex. Several methods exist and we will describe one of them here that uses the Fleishman power transformation method (Fleishman, 1978). A method using copulas is also possible and interested researchers may wish to explore this. Simulation using copulas was successfully accomplished by Khan (2015) . Details of how this can be achieved are found in the technical appendix A9.1.

TABLE 9.10

Distributional Assumptions of Inputs for in Probabilistic Sensitivity Analyis

	Distribution Assumed	Justification
Total costs	Normal	Costs > 0 and some extreme values
EQ-5D pre-progression utility	Beta-binomial	Utilities between 0 and 1
EQ-5D post-progression utility	Beta-binomial	Utilities between 0 and 1
OS	Exponential	Survival times assumed exponential
PFS	Exponential	Progression-free survival exponential

TABLE 9.11

Correlation Matrix Used for Simulating Multivariate Data (Experimental Arm Only)

	Total Costs	PrP-utility	PP-utility	OS	PFS
Total costs	1				
Pre-utility	0.61	1			
Post-utility	0.65	0.89	1		
OS	0.71	0.58	0.62	1	
PFS	0.69	0.55	0.66	0.88	1

Notes: PrP, pre-progression; PP, post-progression.

TABLE 9.12

Output from Multivariate Simulation Using the Fleishman Method for the Experimental Treatment Group for Example 9.9

Patient	Total Costs (£)	Pre-utility	Post-utility	PFS (Months	OS (Months)
1	4,000	0.4	0.2	1.2	1.8
2	8,000	0.8	0.4	2.2	4.4
3	3,500	0.8	0.4	1.1	2.7
Etc. ...	...	...	...	...	...
350	8,500	0.7	0.2	4.9	6.2

For each simulated data set (for each arm), the mean total costs and QALYs are calculated. It is important that the way the mean total costs are computed from each simulated sample uses the same methods in the base case approach. For example, if the mean costs were estimated using a generalized gamma model in the base case analysis, this should be repeated for each data set and not using the simple mean. An example of the structure of the data for each simulation may look like that in Table 9.12 (the data are fictitious). Table 9.13 shows how the data are structured and simulated for both arms.

The data in Table 9.13 can be used to compute the mean ICER along with 95% CI as well as the CEAC.

(iv) Cost-Effectiveness Acceptability Curves

The next step will be to determine the proportion of ICERs below a specified CE threshold (or willingness-to-pay). Recall that an acceptable ICER is defined as:

$$\Delta_C / \Delta_e < \lambda$$

where λ is the CE willingness-to-pay threshold, Δ_c is the difference of the mean costs per arm and Δ_e is the difference of the mean QALYs per arm. From the 10,000 simulated ICERs, we can calculate the proportion of simulations that are below any given λ and we can then plot these

TABLE 9.13

Simulated ICERs from Each Data Set

Simulation K = 1 to 10,000	Mean total cost K (erlotinib)	Mean total cost K (placebo)	Mean QALY K (erlotinib)	Mean QALY K (placebo)	ICER K Erlotinib vs. placebo
1	6,700	5,200	1.80	1.77	50,000
2	8,300	5,200	1.60	1.59	310,000
3	11,700	10,100	1.10	1.0	16,000
Etc...					
10,000					

proportions in ascending order of λ to generate the CEAC. An alternative expression introduced earlier is:

$$INMB = \lambda * \Delta_e - \Delta_C$$

What we require is the probability of the INMB to be >0 for specified values of λ. In Table 9.14, the proportion of times the ICER is less than the CE threshold of £1,000 and £10,000 is zero. As the CE increases to £20,000, one of the simulated ICERs is below £20,000. The process continues and then the probabilities are plotted on the Y-axis and the CE threshold on the X-axis. From this, we can generate the CEAC as shown in Figure 9.9.

TABLE 9.14

Proportion of ICERs below the CE Threshold for First 3 Simulated ICERs

Simulation	ICER (£)	CE threshold (£)	Is ICER > CE Threshold?	Probability ICER < CE Threshold
1	50,000	1,000	No	0
2	310,000	1,000	No	0
3	16,000	1,000	No	0
...				
10,000				
1	50,000	10,000	No	0
2	310,000	10,000	No	0
3	16,000	10,000	No	0
...		Etc.		
10,000				
1	50,000	20,000	No	0
2	310,000	20,000	No	0
3	16,000	20,000	Yes	1/3
...				
10,000				

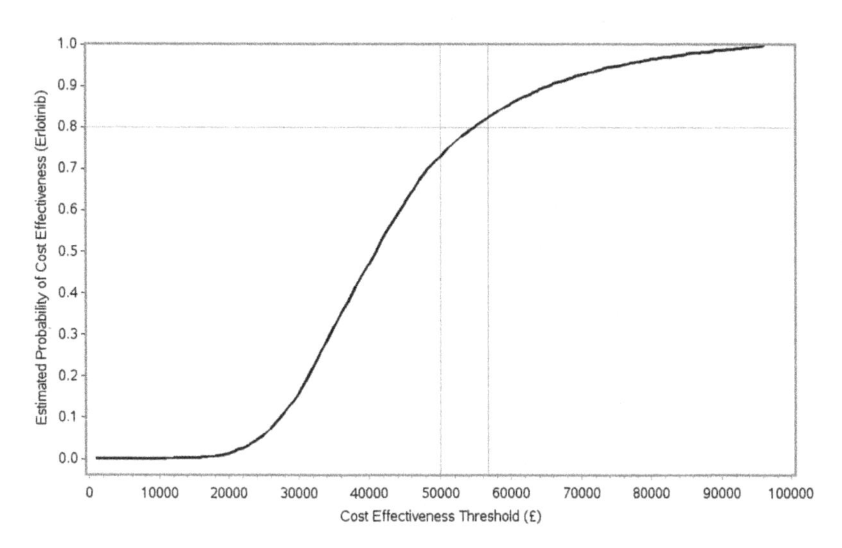

FIGURE 9.9
CEAC showing probability of cost-effectiveness of erlotinib versus placebo.

The CEAC in Figure 9.9 shows the (empirical cumulative) probability of cost-effectiveness for varying thresholds up to £100,000 per QALY. The horizontal line represents the 80% probability of cost-effectiveness. Where this line meets the curve, it tells us that for an 80% chance of cost-effectiveness with the new treatment, the cost per QALY is about £56,000. At a threshold of £30,000 per QALY, the chance of cost-effectiveness is <10%. The vertical line at £50,000 is the threshold for end-of-life treatments in the UK. Hence, if erlotinib qualified for an end of life reimbursement, the chance of cost-effectiveness approximates 70% if society was prepared to pay £50,000 per QALY. At some very large value of CE thresholds there will be a 100% chance that the new treatment (or for that matter any new treatment) is cost-effective, because ultimately if there was a very large budget (money is not a concern), λ tends to infinity.

There is however no universal agreement as to what probability level is acceptable for a new treatment to be cost-effective. The general rule is the higher the probability, the better. In practice, other factors such as disease type, target population type and size, availability, and number of alternative treatments might all play a part in the funding decision. The CEAC threshold is often based on the primary endpoint of a trial. Separate CEACs for subgroups and secondary endpoints could be derived. How results like these are to be interpreted is not always clear (or easy). For example, consider a CEAC for the primary endpoint (survival) that is modestly cost effective (e.g. 65% chance of cost-effective at a threshold of £30,000/QALY). Even if the secondary endpoints generated strong effects, the CEAC for the primary endpoint would not change.

For this reason, one might argue that decisions should not be made on the primary endpoint CEAC alone, unless the CEAC encompasses some secondary efficacy endpoints also (not to mention the correlation between primary and secondary efficacy endpoints).

9.6 Bayesian Sensitivity Analysis

In the above example, Monte-Carlo simulation was used to estimate the (long-run) probability of cost-effectiveness for varying levels of the CE threshold. The Bayesian approach is likely to lead to the same conclusions, depending on prior beliefs about parameters and/or distributions of costs and effects. For example, if the prior distributions are non-informative (i.e. observed data dominate the results over the weak prior beliefs), the usual (frequentist) and Bayesian analyses will give very similar results. If however there is some previous information available, this can be included in the analysis through 'informative priors.'

Different choices for priors can lead to different cost-effectiveness conclusions (Maiwenn et al., 2000; Al & Van Hout, 2000). However, Bayesian analysis, despite giving similar results in the case of using weak prior information gives a different interpretation of the results. In Chapter 4, we noted how, in hypothesis testing, we simply decide one hypothesis over the other as being true. The Bayesian philosophy quantifies the probability of a hypothesis being (credible) true. A clinician is more likely to appreciate the idea of the chance of a hypothesis being true, than deciding one of two hypotheses

TABLE 9.15

Summary of Main Issues in Uncertainty Analyses

Method	Situation/Model	Main Issues
One-way	Decision model/ clinical trial	• Arbitrary amounts varied • Simple • Can result in extreme ICERS
Two-way	Decision model/ clinical trial	• Arbitrary amounts varied • Simple but can become complicated with >2 inputs
Confidence or credible Intervals/ bootstrap CIs	Aggregate patient-level data[a]	• Based on statistical theory • Can result in extreme ICERs • Can lead to different conclusions • In some cases may not be estimable
CEAC	Any	• Simple to interpret • Provides an intuitive approach to estimating the probability of cost-effectiveness • A bit more complicated with >2 treatments • Unclear how secondary endpoints information is incorporated
Scatter plot/CE plane	Any	• Shows uncertainty around the individual ICERs • Can see visually how many ICERs might lie in different quadrants
CE Frontier	Any	• More appropriate when comparing >2 treatments

[a] For bootstrapped CI we start from mean cumulative (total) cost and mean QALY from the observed trial.

to be true. However, unless a prior statistical cost-effectiveness hypothesis is postulated, the Monte-Carlo simulation (or bootstrap) will provide a similar interpretation of the results in the context of a probability.

The interpretation of the confidence interval from a Bayesian analysis is called a credible interval. The credible interval expresses uncertainty about the (posterior) point estimate of the ICER and is interpreted as offering a probability of where the parameter of interest lies: "there is a 95% probability that the credible (confidence) interval will contain the true ICER." Compare this with the more wordy frequentist 95% confidence interval "if you repeated this analysis 1,000 times, then 950 of the confidence intervals would contain the true ICER."

Table 9.15 provides a summary of some key issues in uncertainty analysis.

9.6.1 Limitations of the ICER and Using the INMB

There are several limitations of the ICER. One of the major problems with the ICER, given that it is a ratio, is that when the denominator tends to zero, the ICER becomes infinitely large. Defining a confidence interval in that case becomes problematic. Moreover, for negative values of either the numerator or denominator, the interpretations become trickier. The net monetary benefit (NMB) has been developed as an alternative measure that does not imply a ratio. It is defined as:

$$\text{Net monetary benefit}(\text{NMB}) = \text{E} * \lambda - \mathbf{C} \tag{9.2}$$

Its inverse is the net health benefit

$$(\text{NHB}) = -\text{C} / \lambda + \text{E} \tag{9.3}$$

The incremental Net Monetary Benefit $(\text{INMB}) = \text{NMBT - NMBC} = \lambda * \Delta_E - \Delta_C$

where E = effectiveness (LYG or QALY),

λ = threshold for WTP, and C= total cost of treatment;

Δ_E and Δ_C are the difference in mean effects and difference in mean costs respectively.

As the NMB and NHB are monotonic linear functions it is statistically simpler to calculate confidence intervals compared to an ICER. It has also some nice mathematical properties as highlighted by Messori & Trippoli, (2017). In contrast to the ICER, the NMB can be calculated for a single treatment in the absence of any comparison (absolute NMB). Another feature of NMB is that the incremental NMB (INMB) for the comparison of A versus B can be estimated as the absolute NMB calculated for treatment A minus the absolute NMB calculated for treatment B (Messori & Trippoli, 2017, 2018).

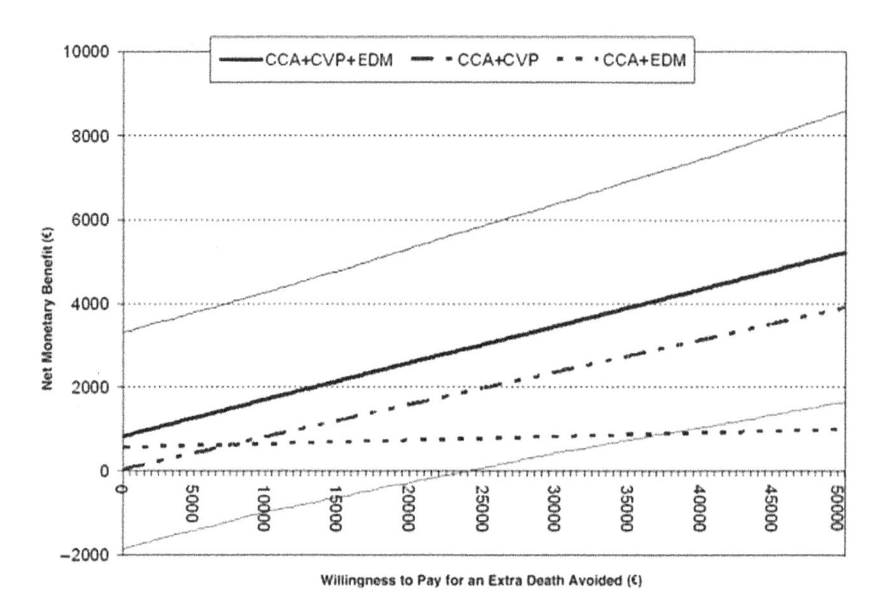

FIGURE 9.10
Using the NMB.

Source: Maeso et al., 2011.

Graphically, the absolute NMB is shown using straight lines, where a higher cost decreases the NMB and therefore shifts the entire line down, and increasing effectiveness increases the slope of the line up from the intercept. Any treatment that has an NMB above 0 is then by definition a candidate for funding. Figure 9.10 shows a comparison of the absolute NMB of three treatments with the CCA+CVP+EDM combination superior (more cost-effective) to the two other modalities (the outer most lines represent 95% CI).

An additional feature of the NMB approach is that it is more amenable to regression analysis with individual patient data, because it can be disaggregated to individual NMBs due to the linearity of the NMB for evaluating the influence of patient, center, or treatment characteristics, which is not the case for the ICER . For regressing the ICER, a bivariate regression (such as seemingly unrelated regression) for deriving ICERs could be used (Willan et al., 2004) as could equivalent Bayesian approaches that take into account the correlation between costs and effects (Hernandez, 2009).

9.7 Presenting and Interpreting Results from Value of Information Analyses

In this and previous chapters, we saw how cost-effectiveness models were used to estimate the INMB and the ICER. In addition, we discussed how the model inputs could be subject to uncertainty analysis either using one, two-way sensitivity analysis and PSA. We also showed how the CEAC was generated from PSA. Value of information (VOI) can be considered as an extension of PSA. However, whereas the CEAC yield estimates of the probability of cost-effectiveness of the new treatment, VOI allows us to quantify the consequences of selecting the wrong treatment and to estimate the expected gain (reduction) in uncertainty from some (further) data collection. In lay terms, does the value of additional information outweigh its cost?

Recall the expected net benefit (ENB) is: effects*λ – costs, where λ is the CE threshold and effects are measures of effectiveness (e.g. QALYs). At the time of a cost-effectiveness analysis and during a review of the evidence for the cost-effectiveness of a new treatment by a reimbursement agency, any decision to reimburse the treatment(s) is based on the highest expected benefit (expected net benefit). There is always a risk that the decision-maker may choose the wrong treatment to reimburse based on current evidence. This is because it is impossible to have complete and perfect information on all aspects (Fenwick et al., 2008; Claxton, 2008).

Since uncertainty almost always exists, the chance of a wrong decision is always possible. For example, an economic evaluation might be performed that results in the new treatment yielding an incremental net benefit (INB) > 0. However, at the time of marketing authorization, the pharmaceutical company might be requested to carry out a post-marketing commitment study to evaluate the longer-term effects (e.g. side effects) of the new treatment. It might transpire from the post-marketing study that the adverse event rates were slightly higher for the experimental/new group or that survival in the real world was not as long as in the clinical trial (as can sometimes be the case). Consequently, when the incremental cost-effectiveness ratio and the INMB were recalculated from the post-marketing study data, they were not as large as initially estimated from the clinical trial, leading to a lower INMB, which would have led to the rejection of the product had that been known from the start.

A decision at the time of the first analysis (before the post-marketing study) might be considered too risky if, for example, the available evidence proves equivocal. In that case, more research to decrease the uncertainty around the expected result (the incremental net benefit, which is the payoff to be maximized) has two consequences:

(i) generating new research costs, and
(ii) delaying the availability of the new treatments for patients while additional research is conducted.

If the new treatment was initially accepted and proved to be more costly or less effective (i.e. lower survival or QALY) the opportunity cost would include the extra cost of treatment over the patient population or the difference in survival over a certain time horizon. The magnitude of the opportunity loss of the initial decision due to the uncertainty about its payoff (the expected incremental net (monetary) benefit or EINB) can be quantified and is known as the expected value of perfect information (EVPI). Basically, this represents the probability of 'being wrong' multiplied by the average cost of being wrong (the opportunity loss).

More formally, the EVPI is the amount the EINB changes (higher or lower) by eliminating the uncertainty (simultaneously) of all parameters/variables (e.g. costs, effects, utilities, adverse event rates, etc.) used in a decision to choose a particular treatment for reimbursement. In some cases, additional information (through more research) on some specific parameters (e.g. efficacy endpoints, like survival or HRQoL) might be sought. Specific parameters might be those whose uncertainty is largest (because there was very little data available before the trial started) and the value (in terms of changes to the EINB) of reducing this will be estimated. When only one parameter is assessed this is called the expected value of partially perfect information (EVPPI) or expected value of perfect parameter estimation. When the per patient EVPI is multiplied by the expected future patient population over a number of years it is called the 'population EVPI.' As such it represents the maximum potential value of further research. If this is close to zero then this means that it is unlikely that the value brought by additional research (to reduce uncertainty) will exceed the cost of that research. Hence, a first step in analyzing the decision is to calculate its population EVPI.

However, in order to have 'perfect information' (i.e. eliminate all sources of uncertainty) we would need a very large, in fact infinite, sample size. Hence, 'perfect information' is an ideal (in as much as having an unlimited sample size is in a clinical trial) to answer a specific question. Therefore, in practice, we try to quantify the uncertainty of decisions (of choosing treatments) by research based on some finite sample size. As such we are interested in the expected value of sample information (EVSI).

The EVSI compares the INB based on trial results given a current sample size (imperfect information based on current data) with that obtained if more data were collected (approaching perfect information – since the greater the sample size, the closer to perfect information one gets).

We may calculate the EVSI for a range of sample sizes for a given research design and compare it to the cost of conducting that research, including the opportunity cost for the patients that will receive the 'inferior' treatment during that study (typically lower survival or QALYs). This is called the expected net benefit of sampling (ENBS). As for the EVPI it can be calculated on a per patient or population level, for all sources of uncertainty or for only some parameters (partial ENBS).

Hence the EVSI is considered to be another approach to estimating the optimal sample size for a future study (Figure 9.11) [22].

The question therefore becomes, for example: "How much value (based on the INB) is there in having more data (with possibly a larger sample size than the one we currently have) so that the current decision does (or does not) not change?" We now show an example of how the EVSI can be calculated and used in the context of sample size calculation. The EVSI is considered to be

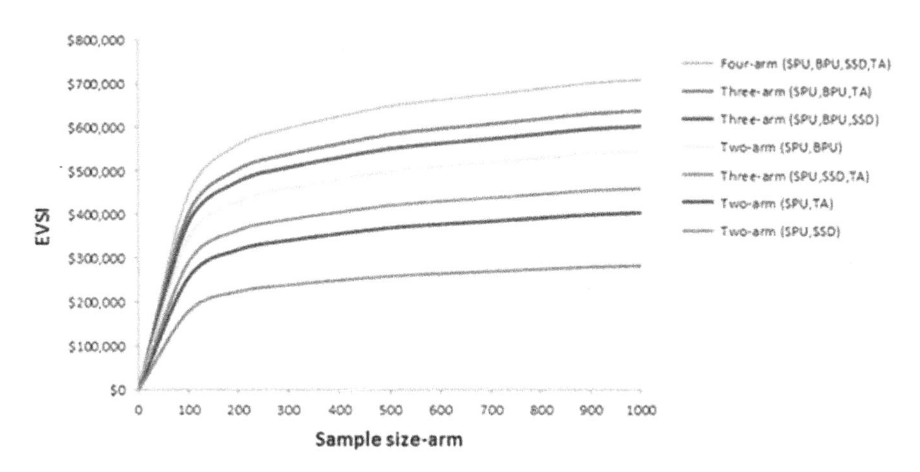

FIGURE 9.11
Sample sizes for varying values of EVSI.

Source: Maeso et al., 2011.

a fully Bayesian approach, but we have removed technical details to ensure focus is on understanding the concept.

Example 9.10: Simple Description of EVSI

We adapt an example from Ades et al. (2004) following their algorithms to compute the EVSI.

A clinical trial has been performed (n = 600; 300 per treatment group). The experimental treatment group (treatment A) was shown to be more cost-effective than the standard treatment (treatment B) with the current expected net monetary benefit (ENMB) of £30,000 for treatment A and £20,000 for treatment B (Table 9.16).

However, it may be the case that a reimbursement agency requests more data in order to better estimate the uncertainty of long-term toxicity data (which can have a significant cost burden). Although the initial decision looks favorable for treatment A (i.e. a higher expected NMB), the payer review group (who are involved in reimbursement) has suggested the sponsor continue to investigate whether AE rates (perhaps using a two arm observational study) might change the current decision (that A is cost-effective compared to B). One question is how much more information should we collect (i.e. what sample size should be used) so that a (currently favorable) decision remains favorable in the future. At what point should we be concerned that the payer will switch a decision (from favorable to unfavorable, or vice versa).

As a starting point, let us assume the payer requests additional data because they believe, from clinical trial data, the longer-term toxicity of chemotherapy is too uncertain. We decide to proceed with a sample size of n = 200 (100 per group), with the primary objective of toxicity, since efficacy has been already demonstrated and there are no major concerns around the uncertainty of OS or PFS.

TABLE 9.16

Model Inputs for EVSI Computations

Treatment	PAE	Cost of treatment (£)	QALY	ENMB[a] (£)
A	0.25	150,000	6	30,000
B	0.10	100,000	4.3	29,000

[a] *Note:* ENMB = –Cost + λ*Effect: ENMB-A = –£150,000 + 6*£30,000; ENMB-B = –£100,000 + 4.3*£30,000 (assuming a CE threshold, λ of £30,000). PAE: probability of adverse event

TABLE 9.17

Example Realization of Value of Sample Information After One Simulation of P^AAE and P^BAE, the Adverse Event Rates for Treatments A and B, Respectively

Simulation Number	Current decision			Posterior decision	VSI
	P^AAE P^BAE	ENB^A	ENB^B [Max]	ENB^A ENB^B [max]	
Prior (trial)	25% 10%	33,000	30,000 33,000	–	37,000
1	28%, 15%	33,000	30,000 33,000	31,000 37,000	– 4,000+
2	...	...	...	...	
...					
10,000					
Mean (EVSI)					6,120

The parameter of particular interest was the (long-term) probability of an adverse event (PAE) , estimated as 25% for treatment A and 10% for B in the initial RCT (which had a sample size of $n = 600$ patients). The question is whether collecting additional data impacts the ENMB. Currently, the decision is in favor of treatment A (ENMB-A > ENMB-B = £30,000 – £29,000 = £1,000) as shown in Table 9.17. A step-by-step approach to a VOI is relegated to the technical appendix (A9.3). We interpret the results.

After the technical process of simulating the possibilities of future long-term toxicity response rates, we compute the maximum of the ENMB between each treatment. For example, if, after the first simulation, we might believe the AE rate is going to be 28% and 15% (higher than that in the trial) for treatments A and B respectively, the posterior mean ENMB for treatment A is now £37,000 and for treatment B is now £31,000 (before these were £33,000 and £30,000 for treatments A and B respectively).

We retain the maximum of these values (i.e. £37,000) – sometimes the ENMB for B may be higher and sometimes (occasionally) lower because we are randomly sampling the AE rate so the costs will vary. This maximum is then compared (subtracted) with the ENMB under the current decision (i.e. £33,000) as shown in Table 9.18. Table 9.18 shows how the data structure might look like after one simulation.

Note: VSI is the value of sample information. The EVSI is the expected value, which is calculated from the average of all the 10,000 VSI values. The VSI is calculated as 33,000 – 37,000 = –4,000.

TABLE 9.18

EVSI and Chance that the ENMB Under the Plan of Additional Data is > ENB Under the Current Decision

Sample Size (n_i)	EVSI (£)	Pr[ENBn=n_i]B > Pr[ENBcurrent]A
50	1,300	0.15
100	2,400	0.22
200	5,280	0.27
400	6,090	0.29
600	6,120	0.33
1,000	6,180	0.38
2,000	6,185	0.39
5,000	6,190	0.40
10,000	6,192	0.40

Based on Table 9.18, after one simulation, a decision-maker (payer) may switch from the initial decision that treatment A was cost-effective (£33,000 vs. £30,000) to it now being not cost-effective (£31,000 vs. £37,000): Treatment B (old, or standard of care) has a greater (posterior) ENMB than treatment A. The process continues for each cycle of the simulation so that we generate a posterior distribution of differences.

For all the 10,000 simulated differences between current ENMB and posterior ENMB, we can compute the mean of all the differences (Table 9.18) to generate the EVSI, which is £6,120. This was evaluated for a sample size of n = 150 per group. This can be repeated for other sample sizes (Table 9.18).

In other words, if we continued to collect further data (e.g. about 300 patients) on long-term toxicity, the ENMB for treatment A will exceed that of treatment B, on average, about 70% of the time (Table 9.19). There may be some chance that treatment B will be less cost-effective than A (Table 9.19) about 27% to 29% of the time. That is, the decision-maker might switch the decision with about a 30% (27% exactly) chance if more data were collected on longer-term toxicity. Hence, the payer may request additional data (on toxicity) to be more certain the ENMB for treatment A is higher than treatment B. Conversely, there is about a 70% chance the payer has made the correct decision and the chance of switching is low. What the threshold chance of switching should be to request further data is unclear and may vary from payer to payer. If collecting further data does not have much chance of changing the decision, then there is less justification for a payer to delay a decision for reimbursement.

The chance of switching a decision appears to plateau after 1,000 patients (Table 9.18). Hence, any further data collected from either clinical trials or observational studies are likely to result in 'erroneous' decisions not greater than 40% of the time, if we had much more information (e.g. data from 10,000 patients). That is, with perfect information of long-term toxicity, a decision-maker could switch their decision with a

TABLE 9.19

Example of a Bootstrap Simulation Showing Probability of Cost-Effectiveness >80%

Simulated Sample	CER (Cost/ QALY)	Below £30,000?
1	19,445	Yes
2	34,215	No
3	33,111	No
4	28,666	Yes
5	19,114	Yes
6	22,875	Yes
7	24,934	Yes
8	27,143	Yes
9	26,165	Yes
10	28,888	Yes

probability of 40%. To reduce this uncertainty, the payer might be justified in requesting more data on toxicity (or even ask the manufacturer to change the price so that value is demonstrated!).

A separate question is whether a probability of 30% (27%) is an acceptable risk level for the decision-maker and the patient. In comparison with a Type I error of 5% for marketing approval, this value might be high. One (perhaps ethical) issue is whether patients should continue to be treated with the new treatment even if there is a risk that the payer might be wrong 30% of the time. The risk is not that the new treatment is not efficacious, but rather that it may not be cost-effective. This risk to the public (declaring that the new treatment is efficacious when in reality it is not) set at 5% (5% Type I error) is unlikely to be given the same weight as a wrong decision on economic grounds. Whether this is right or wrong is a matter for debate.

Example 9.11: Value of Information from Bevacizumab Trial

We now present an example of a value of information analysis reported for bevacizumab used for the treatment of platinum-resistant, recurrent ovarian cancer in a Canadian population (Ball et al., 2018).

BACKGROUND

A cost-utility analysis was undertaken over a 7-year time horizon using a three-state partitioned survival model to compare the effectiveness of bevacizumab plus chemotherapy (BEV) compared to chemotherapy alone. The original trial results were published from the AURELIA Phase III RCT ($n = 361$). which had a primary endpoint of PFS. The published KM curves were taken and using special software, the survival rates for each time point were digitally determined. These were used to determine the transition probabilities for a three-state partitioned survival cost-effectiveness model.

The survival times were assumed to follow a log normal distribution (see Chapter 7) as these fitted the Kaplan-Meier curve estimates best using statistical tests (e.g. Akaike's information criterion) and visual inspection. By 7 years, the expected survival rates are around 0 (the median OS was 13.3 and 16.6 months for chemotherapy and bevacizumab, respectively), which provides some justification for the proposed model.

RESULTS

The results reported the incremental cost per QALY (ICER) as Can $213,424 (£123,064; Can $1/£1 = 0.58) based on a mean incremental QALY of 0.1129. A threshold cost/QALY in oncology reported by the authors was considered to be Can $100,000 (£58,000); and to ensure this threshold could be reached, the authors advised the price (of bevacizumab) should be reduced by 39%.

A value of information analysis was undertaken. The object of this VOI was not, as in the example above, to compute a probability of switching, but rather, to estimate the value of future research when the WTP (cost-effectiveness) threshold was fixed at Can $100,000. The description of the VOI described by the authors is given below:

(i) First, the mean net benefit was calculated over all of the Monte-Carlo simulations in the probabilistic sensitivity analysis.
(ii) Second, the net benefit for each individual Monte-Carlo simulation in each of the treatment arms was calculated, and the maximum net benefit across the treatment arms for each simulation was identified.
(iii) Third, the mean of these maximized net benefit values was then taken.
(iv) Finally, the difference between the mean of the maximized net benefits and the maximum of the mean values was calculated.
(v) The EVPI was estimated to explore the value of conducting future research given a willingness-to-pay ceiling ratio of Can $100,000 (£58,000) per QALY gained and was calculated by multiplying per-patient EVPI by the effective population.
(vi) The estimated 2015 incidence of ovarian cancer multiplied by the proportion of patients with recurrent ovarian cancer yielded an effective per annum population of 2,380.
(vii) In addition, expected value of perfect partial information (EVPPI) analyses were conducted to identify specific parameters for which additional data collection may be worthwhile.
(viii) The EVPI was estimated to be Can $804,818 (£466,794) at a willingness-to-pay threshold of Can $100,000 per QALY gained. Hence, further research may be worth conducting up to a maximum expected cost of Can $804,818 (£466,794).
(ix) Results of the EVPPI analyses showed EVPPI to be the highest for the OS parameter values, suggesting that additional data collection could be worthwhile for collecting further information on OS – for example on longer-term survival.

9.8 Challenges of VOI Analysis in Healthcare Decisions

In practice, few VOI analyses have been conducted up to now in health policy decisions for cancer treatment. One reason is that VOI analysis requires sophisticated simulation methods and presents computational challenges, especially for EVPPI and EVSI (long computation times because of multiple random sampling loops). There is also a lack of automatized dedicated software to make it easier to perform for nonspecialists. It also requires some assumptions about the distribution of the INB (normal or non-normal) and its variance. Most published VOI studies are based on a simulation model (such as the Markov model) rather than on individual patient data (from single or pooled trials), as it is felt that models are able to incorporate more evidence than a single trial.

However, with limited evidence when new treatments are assessed (typically one or two pivotal Phase III trials or a single Phase II trial) VOI analysis can be performed on individual patient data as well. Previous results from Phase II trials or observational studies could then be incorporated in the choice of priors in a fully Bayesian analysis of the pivotal trial(s). In addition, from a policy perspective the decision to adopt (and pay for) the new technology and the cost of conducting additional research are often not borne by the same economic actor (typically a healthcare ministry or agency on the one hand, with a remit for adoption or reimbursement, and a private drug or medical device company, or another official agency, on the other hand). Furthermore, once an adoption/reimbursement decision has been made, reversing it proves very difficult in practice.

As an example, one might cite the Belgian law of 2010 that introduced the possibility of temporary reimbursement for mostly orphan and innovative drugs (so-called Class 1 drugs) and drugs with a high social or therapeutic purpose. Only Class 1 drugs need to complete a cost-effectiveness analysis. The reimbursement price is then, in principle, granted for a limited period of up to three years (renewable twice) during which additional (generally real-life observational) data are to be collected by (and at the cost) of the applicant. Since the year 2010, about 169 contracts have been initiated of which about 60% are active (some firms may be dropped during the procedure because of a lack of agreement between the parties, or for some other reason). Most contracts (called 'article 81 agreement ') find their origin in a difference between the company's asking price for reimbursement and the price proposed by the Drug Reimbursement Commission; or because of drug budget impact consequences (Gerkens, 2017). Not all conventions include an additional research requirement. Firms are generally also reluctant to start a new RCT if they have already performed one, or several, Phase III trials.

Furthermore, it appears that few of these conventions led to much new data collection in practice, although no formal systematic assessment has been published to our knowledge (the details of the conventions are confidential by law in Belgium). In cases where further data collection is requested, VOI and especially (partial) EVSI approaches could be helpful tools. A potential application of VOI could be for an interim analysis decision where the magnitude of the observed effect size is uncertain. VOI using the expected net benefit could be used to evaluate whether collecting additional data is likely to reach a different value proposition based on alternative possibilities of the effect size (in short, is continuing the trial based on the observed effect size likely to lead to a different future cost-effectiveness decision compared to the present).

9.9 Summary

In this chapter we discussed how to present and interpret incremental cost-effectiveness ratios and gave an example of calculating incremental QALYs from a Kaplan-Meier survival curve using the trapezoid rule. We derived QALYs with extrapolated survival data and discussed the relationship between individual costs and QALYs using lung cancer data. Various univariate and multivariate sensitivity analyses were presented in the form of cost-effectiveness acceptability curves (CEACs). We also introduced Bayesian sensitivity analysis techniques and discussed the limitations of ICERs. Finally we introduced the value of information (VOI) concept and its calculation from clinical trial data, giving a detailed example from a bevacizumab trial. We finally discussed, in brief, the challenges of VOI analysis in practice for healthcare decisions.

9.10 Exercises for Chapter 9

1. How would you decide whether a new treatment was cost-effective in the following situations (assume two treatments being compared against each other)?
    a. The primary endpoint was very positive (i.e. a good outcome for the new treatment) and all secondary outcomes were also better for the new treatment.
    b. The primary endpoint was very positive (i.e. a good outcome) and all secondary outcomes were worse for the new treatment.
    c. The primary endpoint was negative and all secondary outcomes were worse for the new treatment.
    d. The primary endpoint was no different between treatments but all secondary outcomes were superior for the new treatment.
    e. Is there a limitation in the way current economic evaluation is performed, based on your answers to the above?

2. What is value of information? When should it be used? Could value of information be used in an interim analysis and, if so, under what circumstances?
3. What is a CEAC and what does it show? What should be an appropriate threshold for a chance of cost-effectiveness in your opinion, and why? justify your answer.
4. What does a cost-effectiveness plane show?

Technical Appendix for Chapter 9

A9.1 Simulation

The process of simulating multivariate correlated data from any distribution requires the use of Fleishman coefficients for pairwise variables to generate the intermediate correlations. For example, with two inputs, total costs, and pre-progression utility, these can be relabeled as X_1 and X_2 respectively. Hence:

$$X_1 = a_1 + b_1 Z_1 + c_1 Z_1^2 + d_1 Z_1^3 \quad (9.1)$$

$$X_2 = a_2 + b_2 Z_2 + c_2 Z_2^2 + d_2 Z_2^3 \quad (9.2)$$

The values of a_i, b_i, c_i, and d_i for (i = 1, 2) are estimated through the power transformation and may be found in Fleishman tables using higher-order moments. Once the values of a_i, b_i, c_i, and d_i are estimated, the intermediate correlation between X_1 and X_2 is determined by using the equation from Vale and Maurelli (1983):

$$R_{x_1 x_2} = \rho\left(b_1 b_2 + 3b_1 d_2 + 3d_1 b_2 + 9d_1 d_2\right) + \rho^2\left(2c_1 c_2\right) + \rho^3\left(6d_1 d_2\right)$$

This is then repeated for each of the pairwise variables to form an 'intermediate correlation matrix.' SAS code based on Fan et al., (2002) can be used to simulate multivariate correlated data where each variable is from any distribution:

The SAS code uses PROC IML for a Newton-Raphson iterative procedure to find the values of a, b, c and d in (9.1) and (9.2). Using the data from Lee et al. (2012), with a sample size of 670, a data set of n = 670 patients was simulated with corresponding costs and effects. This was then repeated 10,000 times (10,000 data sets of size n = 670 with n = 350 on erlotinib and n = 320 on placebo). For each data set the ICER was computed.

A9.2 Bayesian PSA

PSA under a Bayesian context is best understood starting with the bivariate general linear model (GLM). We start with each patient having two responses, one for costs, c_i and one for effects, e_i, contained in the matrix **Y**. In addition, there are two treatment groups (although it can be extended to more than two groups). This is the matrix **X**, where the first column is the intercept and the second column an indicator variable for the treatment group. We also have the parameter matrix β and the error vector ε.

Hence: $Y_{ij} = \mu + \tau_i + \varepsilon_{ij}$ is a standard form of a GLM, where the subscript i = 1, 2 indicates the treatment group and j is the number of observations for each patient in the trial.

Furthermore, μ is a vector $\begin{pmatrix} \mu_c \\ \mu_e \end{pmatrix}$ of the mean costs and effects and τ is a vector of treatment effects for each of costs and effects: $\begin{pmatrix} \tau_c \\ \tau_e \end{pmatrix}$; ε_{ij} is a matrix of residual errors: $\begin{pmatrix} \varepsilon_{11} & \varepsilon_{21} \\ \vdots & \vdots \\ \varepsilon_{1n} & \varepsilon_{2n} \end{pmatrix}$ where the $\varepsilon_{ij} \sim \text{MVN}(0, \beta)$.

If **Y** is $\begin{pmatrix} c_{11} & e_{21} \\ \vdots & \vdots \\ c_{1n} & e_{2n} \end{pmatrix}$, a matrix (of $n \times 2$) of responses for costs and effects, then the model (in a frequentist framework) can be written as below:

Y =		X	β +	ε
Costs	Effects	Intercept group	Parameters	Error
2,000	1.2	1 1	$\mu_1\ \mu_2$	$\varepsilon_{11}\ \varepsilon_{21}$
3,000	1.6	1 1	$\tau_{11}\ \tau_{12}$	$\varepsilon_{12}\ \varepsilon_{22}$
8,000	0.8	1 1		$\varepsilon_{13}\ \varepsilon_{23}$
etc.	etc.	. .		. .
		. .		. .
		. 0		. .
		1 0		$\varepsilon_{1n}\ \varepsilon_{2n}$

The parameters to be estimated are $\mu = \begin{pmatrix} \mu_c \\ \mu_e \end{pmatrix}$ and the variance – covariance matrix Σ. In a Bayesian context, we assume prior distributions for $\mu = \begin{pmatrix} \mu_c \\ \mu_e \end{pmatrix}$, which we can call

$\mu_0 = \begin{pmatrix} \mu_{0c} \\ \mu_{0e} \end{pmatrix}$ and also a prior distribution for Σ,t med $\Sigma_0 = \begin{pmatrix} \sigma_c^2 & \rho\sigma_c\sigma_e \\ \rho\sigma_c\sigma_e & \sigma_e^2 \end{pmatrix}$

TABLE A1

Model Inputs for EVSI Computations

Treatment	PAE	Cost of Treatment (£)	QALY	ENB[a] (£)
A	0.25	150,000	6	30,000
B	0.10	100,000	4.3	29,000

[a] ENB = –Cost + λ*Effect: ENB_A = –£150,000 + 6*£30,000; ENB_B = –£100,000 + 4.3*£30,000 (assuming a CE threshold, λ of £30,000).

The objective is to combine the prior information with the likelihood functions to determine an (updated) estimate of the mean costs and effects. These are called posterior means. Using the posterior means, the (posterior) ICER is then derived. Simulations from the posterior distributions (i.e. posterior mean costs and effects) are carried out (similar to the frequentist method) resulting in 10,000 (for example) posterior mean costs and effects. With this data, the CEAC can be generated as before.

The software in which Bayesian modeling is often carried out in is called WINBUGS, however the PROC MCMC and a PROC GENMOD in SAS are also available for Bayesian analysis.

A9.3 Value of Information

Step 1: First calculate the ENB for each treatment group (Table A1).

Step 2: Determine which parameters will be subject to uncertainty and determine the distribution to be used. The main reason for a future observational study is to get a better estimate of the values of the parameter PAE, the probability of an adverse event (since only one RCT has ever been conducted in this indication). One concern was that data from which the current adverse event rate probability is uncertain and a further observational study with a sample size of n = 300 (150 per group) may help to reduce the uncertainty for the purposes of decision making. Therefore, PAE will be simulated 10,000 times from a beta binomial (BB) distribution. The BB distribution has parameters (α, β), so we need to choose a set of parameters whose mean will result in about 0.25 for treatment A and 0.10 for B, using the fact that:

$$\alpha = \mu * \left[\left(\left(\mu * (1-\mu)\right)/\sigma^2\right) - 1\right] \quad (9.3)$$

$$\beta = (1-\mu) * \left[\left(\left(\mu * (1-\mu)\right)/\sigma^2 - 1\right)\right] \quad (9.4)$$

In this example, an estimate of α = 3 and β = 9 for treatment A (this combination of α and β yields an estimate with mean 0.25, using mean = α/α+β for treatment A, from (9.3)). Simulation from a BB is carried out for each treatment group separately. Data from a BB can be simulated in SAS using the fact that the ratio of two gamma distributed variables is a beta:

$$Z1 = \text{rangam}(\text{seed,alpha});$$

$$Z2 = \text{rangam}(\text{seed,beta});$$

$$X = Z1/(Z1+Z2);\ **\text{gamma}(\text{alpha, beta})$$

Step 3: Once 10,000 values of P_{AE} for each of the treatments have been generated, for each simulated P_{AE}, we then generate data from: binomial (n = 150, P_{AE}), each simulated data set being of sample size n = 150. The likelihood was therefore generated from a binomial (n = 150, P^*_{AE}).

Step 4: The next step is to compute the posterior mean adverse event rate. The prior BB combined with a binomial likelihood yields a posterior mean of P^*_{AE} of the form:

$$a^*/a^*+b^*$$

Example A9.3.1: Beta-Binomial Prior and Binomial Likelihood

Before Any Data is Observed

Before observing any data, θ (i.e. P_{AE} for treatment A) was assumed to be a Beta (2, 2). Since the mean of a Beta $(a,b) = a/(a + b)$, this corresponds to a prior mean of (2/(2 + 2) = 50%).

The form of a prior Beta (1, 3) is : $\dfrac{1}{\text{Beta}(1,3)}\theta(1-\theta)$

In general, a Beta (a,b) density is: $\dfrac{1}{\text{Beta}(a,b)}\ \theta^{a-1}(1-\theta)^{b-1}$

After Data Have Been Observed

Now assume that 10 further patients are observed for any adverse events. These outcomes are assumed to be dichotomous (Yes/No type outcomes). Assume that the 10 subjects have the following observed data:

$$X = (1,0,1,0,0,0,0,1,0,0)$$

where x_i is an indicator variable for 1 if an AE is observed and 0 if not.

For the above realization of AEs, the P_{AE} rate can now be updated by computing the posterior mean. In order to do this we need the likelihood of the 10 outcomes.

$$L(\theta;x) = \prod_{i=1}^{10}\theta^{x_i}(1-\theta)^{1-x_i} = \theta^3(1-\theta)^7$$

We now combine the prior distribution with the likelihood to form the posterior distribution of P_{AE}:

$$P(\theta;x) \propto \theta^3(1-\theta)^7\,\theta(1-\theta) = \theta^4(1-\theta)^8$$

Compare this with: $\dfrac{1}{\text{Beta}(a,b)}\theta^{a-1}(1-\theta)^{b-1}$ (a posterior Beta (5, 9))

Here $a - 1 = 4$ and $b - 1 = 8$, giving $a = 5$ and $b = 9$.

Prior	Beta (2, 2)	2/(2 + 2) = 50%
Posterior	Beta (5, 9)	5/(5 + 9) = 36%

The proportionality symbol (α) means that the full computation of the likelihood with the prior is determined through integrating out the prior × likelihood such that some terms cancel out.

From the computations (integrations), the above results in a posterior Beta (5,9). The mean of a Beta $(a,b) = a/(a+b)$. Therefore, the posterior (mean) PAE, after having observed a further 10 outcomes is 5/(5+9) = 36%. The new (additional) data has revised the estimate of P_{AE} from 50% to 36%.

Hence, we will generate 10,000 posterior mean values $P_i^*{}_{AE}$, where the subscript i is from 1 to 10,000 for each simulated value.

Step 5: For each simulated posterior mean PAE, compute the ENB for each treatment group. That is, we would have 10,000 ENB values for each of treatments A and B. Hence, by formulating a prior distribution based on the original $n = 600$ from the RCT (which is a large amount of data to have an informative prior), and further simulate $n = 300$ ($n = 150$ per treatment group if a two group observational study), we now have 10,000 (updated) ENBs for each of the treatments. We are now in a position for each simulated ENB to compute the impact of the additional $n = 300$ patients through the EVSI.

10

Factors Predictive of HTA Success and the Global Landscape

10.1 Introduction

In this chapter we will discuss reimbursement strategies and experiences across several countries within Europe. In the UK, NICE appears to have one of the most comprehensive and transparent approaches to evaluating cost-effectiveness. We will then discuss briefly some approaches for HTA in other countries, including the US. We consider the potential factors predictive of successful HTAs using available data. Some practical issues in HTAs are also discussed when designing cancer trials for cost-effectiveness.

10.2 Cancer Drugs Rejected by NICE

The National Institute for Health and Care Excellence (NICE) became a legal entity in April 1999 with the aim to create consistent guidelines and to end the rationing of treatment through 'postcode lotteries' (i.e. a random process where some regions could get access to cancer treatments and others could not, thereby increasing inequality) across the UK. NICE provides guidance to the NHS in England on the clinical- and cost-effectiveness of selected new and established technologies. The Institute undertakes appraisals of health technologies at the request of the UK Department of Health. Guidance produced by the Institute on health technologies is also applied selectively in Northern Ireland, Scotland, and Wales (Timmins, Rawlins & Appleby, 2016).

Initially, the technology appraisal was based on examining the values from multiple health technologies (drugs, devices, or other health interventions in the NHS, including advice) for any one condition. The single technology appraisal (STA) process was introduced in early 2005 to assess a single drug or treatment for a single indication. Both the multiple technology appraisal (MTA) and the STA are processes designed to provide recommendations, in

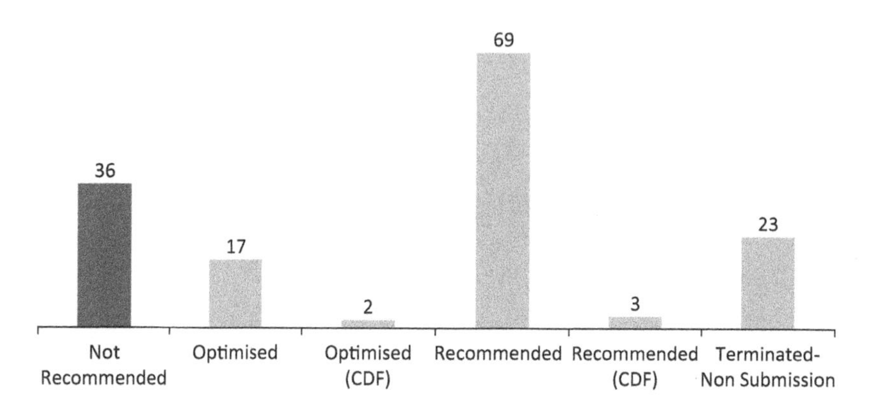

FIGURE 10.1
Breakdown of HTA decisions from 150 cancer products (NICE HTA, April 2018). Note: CDF: cancer drug fund; optimized: the reimbursement guideline only covers a subpopulation of the licensed population; terminated non-submission: manufacturer decided not to submit the evidence.

the form of NICE guidance, on the use of new and existing medicines, products, and treatments in the NHS. The STA process was introduced as a mechanism to provide a prompt appraisal of technologies for use within the NHS in England and Wales so that national guidance for new products could be provided as closely as possible to their launch (i.e. when they would be officially available for prescription or access by patients), and more quickly than the existing MTA process.

According to the data available, as of October 2017, 150 cancer medicines (technologies) were appraised by NICE following the STA process. Figure 10.1 provides a breakdown of outcomes for different decisions reached by NICE.

Of the 150 single technology assessment submissions, almost one-quarter (36/150 or 24%) were not recommended for routine clinical use in England and Wales; 23 appraisals were terminated due to non-submission of evidence by the manufacturers. Reimbursement was granted for 91 out of 150 (61%) of the technologies, either as a recommendation in line with marketing authorization ($n = 69$) for routine use through the cancer drug fund (CDF), or optimized recommendation, which cover only a subgroup.

Table 10.1 lists the drugs not recommended for reimbursement by NICE since 2001, including both STA and MTA recommendations.

10.3 Summary of Criticisms of Economic Models of Cancer

The availability of appropriate and robust data to populate model parameters requires efficacy and safety data regarding disease symptoms, disease progression, adverse events, death, HRQoL, health resource utilization, as well

TABLE 10.1

List of Drugs Not Recommended by NICE between 2001 and 2017

Appraisal Number	Year	Process	Drug	Condition
TA025	2001	MTA	Gemcitabine (second line)	Pancreatic cancer
TA030	2001	MTA	Docetaxel in combination with an anthracycline (first line)	Advanced breast cancer
TA033	2002	MTA	Irinotecan in combination with 5-fluorouracil and folinic acid (5FU/FA) (first-line)	Colorectal cancer (advanced)
TA037	2002	MTA	Rituximab (third and subsequent lines of treatment)	Lymphoma (follicular non-Hodgkin's)
TA054	2002	MTA	Vinorelbine combination therapies	Breast cancer
TA108	2006	STA	Paclitaxel	Breast cancer (early)
TA118	2007	MTA	Bevacizumab in combination with 5-fluorouracil plus folinic acid (with or without irinotecan)	Colorectal cancer (metastatic)
TA118	2007	MTA	Cetuximab in combination with irinotecan	Colorectal cancer (metastatic)
TA119	2007	STA	Fludarabine (monotherapy)	Leukemia (lymphocytic)
TA124	2007	STA	Pemetrexed (second line)	Non-small-cell lung cancer
TA162	2008	STA	Erlotinib (second-line treatment in patients for whom docetaxel is unsuitable; or as a third-line treatment after docetaxel therapy)	Non-small-cell lung cancer
TA172	2009	STA	Cetuximab	Head and neck
TA178	2009	MTA	Bevacizumab (first line)	Advanced and/or metastatic renal cell carcinoma (RCC)
TA178	2009	MTA	Sorafenib (first line)	RCC
TA178	2009	MTA	Temsirolimus (first line)	RCC
TA178	2009	MTA	Sunitinib (second line)	RCC
TA178	2009	MTA	Sorafenib (second line)	RCC

(Continued)

TABLE 10.1 (CONTINUED)

List of Drugs Not Recommended by NICE between 2001 and 2017

Appraisal Number	Year	Process	Drug	Condition
TA184	2009	MTA	Intravenous topotecan	Relapsed small-cell lung cancer
TA189	2010	STA	Sorafenib (first line)	Hepatocellular carcinoma
TA196	2010	STA	Imatinib adjuvant	Gastrointestinal stromal tumors (resectable)
TA202	2010	STA	Ofatumumab	CLL
TA209	2010	MTA	Imatinib (dose escalation to 600 mg/day or 800 mg/day following disease progression on 400 mg/day imatinib)	Gastrointestinal stromal tumors
TA212	2010	STA	Bevacizumab in combination with oxaliplatin and either fluorouracil plus folinic acid or capecitabine	Metastatic colorectal cancer
TA214	2011	STA	Bevacizumab in combination with a taxane (first line)	Metastatic breast cancer
TA219	2011	STA	Everolimus	Advanced renal cell carcinoma
TA227	2011	STA	Erlotinib (first line maintenance treatment)	Advanced/ metastatic NSCLC
TA239	2011	STA	Fulvestrant	Locally advanced or metastatic breast cancer
TA241	2012	MTA	Dasatinib	Chronic myeloid leukemia
TA241	2012	MTA	High dose imatinib	Chronic myeloid leukemia
TA242	2012	MTA	Cetuximab monotherapy or in combination with chemotherapy	Metastatic colorectal cancer
TA242	2012	MTA	Bevacizumab + non-oxaliplatin chemotherapy	Metastatic colorectal cancer
TA242	2012	MTA	Panitumumab monotherapy	Metastatic colorectal cancer
TA250	2012	STA	Eribulin	Advanced or metastatic breast cancer

(Continued)

TABLE 10.1 (CONTINUED)

List of Drugs Not Recommended by NICE between 2001 and 2017

Appraisal Number	Year	Process	Drug	Condition
TA251	2012	MTA	Dasatinib (first-line)	Chronic phase Philadelphia-chromosome-positive chronic myeloid leukemia
TA255	2012	STA	Cabazitaxel in combination with prednisone or prednisolone	Metastatic prostate cancer
TA257	2012	MTA	Trastuzumab in combination with an aromatase inhibitor (first line)	Metastatic breast cancer
TA263	2012	STA	Bevacizumab in combination with capecitabine (first line)	Metastatic breast cancer
TA272	2013	STA	Vinflunine	Advanced or metastatic transitional cell carcinoma of the urothelial tract
TA284	2013	STA	Bevacizumab in combination with paclitaxel and carboplatin	Advanced ovarian cancer
TA285	2013	STA	Bevacizumab in combination with gemcitabine and carboplatin	Advanced ovarian cancer
TA289	2013	STA	Ruxolitinib	Myelofibrosis
TA295	2013	STA	Everolimus in combination with exemestane	Advanced breast cancer
TA296	2013	STA	Crizotinib	Non-small-cell lung cancer (NSCLC)/anaplastic lymphoma
TA299	2013	STA	Bosutinib	Chronic myeloid leukemia
TA307	2014	STA	Aflibercept in combination with irinotecan and fluorouracil-based therapy	Metastatic colorectal cancer
TA309	2014	STA	Pemetrexed	NSCLC
TA338	2015	STA	Pomalidomide in combination with dexamethasone	Multiple myeloma

(Continued)

TABLE 10.1 (CONTINUED)

List of Drugs Not Recommended by NICE between 2001 and 2017

Appraisal Number	Year	Process	Drug	Condition
TA360	2015	STA	Paclitaxel as albuminbound nanoparticles in combination with gemcitabine	Pancreatic cancer
TA371	2015	STA	Trastuzumab emtansine	Metastatic breast cancer
TA374	2015	MTA	Gefitinib	NSCLC
TA378	2016	STA	Ramucirumab alone or with paclitaxel	Gastric cancer or gastro-oesophageal
TA389	2016	MTA	Gemcitabine in combination with carboplatin	Recurrent ovarian cancer
TA389	2016	MTA	Trabectedin in combination with PLDH	Recurrent ovarian cancer
TA389	2016	MTA	Topotecan	Recurrent ovarian cancer
TA399	2016	STA	Azacitidine	Acute myeloid leukemia
TA403	2016	STA	Ramucirumab in combination with docetaxel	NSCLC
TA411	2016	STA	Necitumumab, in combination with gemcitabine and cisplatin	NSCLC
TA414	2016	STA	Cobimetinib in combination with vemurafenib	Melanoma
TA425	2016	STA	High-dose imatinib	Chronic myeloid leukemia
TA440	2017	STA	Pegylated liposomal irinotecan in combination with 5fluorouracil and leucovorin	Pancreatic cancer

STA: Single Technology Appraisal; MTA: Multiple Technology Appraisal.

as data regarding patient drug utilization behaviors (e.g. therapy discontinuation or switching). These inputs are needed to generate cost-effectiveness analyses. Not all of this data, as noted from previous chapters, are routinely collected during clinical trials; data from other diverse sources are used to complement or 'fill in the gaps' in order to build a robust health economic model. More often than not, economic data for health economic models in cancer come from alternative sources such as naturalistic, non-interventional studies (including both prospective and retrospective observational studies). For these reasons, the quality of the final health economic model may not always meet the standards expected for a positive recommendation by reimbursement bodies.

Given that approximately 25% of oncology drugs were not recommended by NICE for a variety of different cancer subtypes and indications, the common criticisms of health economic models that led to their rejection are worthwhile reviewing. In subsequent sections of this chapter, we summarize the research carried out to identify potential factors predictive of successful HTA submissions. We also present the major areas of criticism of health economic models used for cancer drugs. The criticisms are categorized as follows:

- (i) Criticism of clinical evidence. There is a debate as to whether this is the remit of NICE given that the multiple licensing authorities have already given an approval.
- (ii) Criticism of utility data. The use of external data based on unreasonable assumptions is often cited. see recent ISPOR publication on 29 March 2019 http://press.ispor.org/index.php/global-expert-panel-publishes-new-recommendations-on-the-use-of-health-state-utilities-in-cost-effectiveness-models/
- (iii) Criticism of the health economic model and/or analysis. The type of model, its assumptions, and failure to take into account fundamental aspects (e.g. treatment switching) are often cited.

Given the large number of HTAs not recommended for reimbursement, it is difficult to detail every particular feature and the reasons for rejection. Table 10.2 shows the variety of criticisms from a number of NICE-appraised HTAs.

There were some common themes:

- (a) Absence of EQ-5D utility, or inadequate reporting, or assumptions around it.
- (b) Modeling survival data was found problematic, and also based on unjustifiable assumptions.
- (c) Evidence synthesis often inadequate.
- (d) Reliable or immature evidence from overall survival (often the primary endpoint).

(i) Summary of Criticisms of Clinical Evidence from NICE HTAs

TABLE 10.2

Summary of Criticisms Across Most HTAs

Feature	Main Criticisms	Example Review Cited
Clinical evidence		
Population	• Worse performance patients not presented adequately • Differences in baseline characteristics • Target population likely to be older than trial sample	TA374 TA374 TA307
Intervention		
Comparator	• Nivolumab and criotinib were excluded (this is despite the fact that nivolumab was undergoing appraisal at the same time)	TA403
Outcomes	• Absence of benefit in OS • Mean estimate of OS unreliable due to small numbers • Lack of information on censoring. Suggestion that censoring may be informative and reduce validity of Kaplan-Meier and other survival estimates	TA374 TA304 TA389
Trial design		
Experimental design	Trial design good, but unlikely to reflect clinical practice	TA374
Interim analyses	No mature data during interim analyses	TA 202
Health resource/ costs	• Regimen used in trials unlikely to be used in practice • Determined from a retrospective study • Acquisition and administration costs of drug inappropriate • Median values of health resource use applied; whereas means used in cost-effectiveness • Assumption that patients will receive a low number of cycles (which reduces costs); assuming efficacy is not impacted	TA374 TA304 TA304 TA304 TA389
HRoL (utility)	• Unpublished or lack of peer review • Treatment-related AE utilities used not related to population • Estimated from a separate cross-section study • Utility value in progressive disease state too high • No adjustment of utility of patient aging over time • Insufficient review of utility data • Utility estimated from a separate trial • Validity of EQ-5D translation • Small differences in EQ-5D • Statistical comparisons of EQ-5D not provided • External EQ-5D data (mis-reported) • Contradictory assumptions on EQ-5D: on the one hand, assuming a constant EQ-5D post-progression while, on the other hand, using systematic reviews showing utility declined during subsequent therapy	TA374 TA374 TA374 TA304 TA304 TA389 TA389 TA403 TA403 TA403 TA403 TA403

(Continued)

TABLE 10.2 (CONTINUED)

Summary of Criticisms Across Most HTAs

Feature	Main Criticisms	Example Review Cited
Economic model		
Assumptions	• Nonproportional hazards not accepted: survival curves considered to converge after 5 years. • Assumptions around model too simplistic • Proportional hazards assumption violated • Similarity of treatment effects between studies in meta-analyses not justified • Unjustifiable assumption of PH: "no theoretical reason to believe PH assumption holds for two treatments that differ in their mode of action"[1]	TA304 TA304 TA389, TA403 TA403 TA403
Model structure	• Partitioned survival model • 3 state Markov model	TA374, TA403, TA304, TA374 TA304
Confounding	Post-progression therapy use/crossover bias	TA389
Prediction of survival	• Piecewise model preferred • Extrapolation is uncertain (small numbers): projected curve separation is unreliable • Truncation of projected OS advised	TA374 TA304 TA304
Estimate of treatment effects	Hazard ratios were adjusted when used in the economic model, ERG used unadjusted	TA389
Subgroup analyses	Lack of statistical significance	TA307
New comparator	Nivolumab not yet appraised, but expected as a comparator	TA403
Systematic review	• Insufficient evidence or further evidence needed • No previous published cost-effectiveness analyses • Insufficient data for a pairwise meta-analysis • Network meta-analyses (NMA) performed, but limited data • Exclusion of some studies in the NMA	TA374 TA304 TA389 TA389 TA403
Analysis	• Statistical heterogeneity across the different studies not adequately addressed • Sparse data resulting in lack of convergence for statistical models	TA403 TA403

Note: [1] One normally tests for a rejection of PH (i.e. in the absence of data we assume PH). Here the ERG assumes a starting position of non-PH unless evidence is bought forward contrary to this hypothesis. For example, for both cytotoxic (drugs that kill cancer cells) and cytostatic drug s (drugs that arrest the growth of cancer cells), the relationship between OS and tumor response might be poor; it does not follow that it is a necessary condition that the survival rates of the two drugs when compared are proportional (i.e. parallel survival curves).

The robustness of clinical evidence is frequently questioned by NICE appraisal committees and 'independent' evidence review groups (ERG). As discussed in detail in Chapter 2, the endpoints in oncology clinical trials are often well defined and primarily related to survival. Most regulatory authorities require evidence of clinical efficacy for new drug registration in terms of benefits from OS, either directly or indirectly using surrogate endpoints such as PFS.

On many occasions, the evidence for improvement in OS and/or HRQoL is limited at the time of initial drug registration. Only 57% (39/68) of cancer drugs approved by the European Medicines Agency (EMA) between 2009 and 2013 showed evidence of improved survival or HRQoL at the time of market entry (Davis, 2017). Showing benefits in OS, simply put, takes longer and it is more expensive to follow up patients until death. Kim and Prasad (2015, 2016) show something similar. Hence, it should come as no surprise that the clinical benefit based on OS at the time of initial regulatory approval is inadequate or uncertain at best. In some cases, it may even be difficult to measure meaningful OS improvements, because patients are likely to experience crossover and receive multiple lines of treatment following disease progression.

PFS is an often used surrogate endpoint accepted by several regulatory authorities and also some reimbursement bodies. In Germany, the Institute for Quality and Efficiency in Health Care (IQWiG) is likely to endorse the combination of PFS with improved HRQoL (not necessarily the EQ-5D) as an acceptable 'benefit' for their assessments. However, for countries where cost-effectiveness assessments are carried out, such as England and Wales (NICE), Scotland (SMC), and Australia (PBAC), both OS and HRQoL data may be required. In the absence of OS and HRQoL data (e.g. using tumor response), drug manufacturers are likely to be required to conduct economic modeling in order to *extrapolate* available clinical data to show a meaningful improvement in survival and HRQoL.

A lack of head-to-head clinical data comparing investigational treatments with all possible comparators is one of the larger problems in developing economic models, as noted in Table 10.2. For example, most payers and reimbursement bodies around the world require comparisons with the most appropriate comparators for their health economic evaluations. In some cases, for an emerging treatment, no published data are available, yet the decision-making body will request it. This might seem like an unfair request, however it will be important at some point to ensure optimal decisions can be made on cost-effectiveness. Hence relegating the comparison to a future date only delays the inevitable.

Local decision-makers are often interested to know what extent the trial data are reflected in or applicable to the target population. Multinational trials should try to account for some features of the target population. For some rare tumors this might be difficult, because each country will only have a few patients. Oncology clinical trials recruit fewer patients than some of the other non-oncology indications such as respiratory or cardiovascular disease. According to one study, based on data from Clinicaltrials.gov, 98% of oncology-related clinical trials registered from 2007 to 2010 have 1,000 participants or fewer, and 75% have 100 or fewer participants (Miller et al., 2014). Due to the global nature of these trials, there may only be a limited number of patients enrolled from a particular country or region.

Some multinational trials may be nonrandomized, single arm, Phase I/II studies, with no comparators. In some cases, RCTs may not include all the potential treatment options that may be considered the standard of care in a particular country. In fact, the NICE scoping document (NICE – Guide to Technology Appraisal Process, January 2019), which is prepared in collaboration with the manufacturer prior to the STA submission, often includes more comparators than those included in the control arm of registration clinical studies. In the absence of head-to-head trials versus all possible comparators, published data is used for clinical and cost-effectiveness modeling, which leaves the models open to criticisms and increased uncertainty (see Table 10.2).

Example 10.1: Case Study – TA428 (NICE, TA428, 2017): Pembrolizumab for PD-L1-Positive Non-Small-Cell Lung Cancer after Chemotherapy

BACKGROUND

Pembrolizumab received marketing authorization for treating locally advanced or metastatic NSCLC in adults whose tumors express PD-L1 (defined as a tumor proportion score (TPS) $\geq$ 1%) and who have had at least one chemotherapy regimen. Patients with the actionable tumor mutations positive (EGFR positive or anaplastic lymphoma kinase (ALK) positive tumor) should also have had an approved therapy for these mutations (e.g. erlotinib, which is used for EGFR +ve patients) before having pembrolizumab.

CLINICAL TRIAL EVIDENCE

The manufacturers submission was based on two trials:

(i) The KEYNOTE-010, and
(ii) KEYNOTE-001

The KEYNOTE-010 population consisted only of patients with PD-L1-positive NSCLC. KEYNOTE-010 was powered to detect a difference between pembrolizumab and docetaxel in the population with a TPS of 50% or more, and in the overall TPS 1% or more population, but not for the TPS 1 to 49% population. The TPS is a biomarker to score patients at different levels of expression of the program cell death ligand-1 (PD-L1) expression on the cancer cells. The patients, whose tumors express high levels of PD-L1 are scored high on the TPS, are more likely to respond to pembrolizumab treatment.

The inclusion criteria in KEYNOTE-010 required patients to have an Eastern Cooperative Oncology Group (ECOG) performance status of 0 or 1. The median overall survival was 10.5 months for pembrolizumab compared with 8.6 months for docetaxel in the ITT population. This difference was statistically significant.

KEYNOTE-001 was a nonrandomized cohort study of pembrolizumab that retrospectively identified PD-L1 status and used the docetaxel arm of KEYNOTE-010 as a comparator.

The manufacturer's base case ICER using a simple discount (confidential discount from the list price) was £48,667 per QALY. In the pivotal trial, treatment continued until disease progression and, given the long-term benefit of immunotherapy drugs such as pembrolizumab, some patient continued to benefit from treatment for a longer period of time, incurring costs to the NHS. However, NICE recognized that with no treatment stopping rule (i.e. a hard stop once a patient received treatment for a certain number of cycles) the ICER was likely to be higher. Following further analysis to address uncertainties in the model, the NICE appraisal committee concluded that based on the trial data, pembrolizumab had an important extension-to-life benefit for people with locally advanced or metastatic NSCLC whose tumors express PD-L1 compared with docetaxel.

In order to meet the NICE cost-effectiveness threshold, the manufacturer proposed that the treatment should be stopped at two years instead of the treatment-till-progression approach employed in the clinical trials. During the appraisal committee meeting, NICE identified the following areas of uncertainty:

- Optimal duration of treatment
- Magnitude of OS gain
- Long-term treatment effect

NICE concluded that it was aware of several ongoing clinical trials that could reduce this uncertainty and, if pembrolizumab was recommended for routine commissioning, relevant data would be collected by the systemic anti-cancer therapy (SACT) data set (see Chapter 8 on RWD). NICE concluded that uncertainty about the long-term treatment effect would fall as more information (data) became available on the optimal duration of treatment of PD-1 inhibitors in the next two years.

WHAT HAPPENED NEXT?

NICE will review the data available from ongoing clinical trials and the data collected within the SACT data set in two years' time to issue the final guidance whether pemobrolizumab should be made available for routine use outside CDF. In this example, too, reliance on data outside a clinical trial (the SACT database) is of interest as noted in Chapter 8 on real-world evidence.

10.4 Factors Predictive of Successful HTAs in Cancer

We noted earlier in Section 10.1, NICE issued not-recommended guidance for 24% of STA cancer drugs. In contrast, during the same period, the overall not-recommended guidance for oncology and non-oncology technologies was 18%. This gives one the impression that oncology drugs are more likely to be issued with a negative reimbursement decision and there may be some bias, systematic or otherwise, in how cancer drugs are viewed for reimbursement in the UK.

Although a shadow price of a QALY is not described as a single threshold, according to the most recent and definitive statement from NICE (2013), technologies costing less than £20,000 cost per QALY gained are usually considered cost-effective. Treatments for children, disadvantaged populations, and severe diseases may be treated more favorably (NICE 2008, 2013; Rawlins et al., 2010). A drug with orphan designation does not play any role in the NICE cost-effectiveness assessment (Littlejohns and Rawlins, 2009). Although NICE has become increasingly explicit and transparent about its decision-making process, areas of considerable uncertainty remain. This issue is not limited to NICE but also to some European countries:

> there remains a lack of transparency around critical elements, such as how multiple factors or criteria are weighed during committee deliberations.
>
> **(Stafiniski et al. 2011)**

For example, Bossers et al. (2015) , analyzed single technology assessments conducted by NICE, Scottish Medicines Consortium (SMC), Zorginstituut Nederland (ZIN), Haute Autorité de Santé (HAS), and Gemeinsamer Bundesausschuss (G-BA) as well as the clinical, economic, and societal data underlying these assessments. This analysis revealed that in most countries clinical factors appeared to be predictive factors for successful reimbursement, whereas in countries such as the UK, where cost-effectiveness analyses are performed, economic factors appeared to be predictive. These findings confirm the previous results of Devlin and Parkin (2004), who showed cost-effectiveness was a key driver for NICE decisions – and not necessarily the clinical rationale, although other factors such as uncertainty and burden of disease were also significant. Table 10.3 presents the results of research in this area.

Dakin et al. (2015), investigated the following factors: clinical and economic evidence; characteristics of patients, disease, or treatment; and contextual factors potentially affecting decision-making. Their analysis showed that the ICER alone correctly predicted 82% of all NICE decisions between 1999 and 2011. There was no evidence that the cost per QALY threshold

TABLE 10.3

Research Findings on Factors Predictive of Cost-Effectiveness

HTA Body	Variables	Reference
NICE	Cost-effectiveness, clinical evidence, technology type, and patient group	Dakin et al. (2006)
NICE	Cost-effectiveness, statistical superiority of primary endpoint, number of pharmaceuticals, and the appraisal year	Cerri et al. (2014)
NICE	ICER, uncertainty, availability of other therapies, and severity of illness	Tappenden et al. (2007)
AWMSG	Cost-effectiveness	Linley and Hughes (2012)
SMC	Cost-effectiveness	Msheila et al. (2013)
APBAC	Cost-effectiveness	Harris et al. (2008)

Note: AWMSG: All Wales Medicines Strategy Group; SMC: Scottish Medicines Consortium; APBAC: Australian Pharmaceutical Benefits Advisory Committee

has significantly changed over time. No other variables were statistically predictive of a decision to reimburse. This essentially means that all focus should be to reduce the ICER. This is an expected conclusion as it is logical that the lower (or higher) the ICER, the higher (or lower) the chance of a reimbursement decision. Technologies costing £27,000, £40,000, and £52,000 per QALY were reported to have probabilities of rejection at around 25%, 50%, and 75% respectively (which is also logical, as the higher the ICER, the greater the likelihood that it will be rejected). A more interesting question however, is what the predictors of successful reimbursement for cancer drugs are, based on a range of evidence. In particular, are there any features, such as lower incremental costs, QALYs, or the size of the study, that are predictive of this?

Table 10.4 shows data extracted from HTA reports showing the decision (recommend/not recommend) in relation to:

(i) ICER
(ii) Incremental QALY
(iii) Incremental cost
(iv) Hazard ratio
(v) Performance status (ECOG)
(vi) Sample size

Other factors could also be included, such as mean survival difference, type of model (partitioned survival or Markov model), HRQoL (condition-specific), year of appraisal, and tumor type. However, for simplicity we used the six factors above. The submissions cover multiple tumor types and in some

TABLE 10.4

An Extract of UK HTA Decisions for Cancer Drugs

Drug	Condition	Categorization	ICER	INC_QALY	INC_ COST_best	Hros	ECOG	Sample Size
Temozolomide	Brain cancer (recurrent)	Recommended	42920	0.2	3863	1.44	n/a	n/a
Bevacizumab (first line)	Advanced and/or metastatic renal cell carcinoma	Not Recommended	171301	0.26	45435	1.27	0-1	649
Temsirolimus (first line)	Advanced and/or metastatic renal cell carcinoma	Not Recommended	81687	0.24	19276	1.28	n/a	626
Sunitinib (second line)	Advanced and/or metastatic renal cell carcinoma	Not Recommended	71462	0.44	31185	1.54	0-1	750
Sorafenib (second line)	Advanced and/or metastatic renal cell carcinoma	Not Recommended	102498	0.23	24001	1.38	0-2	903
Sunitinib	Unresectable and/ or metastatic	Recommended	32636	0.5	16337	1.14	0-4	361
Pemetrexed in combination with cisplatin (first line)	Locally advanced or metastatic	Recommended	33065	0.041	1364	1.19	0-1	1725
Sorafenib (first line)	Advanced and metastatic hepatocellular carcinoma	Not Recommended	64754	0.36	23232	1.45	0-2	602

(Continued)

TABLE 10.4 (CONTINUED)

An Extract of UK HTA Decisions for Cancer Drugs

Drug	Condition	Categorization	ICER	INC_QALY	INC_COST_best	Hros	ECOG	Sample Size
Pemetrexed (maintenance treatment)	Non-small-cell lung cancer	Recommended	33732	0.271	9137	1.43	0-1	663
Gefitinib (first line)	Locally advanced or metastatic	Recommended	20744	0.177	3666	1.09	0-2	1217
Gefitinib (first line)	Locally advanced or metastatic	Recommended	19402	0.187	3637	1.09	0-2	1217
Gefitinib (first line)	Locally advanced or metastatic	Recommended	35992	0.223	8023	1.09	0-2	1217
Gefitinib (first line)	Locally advanced or metastatic	Recommended	28663	0.145	4138	1.09	0-2	1217
Bevacizumab in combination with a taxane (first line)	Metastatic breast cancer	Not Recommended	77314	0.259	30469	1.15	n/a	736
Bevacizumab in combination with a taxane (first line)	Metastatic breast cancer	Not Recommended	57753	0.273	31416	1.15	n/a	736
Bevacizumab in combination with a taxane (first line)	Metastatic breast cancer	Not Recommended	60101	0.259	27358	1.15	n/a	736
Erlotinib (first-line maintenance treatment)	Advanced or metastatic non-small cell lung cancer	Not Recommended	44812	0.1591	7129	1.23	0-1	487

(Continued)

TABLE 10.4 (CONTINUED)

An Extract of UK HTA Decisions for Cancer Drugs

Drug	Condition	Categorization	ICER	INC_QALY	INC_ COST_best	Hros	ECOG	Sample Size
Fulvestrant	Treatment of locally advanced breast cancer	Not Recommended	31982	0.383	12239	1.19	n/a	736
Cetuximab monotherapy or in combination with chemotherapy	Treatment of metastatic colorectal carcinoma	Not Recommended	88000	0.6	53100	1.29	0-2	572
Bevacizumab in combination with non-oxaliplatin (fluoropyr	Treatment of metastatic colorectal carcinoma	Not Recommended	98000	0.25	24500	1.29	0-2	572
Panitumumab monotherapy	Treatment of metastatic colorectal carcinoma	Not Recommended	150000	0.19	29000	1.29	0-2	572
Eribulin	Treatment of locally advanced or metastatic breast cancer	Not Recommended	46050	0.1213	5586	1.23	0-2	488
Eribulin	Treatment of locally advanced or metastatic breast cancer	Not Recommended	27183	0.1904	5177	1.23	0-2	78

(Continued)

TABLE 10.4 (CONTINUED)

An Extract of UK HTA Decisions for Cancer Drugs

Drug	Condition	Categorization	ICER	INC_QALY	INC_ COST_best	Hros	ECOG	Sample Size
Eribulin	Treatment of locally advanced or metastatic breast cancer	Not Recommended	35602	0.1136	4041	1.23	0-2	139
Eribulin	Treatment of locally advanced or metastatic breast cancer	Not Recommended	47631	0.2683	12779	1.23	0-2	43
Ipilimumab	Previously untreated advanced melanoma	Recommended	31559	0.75	23766	1.38	0-1	502
Dabrafenib	Unresectable or metastatic BRAF melanoma	Recommended	112727	0.45	55000	1.31	0-1	250
Pembrolizumab	Treating advanced melanoma	Recommended	46662	n/a	n/a	1.13	0-1	540
Cabozantinib	Medullary thyroid cancer	Recommended	31546	1.34	42215	1.01	n/a	331

Source: Data from https://www.nice.org.uk/guidance.

cases several comparisons. We used the HTA-accepted model whenever possible. In some cases data were not available (n/a).

If we summarize the average (mean) of each parameter by whether the drug was recommended or not, we observe from Table 10.5 the mean values that separate recommended from non-recommended drugs for each of the parameters. So, for example, we might expect that for recommended drugs, the mean ICER should be around £39,000, and the median incremental QALY around 0.389. For incremental cost and the treatment effect (the hazard ratios were inverted to reflect the treatment effect of the experimental drug) the average values were £15,558 and 0.794 respectively. Larger studies also seemed more strongly associated with a positive recommendation, on average. If we model the probability of recommendation for these parameters (Table 10.6), we note that, as expected, the ICER is statistically predictive with small p-values for other parameters. Interestingly, larger sample sizes seem to influence a recommendation. This might be a reason to consider powering trials for cost-effectiveness. Due to the small sample of HTAs used in this analysis, there remains much uncertainty. As future analyses will use more data, we should expect to have some patterns emerging (this is an area of current research). This example is merely intended to show how data can be used to provide a more informed framework for investigating reimbursement decisions.

10.5 The Changing Pace of the Reimbursement Environment

There have been large increases in the costs of cancer care worldwide and there is real concern that cancer treatment is becoming unsustainable. Drug budgets are being tightened, resulting in increased payer management of drug pricing and restricted reimbursement decisions. The oncology clinical development market has become crowded, and therefore clear differentiation is essential to demonstrate value. Most reimbursement bodies around the world routinely reject drugs that fail to demonstrate benefit in terms of survival and/or HRQoL (see Table 10.1 for example).

In Germany, the ability to negotiate price is based on assessment of 'benefit' and drugs without assigned 'benefit' are automatically forced to be priced at the cost of the existing standard of care, without any negotiation. Even in countries such as the US, where drug prices can be set without government restrictions, the cost of cancer is rapidly becoming a hot political topic. According to the American Institute of Cancer Research, cancer costs the world more money than any other disease group – about $895 billion a year. In addition to the cost of drugs, we must add the costs of diagnosis, radiotherapy, imaging, pathology, surgery, and end-of-life care. The US National Bureau of Economic Research reports that the prices of cancer drugs have

TABLE 10.5

Sample Parameters Related to Recommendation

Decision	#HTAs	Parameter	*n*	Mean	Median	Min.	Max.
Recommended	12	ICER	12	39,137	32,850	19,402	112,727
		INC QALY	11	0.389	0.223	0.041	1.340
		INC cost	11	15,558	8,023	1,364	55,000
		Sample size	11	840	663	250	1,725
		HR for OS	12	0.794	0.813	0.649	0.869
Not recommended	18	ICER	18	71,804	62,427	27,183	171,301
		INC QALY	17	0.270	0.259	0.113	0.60
		INC cost	17	22,701	24,001	4,041	53,100
		Sample size	18	601	614	43	1,401
		HR for OS	18	0.845	0.881	0.694	0.99

Notes: INC: incremental; HR: hazard ratio for overall survival (OS).

TABLE 10.6

Statistical Predictors of a Recommendation

Parameter	*p*-Value
Incremental cost	0.242
Incremental QALY	0.261
ICER	0.039
HR	0.101
Sample size	0.130

increased 10% every year between 1995 and 2013. In the US, the freedom to price means top-selling drugs are on average three times higher than in the UK. With new immunotherapy drugs given as monotherapy or in combination with other drugs, the costs increase (you have to pay for more than one drug) to more than £100,000 per year per patient. The 'financial toxicity' of these drugs is a real concern for patients and healthcare systems alike across the world.

Since 2012, there has been an increased focus in the US on spiraling cancer drug prices, with oncologists calling for new regulations to keep prices in check. Even American patients are concerned – 77% believe drug costs are unreasonable and 73% think the pharmaceutical industry cares more about profits than people. Professional bodies such as the American Society of Clinical Oncology (ASCO) and the European Society of Medical Oncology (ESMO) are becoming more vocal about the price and effectiveness of new therapies. In June 2015, ASCO unveiled its conceptual framework to assess the value of new cancer treatment options, and ESMO issued guidance on assessment of meaningful clinical benefit of new anti-cancer therapies.

In contrast to other countries, the US has a more fragmented approach to HTA, with different organizations applying varying methodologies. Recently, the Institute of Clinical and Economic Review initiated an emerging therapy assessment program with the goal of creating a transparent method for analyzing and judging value. The institute's budget impact assessment considers the effect of a drug on net health spending over five years, taking into account assumptions about the product's projected uptake. Given those assumptions, it then calculates a drug price such that annual net spending on that drug would not exceed roughly US $900 million, a number derived from assumptions about how fast the US economy is growing and the number of new medications approved each year. The greatest impact of these reports thus far has been to exert pressure on manufacturers when drug prices exceed the institute's threshold of value and societal affordability, although not all the drugs evaluated so far have been determined to be overpriced. Although, a not-for-profit organization, without any legal authority to set prices, its assessments have come under increasing criticism from the drug manufacturers.

10.6 Reimbursement and Payer Evidence Requirements across Different Countries

Over the last three decades, HTA has become more visible and disseminated in Europe, North America, Australia, and, more recently, in developing countries where health policies are being revised (Banta et al., 2009). Almost all of these HTA agencies require health economic evaluation to support reimbursement decisions. Some agencies recommend cost utility analyses while others require cost-effectiveness analyses. In terms of evidence requirements, almost all agencies recommend at least one main comparator. This comparator is often the standard of care or current practice. Recommendations regarding the time horizon depend on the duration of disease, but this is often only useful for a societal perspective, although some HTA agencies such as NICE recommend choosing a time horizon depending on relevant costs and benefits. There are also considerable variations regarding costs that should be included and these vary depending on the chosen perspective. Many agencies, such as NICE, Canadian Agency for Drugs and Technologies in Health (CADTH), and Agency for Healthcare Research and Quality (AHRQ) also include direct costs outside the healthcare system.

Additionally, indirect costs included in the societal perspective differ. Some agencies include only the productivity loss (e.g. IQWiG), while others also include the time cost of families (e.g. Pharmaceutical Benefits Board, Sweden). In Europe, some countries (e.g. the UK, the Netherlands, and Sweden) have well-established procedures for considering cost-effectiveness in reimbursement decisions and require cost per QALY, while others (e.g. France) consider health economic information less formally although cost-effectiveness analysis may be recommended in manufacturers' submissions (Sorenson et al., 2008). IQWiG specifies the type of clinical outcomes, mortality, morbidity, and validated surrogates as the outcomes required, and not the type of analysis.

In the US, while there has been some progress, the trend toward using cost-effectiveness analysis has been slower to develop. American HTA organizations tend to separate the evaluation of clinical evidence from economic evidence. Outside Europe, PBAC in Australia, CADTH in Canada, and AHRQ in the US also conduct economic evaluation of new drugs for their respective territories.

Understanding payers and payer systems is a key element to understanding global market access, drug pricing, and reimbursement. There are a number of different payer systems and price control mechanisms around the world that range from national to regional bodies. NICE (UK) provides national level guidance regarding reimbursement of new cancer drugs within England and Wales, while regional budgets are controlled by clinical commissioning groups (CCGs). Similarly, in Canada, national agencies control certain aspects of drug pricing, and regional provinces are left to decide budget impact and inclusion of new drugs in formularies. In Italy and Spain, there is tight control exerted by the national authorities over drug pricing and reimbursement, however, regional bodies can exert additional control over drug utilization in their own regional healthcare budgets. In Germany and the Netherlands, a large number of independent sick funds control the implementation of healthcare budgets in addition to the national funding and control structure.

For payers worldwide, open consideration of economic efficiency raises challenges. Nevertheless, the lack of procedures for considering economic evidence in a transparent way also creates problems. Recently, the governments of Belgium, the Netherlands, Luxembourg and Austria have joined forces to try to find a more sustainable way to provide access to costly drugs (Beneluxa.org, accessed January 2019). The coalition aims to provide interested parties with a central information point about collaboration and its different strands: horizon scanning, information sharing, health technology appraisals, and joint price negotiations. In the future, this site intends to make available documents, such as the terms of reference of the coalition and scientific reports, and will be regularly updated.

10.6.1 Canada

Since 2003, new drugs are reviewed by the Common Drug Review (CDR) process to evaluate if they qualify for provincial formulary considerations. Oncology drug review is carried out by the pan-Canadian Oncology Drug Review (pCODR). Both CDR and pCODR review drugs through expert committees and are managed by CADTH. Cost-effectiveness assessment is required in addition to comparative drug effectiveness as well as safety assessment and potential budget impact.

10.6.2 France

In theory, France has a free pricing system for non-reimbursed drugs (see https://www.ispor.org/HTARoadMaps/France.asp), however, prices for reimbursed drugs are controlled through the Economic Committee of Health Products (CESP). Medical/economic reviews are required for all new drugs for which the company claims an ASMR (medical improvement score) rating of I, II or III, has expected sales above 20 million euros, and is evaluated by the CEESP (Commission d'Évaluation Économique et de Santé Publique) of the HAS. The ASMR is established by the transparency commission (*commission de la transparence*) as part of the remit of the HAS. The CESP considers assessments in euros per QALY but there are no predefined ICER thresholds (Figure 10.2).

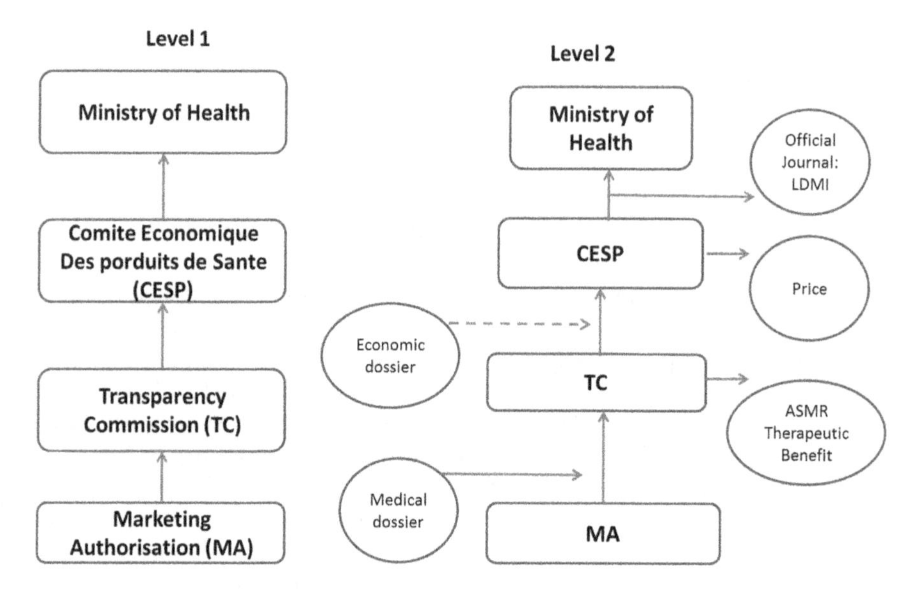

FIGURE 10.2
French system.

Source: Adapted from ISPOR. Accessed from https://tools.ispor.org/htaroadmaps/France.asp.

10.6.3 Germany

Outlines the decision-making process in Germany (ISPOR, 2009). Following dossier submission, G-BA commissions IQWiG to prepare an added benefit of new drug versus one or more existing comparators. Drugs without added benefit are price referenced against the identified comparative benchmarks, without negotiation. Health economic evaluations are not mandated for reimbursement evaluation, but can be undertaken by the manufacturers at their discretion Figure 10.3.

As stated by IQWiG: first, because

> The G-BA is responsible for the overall procedure of early benefit assessment and the pharmaceutical companies submit their dossiers to the G-BA. The G-BA usually commissions IQWiG with the scientific report. After publication of the report, the G-BA conducts a commenting procedure. This can provide supplementary information and can consequently also lead to a modified result of the assessment. The assessment procedure is only complete with a formal decision by the G-BA on the added benefit and on the extent of added benefit. The further procedure depends on this decision and can, in simple terms, take two directions. If no added benefit can be determined, a reference price is allocated to the new drug (or a price that is not allowed to be higher than that of the comparator therapy). The latter is the case if no suitable reference price group exists. If an added benefit has been determined, then price negotiations

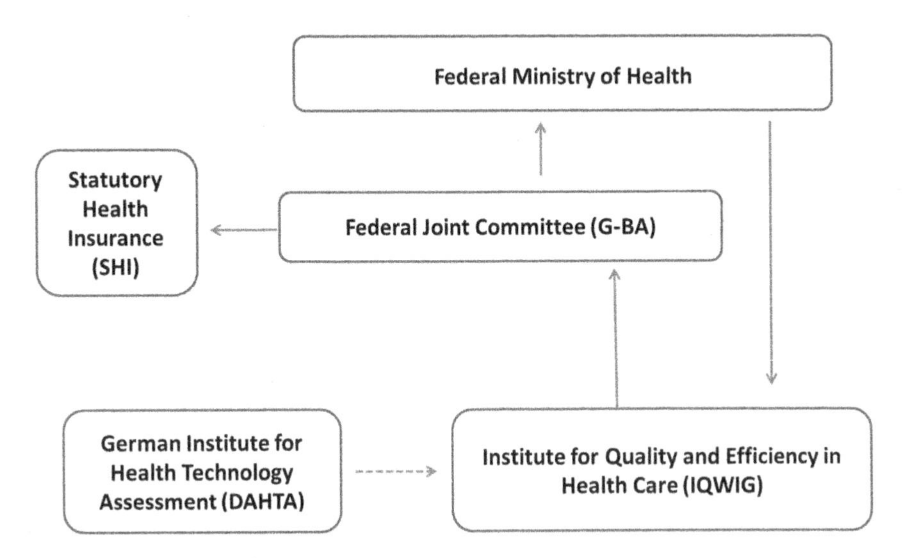

FIGURE 10.3
German process adapted from ISPOR.

Source: IQWiG https://www.iqwig.de/en/about-us/10-years-of-iqwig/amnog-since-2011.6333.html.

are conducted between the Umbrella Organization of Statutory Health Insurance ('GKV-Spitzenverband') and the pharmaceutical company.

Since the introduction of AMNOG, a health economic evaluation is (only) planned for the situation where, after a regular early benefit assessment, price negotiations fail, and an arbitral verdict does not lead to the setting of a price either. Then the pharmaceutical company or the Umbrella Organization of Statutory Health Insurance ('GKV-Spitzenverband') can apply for a health economic evaluation.

10.6.4 Italy

Health economic evaluations in Italy have only limited impact on pricing and reimbursement decisions. However, the budget impact model as well as patient and clinical outcome data play a more important role. At the regional and hospital level, budget impact analyses are particularly important. Another unique aspect of the reimbursement mechanism in Italy is the preference for risk-sharing schemes for oncology drugs. For example, Bayer agreed to provide 50% discount on nexevar for the initial two months of treatment. Once response to treatment is established, only patients who have been deemed to respond to treatment with nexevar will be covered for 100% reimbursement.

10.6.5 Spain

The Spanish National Health Service (Sistema Nacional de Salud, SNS) provides universal health coverage to, essentially, the whole Spanish population.

However, there is limited influence of health economic data on pricing and reimbursement. A recent EUnetHTA report describes it as:

> The Agencia Española de Medicamentos y Productos Sanitarios (AEMPS) is the Spanish Medicines Agency which is part of the Spanish Ministry of Health, Social Services and Equality. As part of its remit it produces health technology assessments of medicinal products called therapeutic positioning reports. Therapeutic positioning reports identify the therapeutic value of a product compared to alternatives. The reports provide advice to the DG Pharmacy to inform national pricing and reimbursement decisions. The reports also provide advice to the 17 regional health authorities about procurement and selection of medicinal products and to other decision makers at a healthcare level (hospitals, prescribers, etc.) about the use of medicinal products.

About 50 therapeutic positioning reports are produced by AEMPS each year:

> Reports produced by AEMPS include clinical effectiveness. The process is completed sequentially where clinical effectiveness information is compiled and an economic assessment is performed after price setting. Because AEMPS is a medicines agency supporting licensing of medicines, they have access to the regulatory documents that underpin the marketing authorisation procedure. AEMPS use these documents to complete the assessment of therapeutic effectiveness themselves without using additional evidence, unless significant evidence exists outside the regulatory submission identified by the organisation itself, provided by the marketing authorisation holder, or other stakeholders involved in the procedure (including scientific societies and patients associations).
>
> **(Source: EUnetHTA WP7 research and analysis activity 1: Annex 2 Case studies)**

10.6.6 Australia

Australia was one of the first countries to implement a cost-effectiveness requirement as a part of pricing and reimbursement approval. Australia's Medicare provides comprehensive healthcare coverage for all residents and prices of drugs that are reimbursed are controlled by the Pharmaceutical Benefits Scheme (PBS). Listing on PBS is subject to review by the Pharmaceutical Benefits Advisory Committee (PBAC). The subcommittee of the PBAC reviews pharmacoeconomic submissions that manufacturers need to submit in order to qualify for reimbursement. Based on the innovation status of the drug, the committee determines whether the manufacturer is required to submit incremental cost-effectiveness or cost-minimization in comparison with the appropriate reference comparator(s).

Generally, manufacturers of a new drug with substantial incremental costs are required to justify this higher cost by demonstrating robust cost-effectiveness. Australian reimbursement authorities may use higher cost-effectiveness thresholds for cost-effectiveness assessment of oncology drugs.

10.6.7 United Kingdom

Under intense pressure from the public, clinicians, and the pharmaceutical industry, the NHS in England has made a number of attempts to reassess its approach to cancer drugs reimbursement. The first of these changes was the introduction of end-of-life criteria. In January 2009, NICE introduced supplementary advice to improve NHS access to end-of-life treatments. The advice meant that treatments for patients with a short life expectancy can exceed NICE's cost effectiveness threshold of £30,000 per QALY, provided that: they are for patients with a short life expectancy; they extend life by at least three months compared with current NHS treatment; and they apply to small patient populations. In addition to end-of-life criteria, the Cancer Drug Fund (CDF) was established in April 2011, which provided a budget and funding approval mechanism for cancer drugs rejected by NICE. The CDF came under intense criticism for lack of value and was subsequently reformed in 2016 (Agrawal et al., 2017). The new arrangements put it on a more sustainable footing with three key objectives:

- Patients have faster access to the most promising new cancer treatments.
- Taxpayers get better value for money in drug expenditure.
- Pharmaceutical companies that are willing to price their products responsibly can access a new, fast-track route to NHS funding for the best and most promising drugs.

10.7 Pricing and Reimbursement Environment in the United States

Healthcare in the US is administered through private insurance or managed care organizations (MCO). Managed care plans are a type of health insurance. They have contracts with healthcare providers and medical facilities to provide care for members at reduced costs. In addition, government-run Medicare and Medicaid bodies also administer healthcare in the US.

The US does not have a centralized reimbursement system and drug prices can be set without government restrictions, although there are some post-launch limitations in pricing freedom for the government-managed sectors.

In the private sector, each drug manufacturer has the freedom to determine the optimal price for their drugs. They can also adjust prices over time, for example linking them to inflation rates or other factors (e.g. competitor drugs or new data availability).

The Institute for Clinical and Economic Review (ICERev) (not to be confused with the incremental cost-effectiveness ratio!) is the first organization in the US to address drug prices using cost-effectiveness methods, and to gain the attention of important stakeholders. An ICERev report is composed of six main parts: comparative clinical-effectiveness, incremental cost-effectiveness, potential benefits or disadvantages that lie outside the scope of clinical- or cost-effectiveness, contextual considerations, budget impact analysis, and a section in which the value-based price benchmark is calculated (see: https://icer-review.org/methodology/). However, it must be pointed out that ICERev is a non-profit organization and does not have any influence over stakeholders involved in setting drug prices in the US.

10.8 Value-Based Pricing (VBP) for Cancer Drugs

Under the PPRS reform discussions in the UK from 2010 to 2013 there was a call for a move to a value-based pricing system, where price is directly linked to the value a drug provides. The idea gained tremendous traction with health economists around the world because of the underlying appeal of linking drug price to the value of drug.

The initial VBP proposal included the following elements (DOH, White Paper, 2010).

1. Flexibility to establish value by incorporating burden of illness and societal benefits as modifiers to the cost-effectiveness cut-off criteria operated by NICE.
2. Price control at the established value of the new drug instead of a limit on reimbursement at that established value under the existing system.

Such a system was due to be introduced in the UK but complexity in the negotiations has seen this, and its iteration, value-based assessment, shelved. The underlying reasons included lack of agreement on the 'value' (DOH, White Paper, 2010; Cohen, 2017). Fundamentally, value is defined as the health outcomes achieved per unit of currency spent, but there is no universally accepted definition of what good value—or even acceptable value—means in cancer care. Value means something different to each stakeholder, whether a patient with cancer or a caregiver, a physician treating patients with cancer, a healthcare payer, or another medical decision-maker. Another important consideration is that the oncology drug development paradigm requires drug manufacturers to demonstrate efficacy and safety in later lines of treatment first because it is considered unethical to experiment new treatment options in earlier lines. The incremental benefit in later lines of treatment is much smaller and therefore a new drug may not be able to demonstrate its 'value' at the time of initial approval and launch, restricting reimbursement decisions.

Table 10.7 shows a case study outlining the approval history of rituximab in patients in follicular lymphoma. Rituximab was evaluated and approved initially in patients who were resistant to prior treatment options, and later trials gradually expanded the indication to earlier lines of treatment and regimens. It is also evident from the data that efficacy benefit was greatest in the first-line setting; however, these data did not become available until more than 12 years after the initial approval.

Example 10.2: Case Study – Evolution of Rituximab Approvals from Last-Line to Front-Line Treatment in Patients with Follicular Lymphoma

This creates a major problem for manufacturers, as a lack of demonstrated benefit at the time of initial approval may force reimbursement and price below the ultimate value, and increasing price later to reflect 'value' is only theoretically possible. For example, the UK has introduced

TABLE 10.7

Approval History of Rituximab in Patients in Follicular Lymphoma (Rituximab Was Evaluated and Approved Initially)

Approval Date	Patient Population	Summary of Clinical Data From Approved Label (SPC)
June 1998	Chemoresistant or in second or higher relapse after chemotherapy	Response rate: 48%
March 2004	Previously untreated (in combination with one particular type of chemotherapy only)	Median time to progression: 14.7 months
July 2006	Maintenance treatment in relapsed or refractory, but responding to induction chemotherapy	Median PFS was 42.2 months in the rituximab maintenance arm compared to 14.3 months in the observation arm
January 2008	Previously untreated	To expand use to combination with all types of chemotherapy based on three different trials in combination with chemotherapy
October 2010	Previously untreated	Median PFS: not reached in rituximab arm vs. 48 months for control arm

Note: SPC: summary of product characteristics.

a formal mechanism to reprice a drug on that basis; however it has never led to an actual increase (Table 10.7).

At the time of publishing of this book, the future of VBP in the UK is still unknown. The terminology seems to have shifted to 'value-based assessment,' however, there is no progress to report on that front either. The uncertainties around the exit of the UK from the European Union ('Brexit') has created uncertainties for both reimbursement and market authorization bodies.

10.9 Risk-Sharing Scheme

Risk-sharing schemes operate on the basic principle that in return for drug manufacturers' guarantee of a price reduction, the new drug will be added to the list of reimbursed drugs (Carlson et al., 2017; Carlson et al., 2010; Gonclaves et al., 2018). These schemes are increasingly common in European countries and Australia where there are centralized reimbursement mechanisms in place, giving payers powers over market access.

In Italy, the risk-sharing deals are used to avoid paying for patients who do not respond to treatment. In the UK, the term patient-access scheme (PAS) is routinely used to describe these arrangements. Table 10.8, lists the oncology treatments approved by NICE with associated patient-access schemes. It is evident from the table that the majority of currently reimbursed drugs have a PAS associated as the condition for reimbursement. As of October 2017, 65 oncology treatments have a PAS associated with positive reimbursement decisions, representing almost two-thirds of total treatments reimbursed by NICE to date. Companies offer these deals in order to bring the ICER within accepted cost-effectiveness threshold.

Figure 10.4 presents the breakdown of different types of PASs. PASs are usually initiated by the drug manufacturers in order to resolve the

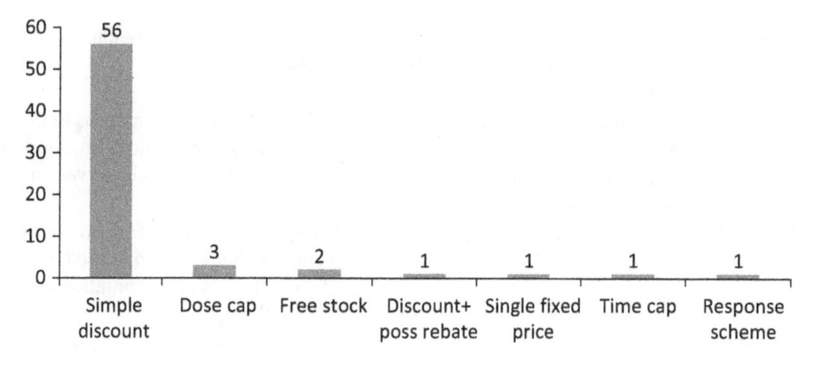

FIGURE 10.4
Breakdown of different types of PAS.

TABLE 10.8

A List of Oncology Treatments Approved by NICE with Associated Patient-Access Schemes

Treatment	Indication	Type of scheme
Bortezomib	Multiple myeloma	Response scheme
Sunitinib	Renal cell carcinoma	Free stock
Lenalidomide	Multiple myeloma	Dose cap
Sunitinib	Gastrointestinal stromal tumor	Free stock
Trabectedin	Advanced soft tissue sarcoma	Dose cap
Gefitinib	Non-small-cell lung cancer	Single fixed price
Pazopanib	Advanced renal cell carcinoma	Discount plus rebate
Azacitidine	Myelodysplastic syndromes, chronic myelomonocytic leukemia and acute myeloid leukemia	Simple discount
Mifamurtide	High grade resectable non-metastatic osteosarcoma	Simple discount
Nilotinib	Imatinib-resistant chronic myeloid leukemia	Simple discount
Nilotinib	First-line treatment of chronic myeloid leukemia	Simple discount
Fingolimod	Highly active relapsing-remitting multiple sclerosis	Simple discount
Erlotinib	First-line treatment of locally advanced or metastatic EGFR-TK mutation-positive non-small-cell lung cancer	Simple discount
Denosumab	Skeletal related events in adults with bone metastases from solid tumors	Simple discount
Ipilimumab	Advanced melanoma, second line	Simple discount
Vemurafenib	Metastatic mutation positive melanoma	Simple discount
Pixantrone	Multiple relapsed or refractory aggressive non-Hodgkin's B-cell lymphoma	Simple discount
Afatinib	Locally advanced or metastatic non-small-cell lung cancer with activating epidermal growth factor	Simple discount
Enzalutamide	Metastatic hormone-relapsed prostate cancer in adults whose disease has progressed during or after docetaxel-containing chemotherapy	Simple discount
Ipilimumab	Adults with previously untreated advanced (unresectable or metastatic) melanoma	Simple discount
Dabrafenib	Unresectable or metastatic melanoma with a BRAFV600 mutation	Simple discount
Lenalidomide	Myelodysplastic syndromes associated with an isolated deletion 5q cytogenetic abnormality	Dose cap
Axitinib	Advanced renal cell carcinoma after failure of prior systemic treatment	Simple discount
Obinutuzumab	Untreated chronic lymphocytic leukemia	Simple discount
Ofatumumab	Untreated chronic lymphocytic leukemia	Simple discount
Nintedanib	Previously treated locally advanced, metastatic, or locally recurrent non-small-cell lung cancer	Simple discount
Pembrolizumab	Advanced melanoma after disease progression with ipilimumab	Simple discount

(*Continued*)

TABLE 10.8 (CONTINUED)

A List of Oncology Treatments Approved by NICE with Associated Patient-Access Schemes

Treatment	Indication	Type of scheme
Pembrolizumab	Advanced melanoma not previously treated with ipilimumab	Simple discount
Erlotinib	Non-small-cell lung cancer that has progressed after prior chemotherapy	Simple discount
Enzalutamide	Metastatic hormone-relapsed prostate cancer before chemotherapy is indicated	Simple discount
Panobinostat	Multiple myeloma after at least 2 previous treatments	Simple discount
Olaparib	Maintenance treatment of relapsed, platinum-sensitive, BRCA mutation-positive ovarian, fallopian tube, and peritoneal cancer after response to second-line or subsequent platinum-based chemotherapy	Time cap
Ruxolitinib	Disease-related splenomegaly or symptoms in adults with myelofibrosis.	Simple discount
Cabazitaxel	Hormone-relapsed metastatic prostate cancer treated with docetaxel.	Simple discount
Ceritinib	Previously treated anaplastic lymphoma kinase positive non-small-cell lung cancer	Simple discount
Trametinib	In combination with dabrafenib for treating unresectable or metastatic melanoma	Simple discount
Dabrafenib	In combination with trametinib for treating unresectable or metastatic melanoma	Simple discount
Bosutinib	Previously treated chronic myeloid leukemia	Simple discount
Trifluridine and tipiracil hydrochloride	Previously treated metastatic colorectal cancer	Simple discount
Crizotinib	Untreated anaplastic lymphoma kinase-positive advanced non-small-cell lung cancer	Simple discount
Talimogene laherparepvec	Unresectable metastatic melanoma	Simple discount
Radium-223 dichloride	Hormone-relapsed prostate cancer with bone metastases	Simple discount
Nivolumab	Previously treated advanced renal cell carcinoma in adults	Simple discount
Everolimus	Advanced breast cancer after endocrine therapy	Simple discount
Crizotinib	Untreated anaplastic lymphoma kinase-positive advanced non-small-cell lung cancer	Simple discount
Eribulin	Breast cancer (locally advanced, metastatic)	Simple discount
Pertuzumab	Neoadjuvant treatment of breast cancer	Simple discount
Dasatinib	Imatinib-resistant or intolerant chronic myeloid leukemia	Simple discount

(*Continued*)

TABLE 10.8 (CONTINUED)

A List of Oncology Treatments Approved by NICE with Associated Patient-Access Schemes

Treatment	Indication	Type of scheme
Nilotinib	Imatinib-resistant or intolerant chronic myeloid leukemia	Simple discount
Dasatinib	Untreated chronic myeloid leukemia	Simple discount
Nilotinib	Untreated chronic myeloid leukemia	Simple discount
Pomalidomide	Multiple myeloma previously treated with lenalidomide and bortezomib	Simple discount
Pembrolizumab	PD-L1-positive non-small-cell lung cancer after chemotherapy	Simple discount
Everolimus	Renal cell carcinoma	Simple discount
Ibrutinib	Previously treated chronic lymphocytic leukemia and untreated chronic lymphocytic leukemia with 17p deletion or TP53 mutation	Simple discount
Cetuximab	Previously untreated metastatic colorectal cancer	Simple discount
Panitumumab	Previously untreated metastatic colorectal cancer	Simple discount
Everolimus	Unresectable or metastatic neuroendocrine tumors in people with progressive disease	Simple discount
Blinatumomab	Previously treated Philadelphia-chromosome-negative acute lymphoblastic leukemia	Simple discount
Ponatinib	Chronic myeloid leukemia and acute lymphoblastic leukemia	Simple discount
Carfilzomib	Previously treated multiple myeloma	Simple discount
Nivolumab	Relapsed or refractory classical Hodgkin lymphoma	Simple discount
Cabozantinib	Previously treated advanced renal cell carcinoma	Simple discount
Obinutuzumab	Rituximab refractory follicular lymphoma	Simple discount
Nab-paclitaxel	Adenocarcinoma of the pancreas	Simple discount

cost-effectiveness issues following initial negative advanced consultation document (ACD) issued by NICE. It is evident from Table 10.8 and Figure 10.4 that almost all of these negotiations involved price reductions by offering confidential simple discounts. However, some of the treatments approved by NICE have innovative PASs associated with the approval.

Example 10.3: Case Study 1 – Bortezomib for Multiple Myeloma – Response-Based PAS

In 2006, NICE declined to recommend bortezomib for the treatment of patients with multiple myeloma, as bortezomib wasn't considered cost-effective (cost per QALY > £30,000). Under the risk-sharing scheme, the company proposed to reimburse the treatment cost for patients with a more than 50% reduction. The M-spike is a sign of abnormal gamma immunoglobin 50% reduction in serum M-protein (a criteria for measuring response to treatment in these patients). Following this arrangement, NICE reversed their initial negative reimbursement ruling and made the drug available for routine use within the NHS.

Example 10.4: Case Study 2 – Lenalidomide for Multiple Myeloma – Dose Cap

Another innovative deal also involved patients with multiple myeloma where, in 2009, NICE declined to reimburse lenalidomide for patients who previously received at least two prior treatments, based on the high cost of drug acquisition (as patients with lenalidomide are treatment-until-progression). The company proposed to provide the drug free of charge beyond two years, i.e. the NHS will pay for first two years of treatment and the company will provide free drugs for patients who continue to derive benefit following two years of treatment.

10.10 The Future of Cost-Effectiveness of Cancer Treatments

There are several areas of future research in cost-effectiveness in cancer. These can be split into methodological aspects, in terms of improving technical methodology in economic evaluation, and how the reimbursement environment may impact on how economic evaluation is conducted.

10.10.1 Future Research: Methodology

Cost-effectiveness in clinical trials still offers many challenges for researchers in health economic evaluation. The methods used in health economic evaluation are not always understood by researchers and payer review groups. For example, the methods described for handling crossover in cancer trials can be very complex, and can take time for even an experienced statistician to appreciate. The use of Bayesian methods in clinical trials still poses problems, since many statisticians are used to designing clinical trials using classical (frequentist) methods and are accustomed to using software such as SAS®. It is only relatively recently that Bayesian computation has become slightly more feasible. Figures 10.5 and 10.6 give some examples of challenges in trial design and analysis for the future.

Statistical support for payer and reimbursement activities are often separated from the clinical drug development programme. This should start from early phase trials. Moreover, statistical knowledge and experience of payer evidence requirements is invested in a few statisticians and clinical trial staff whereas the concept of demonstrating value of treatments is more of a 'mindset' about adding value and not just an isolated (statistical) function. Often,

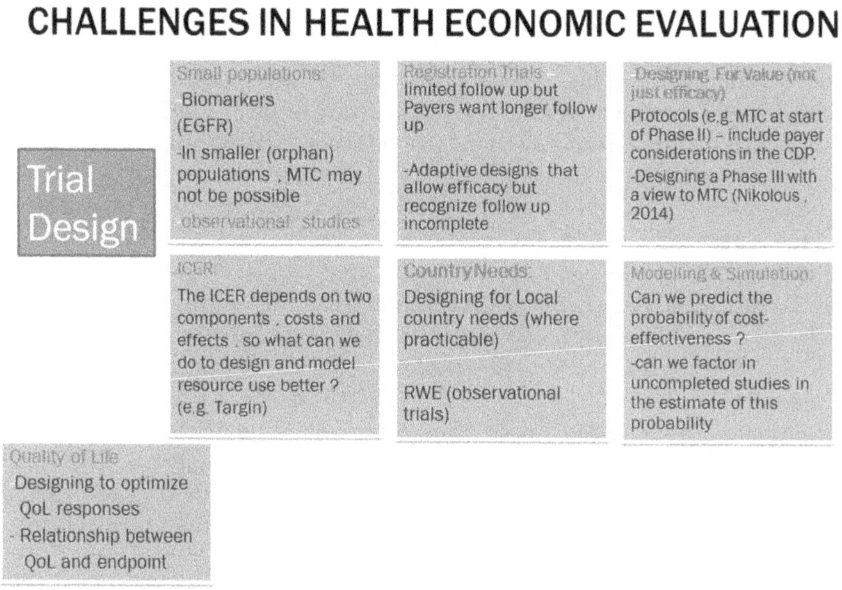

CHALLENGES IN HEALTH ECONOMIC EVALUATION

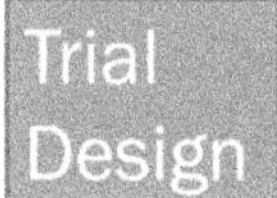

Small populations:
Biomarkers
(EGFR)
-In smaller (orphan) populations , MTC may not be possible
-observational studies

Registration Trials -
limited follow up but Payers want longer follow up
-Adaptive designs that allow efficacy but recognize follow up incomplete

-Designing For Value (not just efficacy)
Protocols (e.g. MTC at start of Phase II) - include payer considerations in the CDP.
-Designing a Phase III with a view to MTC (Nikolous , 2014)

ICER:
The ICER depends on two components , costs and effects . so what can we do to design and model resource use better ?
(e.g. Targin)

Country Needs:
Designing for Local country needs (where practicable)
RWE (observational trials)

Modelling & Simulation:
Can we predict the probability of cost-effectiveness ?
-can we factor in uncompleted studies in the estimate of this probability

Quality of Life
Designing to optimize QoL responses
- Relationship between QoL and endpoint

FIGURE 10.5
Some challenges in designing trials for health economic evaluation.

CHALLENGES IN HEALTH ECONOMIC EVALUATION

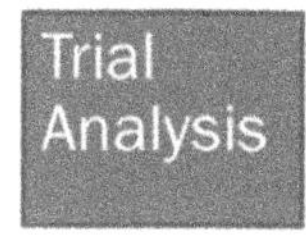

Modelling
-Modelling Costs (censored)
-Sensitivity analysis
-Mapping Functions
-MTC (Bayesian or Frequentist)
-Joint Modelling
-PSA (Copulas, Khan 2013)
- Value of Information
-Secondary endpoints in the value argument
-QoL (Beta Models, Khan, 2014) - Value Metrics (esp. Oncology)
-Crossover

Observational/Epidemiological
-Propensity Models
-Instrumental Variable Method (selection bias)
-Adaptive Analysis
-Combining RWE and trial data

Computing & Predictive Analytics
-Software for extrapolation
-Cubic Splines (Dewar & Khan, 2014)
-Sample Sizes (Sarker, Whitehead, Khan, 2012)
-Combining real world data with patient level data using analytical method:
o identify rare disease groups
o personalized risk
o identify under-diagnosis
- BIG DATA philosophy

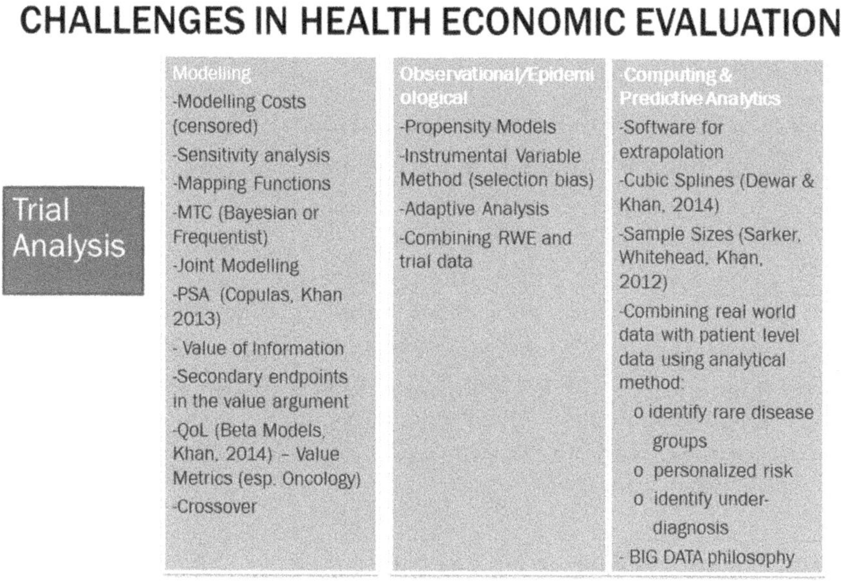

FIGURE 10.6
Some challenges in analyzing data for health economic evaluation.

payer evidence considerations are thought about at the start of the Phase III trial, whereas there is a need to think about what combination of possible studies will result in a high probability of market access; or what combination of studies will be likely to demonstrate value. The other challenge is that the statistical tools for estimating value are not clear or are unknown to statisticians – unfamiliarity with G-estimation techniques for handling crossover or VOI methods are areas where training and courses have only become available relatively recently for applications in clinical trials. Value analysis/reimbursement analysis/health economic analysis plans (HEAPs), in addition to statistical analysis plans (SAPs), which identify clearly those endpoints necessary for demonstrating value and those as direct inputs into a health economic model, are needed to be written collaboratively.

Several other technical issues or interesting areas of research that require additional work include sample sizes based on value of information (VOI), value-based pricing models, cost-effectiveness based on more than one endpoint, extrapolation in the presence of switching treatment (in cancer trials), and also simulation in the presence of crossover for PSA. Applications of flexible parametric models are still limited; improvements in mapping functions for HRQoL and, particularly, some generic measures, where the ability of generic instruments to detect meaningful treatment effects, is of concern. The use of platform and basket trials and the challenges these bring for economic evaluation is also an area of research where much methodological innovation is required. In short, there is no shortage of methodological areas for statisticians, health economists, and researchers in health economic evaluation to develop, whether in academia or industry. More recently, Neumann et al. (2018) identify some areas:

(i) Modeling (Comparative Modeling and Model Transparency).
(ii) Health outcomes (valuing temporary health and path states, as well as health effects on caregivers).
(iii) Incorporating societal perspectives.
(iv) Evidence synthesis (developing theory on learning across studies and combining data from clinical trials and observational studies).
(v) Estimating and using cost-effectiveness thresholds (empirically representing two broad concepts: opportunity costs and public willingness to pay).
(vi) Reporting and communicating CEAs (written protocols and a quality scoring system).

10.10.2 Future Reimbursement Landscape

In October 2016, NICE and NHS England (NHS-E) put out new proposals for consultation on how they would like to work closely to "simplify and speed up" new technology appraisals. The document includes the following proposals:

(a) A new budget impact threshold.
(b) Restructuring of QALY assessment for highly specialized treatments for very rare diseases.
(c) Fast-track appraisals for drugs that have a cost per QALY of below £10,000.

Budget Impact Threshold

The "special arrangements" will be triggered when a drug appraised by NICE is expected to exceed a budget impact threshold of £20 million. NICE would calculate the drug's potential budget impact by estimating its net annual cost to the NHS. NHS-E is responsible for allocating funding for new products, some of which have a high budget impact. In order to deal with this responsibility and avoid risking access to other forms of care, NHS-E wants to put in place new arrangements for managing the budget impact. If an agreement was struck that lowered the drug's budget impact below the threshold, the standard 90-day funding requirement for a NICE-assessed drug would apply. If not, then NHS England could ask NICE to alter the standard funding requirement to allow for a longer period of phased introduction. According to current regulations NICE recommendations have to be complied with no more than three months after the final guidance is published.

10.10.2.1 Automatic Funding for Highly Specialized Drugs for Rare Diseases

The document suggests that treatments for very rare conditions would be automatically funded if they have an incremental cost-effectiveness ratio of up to £100,000 per QALY. The proposed limit is five times higher than the lower end of NICE's standard threshold of less than £20,000 per QALY. Treatments deemed to have a high value and low cost are likely to be the most successful, while those with a low benefit and higher cost will be less likely to win a recommendation. If the drug's ICER did exceed £100,000 per QALY, it would not be subject to the funding requirement, but would be considered for funding through NHS England's annual specialized commissioning process (Adkins et al., 2017).

10.10.2.2 Fast-Track Appraisals

According to the proposal, any products with £10,000 or less per QALY will be fast-tracked with 11 weeks' reduction (32 weeks, down from 43 weeks) to the final guidance. However, between 2007 and 2014, around 15% of NICE's technology appraisals fell at or below £10,000 per QALY. The introduction of a fast-track process would enable them to be routed through a lighter touch appraisal process, "speeding up access for patients," as stated in the document. Any policy changes as a result of this consultation may have profound implications for the pricing and reimbursement of technologies assessed by NICE in future.

10.11 Summary

An analysis of NICE Single Technology Assessments in Oncology since 2001 shows that 61% were granted complete or partial reimbursement. Criticism of the rejected submissions covered a wide range of aspects including health resources/costs, HRQoL measures, clinical-effect predictions, and other lack of evidence. The vast majority, if not all, of submissions relied upon simulation modeling. Problems or lack of sufficient evidence about OS and PFS were often highlighted by the review groups. An analysis of the accepted oncology submissions showed a mean of £39,000 and a median incremental QALY of 0.39 or about 4.7 months. A short review of the payer requirements across different countries shows a highly variable situation, with the administrative processes, evidence, and cost criteria and requirements with no common trend. A general trend was, however, the increase in risk-sharing schemes (often including a discount price) for new, costly cancer drugs in various European countries.

10.12 Exercises for Chapter 10

1. Explain the difference between an MTA and an STA. What factors does NICE consider when making HTAs?
2. What factors might predict the recommendation of a cancer drug by reimbursement authorities?
3. Compare and contrast the different reimbursement strategies across countries worldwide. Is there a general pattern?
4. Identify some future areas of research in cost-effectiveness. Why are some of these important for cancer drugs in particular?

References

Abernethy, A., Abrahams, E., Barker, A. et al. (2014). Turning the tide against cancer through sustained medical innovation: The pathway to progress. *Clinical Cancer Research*; 20(5):1081–1086.

Ades, A.E., Lu, G., & Claxton, K. (2004). Expected value of sample information calculations in medical decision modeling. *Medical Decision Making*; 24(2):207–227.

Ades, A.E., Lu, G., & Madan, J.J. (2013). Which health-related quality-of-life outcome when planning randomized trials: Disease-specific or generic, or both? A common factor model. *Value in Health*; 16(1):185–194.

Ades, A.E., Madan, J., & Welton, N.J. (2011). Indirect and mixed treatment comparisons in arthritis research. *Rheumatology*; 50(suppl 4):iv5–iv9.

Adkins, E.M. , Nicholson, L., Floyd, D. et al. (2017). Oncology drugs for orphan indications: How are HTA processes evolving for this specific drug category? *ClinicoEconomics and Outcomes Research*; 9:327–342.

A'Hern, R.P. (2016). Restricted mean survival time: An obligatory end point for time-to-event analysis in cancer trials? *Journal of Clinical Oncology*; 34(28):3474–3476.

Aggarwal, A., Fojo, T., Chamberlain, C. et al. (2017). Do patient access schemes for high-cost cancer drugs deliver value to society?—lessons from the NHS Cancer Drugs Fund. *Annals of Oncology*; 28(8):1738–1750.

Agresti, A. (2013). *Categorical Adata Analysis*, 3rd Edition. John Wiley Press.

Ajani, J.A. (2007). The area between the curves gets no respect: Is it because of the median madness? *Journal of Clinical Oncology*; 25(34):5531.

Al, M.J., & Van Hout, B.A. (2000). A Bayesian approach to economic analyses of clinical trials: The case of stenting versus balloon angioplasty. *Health Economics*; 9(7):599–609.

Albertsen, P.C., Hanley, J.A., Gleason, D.F. et al. (1998). Competing risk analysis of men aged 55 to 74 years at diagnosis managed conservatively for clinically localized prostate cancer. *JAMA*; 280(11):975–980.

Almirall, D., Ten Have, T.T., & Murphy, S.A. (2010). Structural nested mean models for assessing time-varying effect moderation. *Biometrics*; 66(1):131–139.

Amdahl, J., Manson, S.C., Isbell, R. et al. (2014). Cost-effectiveness of pazopanib in advanced soft tissue sarcoma in the United Kingdom. *Sarcoma*; 2014:481071.

American Lung Association. (n.d.). Lung cancer fact sheet. Retrieved from: www.lung.org/lung-health-and-diseases/lung-disease-lookup/lung-cancer/resource-library/lung-cancer-fact-sheet.html.

American Cancer Society. (2018). Breast cancer survival rates. Retrieved from: www.cancer.org/cancer/breast-cancer/understanding-a-breast-cancer-diagnosis/breast-cancer-survival-rates.html.

Amico, M., & Van Keilegom, I. (2018). Cure models in survival analysis. *Annual Review of Statistics and Its Application*; 5(1):311–342.

Andersen, P.K., Esbjerg, S., & Sorensen, T.I. (2000). Multi-state models for bleeding episodes and mortality in liver cirrhosis. *Statistics in Medicine*; 19(4):587–599.

Andersen, P.K., Hansen, L.S., & Keiding, N. (1991). Assessing the influence of reversible disease indicators on survival. *Statistics in Medicine*; 10(7):1061–1067.

Andersen, P.K., Hansen, M.G., & Klein, J.P. (2004). Regression analysis of restricted mean survival time based on pseudo-observations. *Lifetime Data Analysis*; 10(4):335–350.

Andersen, P.K., & Keiding, N. (2002). Multi-state models for event history analysis. *Statistical Methods in Medical Research*; 11(2):91–115.

Anderson, D.F., & Kurtz, T. (2015). *Stochastic analysis of biochemical systems*, Stochastics in biological systems series, Volume 1.2. Springer International Publishing, p. 592.

Anglemyer, A., Horvath, H.T., & Bero, L. (2014). Healthcare outcomes assessed with nonexperimental designs compared with those assessed in randomised trials. *Cochrane Database of Systematic Reviews*; 4:MR000034.

Ara, R., & Wailoo, A. (n.d.). NICE DSU technical support document 12: The use of health state utility values in decision models. Retrieved from: www.nicedsu.org.uk/.

Araújo, A., Parente, B., Sotto-Mayor, R. et al. (2008). An economic analysis of erlotinib, docetaxel, pemetrexed and best supportive care as second or third line treatment of non-small cell lung cancer. *Revista Portuguesa de Pneumologia (English Edition)*; 14(6):803–827.

Armero, C., Cabras, S., Castellanos, M.E., et al. (2016). Bayesian analysis of a disability model for lung cancer survival. *Statistical Methods in Medical Research*; 25(1):336–351. Epub 2012 July 5.

Asukai, Y., Valladares, A., Camps, C. et al. (2010). Cost-effectiveness analysis of pemetrexed versus docetaxel in the second-line treatment of non-small cell lung cancer in Spain: Results for the non-squamous histology population. *BMC Cancer*; 10(1):26.

Australian Government Department of Health. (2010). Pemetrexed disodium, powder for I.V. infusion, 100 mg (base) and 500 mg (base), Alimta®. The Pharmaceutical Benefits Scheme. Retrieved from: www.pbs.gov.au/info/industry/listing/elements/pbac-meetings/psd/2010-03/pbac-psd-Pemetrexed-mar10.

Australian Government Department of Health. (2013a). Afatinib, tablet, 20 mg, 30 mg, 40 mg and 50 mg, (as dimaleate), Giotrif® (first line) – July 2013. The pharmaceutical benefits scheme. Retrieved from: www.pbs.gov.au/info/industry/listing/elements/pbac-meetings/psd/2013-07/afatinib-first-line.

Australian Government Department of Health. (2013b). Erlotinib, tablets, 25 mg, 100 mg, 150 mg (as hydrochloride), Tarceva® – July 2013. The pharmaceutical benefits scheme. Retrieved from: www.pbs.gov.au/info/industry/listing/elements/pbac-meetings/psd/2013-07/erlotinib.

Australian Government Department of Health. (2013c). Gefitinib, tablet, 250 mg, Iressa® – July 2013. The pharmaceutical benefits scheme. Retrieved from: www.pbs.gov.au/info/industry/listing/elements/pbac-meetings/psd/2013-07/gefitinib.

Bagust, A., & Beale, S. (2014). Survival analysis and extrapolation modeling of time-to-event clinical trial data for economic evaluation: An alternative approach. *Medical Decision Making*; 34(3):343–351. Epub July 30.

Ball, G., Xie, F., & Tarride, J.E. (2018). Economic evaluation of bevacizumab for treatment of platinum-resistant recurrent ovarian cancer in Canada. *PharmacoEconomics Open*; 2(1):19–29.

Bang, H., & Tsiatis, A.A. (2000). Estimating medical costs with censored data. *Biometrika*; 87(2):329–343.

Bang, H., & Zhao, H. (2014). Cost-effectiveness analysis: A proposal of new reporting standards in statistical analysis. *Journal of Biopharmaceutical Statistics.*

Bang, H., & Zhao, H. (2016). Median-based incremental cost-effectiveness ratios with censored data. *Journal of Biopharmaceutical Statistics*; 26(3):552–564. Epub 2015 May 26.

Banta, D., & Almeida, R.T. (2009). The development of health technology assessment in Brazil. *International Journal of Technology Assessment in Health Care*; 25(Suppl 1):255–259.

Bartha, E., Arfwedson, C., Imnell, A. et al. (2013). Randomized controlled trial of goal-directed haemodynamic treatment in patients withproximal femoral fracture. *British Journal of Anaesthesia*; 110(4):545–553.

Basch, E., Deal, A.M., Dueck, A.C. et al. (2017). Overall survival results of a trial assessing patient-reported outcomes for symptom monitoring during routine cancer treatment. *JAMA*; 318(2):197–198.

Batchelor, T.T., Mulholland, P., Neyns, B. et al. (2013). Phase III randomized trial comparing the efficacy of cediranib as monotherapy, and in combination with lomustine, versus lomustine alone in patients with recurrent glioblastoma. *Journal of Clinical Oncology*; 31(26):3212–3218.

Batty, A., Winn, B., Lebmeier, M. et al. (2012). A comparison of patient and general-population utility values for advanced melanoma in health economic modelling. *Value in Health*; 15:A277–575.

Bebu, I., Luta, G., Mathew, T. et al. (2016). Parametric cost-effectiveness inference with skewed data. *Computational Statistics and Data Analysis*; 94:210–220.

Beck, N., & Jackman, S. (1998). Beyond linearity by default: Generalized additive models. *American Journal of Political Science*; 42(2):596–627.

Beckett, P., Calman, L., & Darlison, L. (2012). 91 *Follow-up of patients with advanced NSCLC following 1st line chemotherapy – A British Thoracic Oncology Group National survey*; L. Darlison, P. Beckett, L. Calman, C. Mulatero, K. O'Byrne, M. Peake, D. Talbot; *Lung Cancer*; 75(Suppl 1): S30–S31.

Benelexua Initiative on Pharmaceutical Policy. (n.d.). Retrieved from: www.beneluxa.org/.

Berthelot, J.M., Will, B.P., Evans, W.K. et al. (2000). Decision framework for chemotherapeutic interventions for metastatic non-small-cell lung cancer. *Journal of the National Cancer Institute*; 92(16):1321–1329.

Beusterien, K.M., Szabo, S.M., Kotapati, S. et al. (2009). Societal preference values for advanced melanoma health states in the United Kingdom and Australia. *British Journal of Cancer*; 101(3):387–389.

Billingham, L.J., Bathers, S., Burton, A. et al. (2002). Patterns, costs and cost-effectiveness of care in a trial of chemotherapy for advanced non-small cell lung cancer. *Lung Cancer*; 37(2):219–225.

Biomarkers Definitions Working Group. (2001). Biomarkers and surrogate endpoints: Preferred definitions and conceptual framework. *Clinical Pharmacology and Therapeutics*; 69(3):89–95.

Blazeby, J.M., Avery, K., Sprangers, M. et al. (2006). Health-related quality of life measurement in randomized clinical trials in surgical oncology. *Journal of Clinical Oncology*; 24(19):3178–3186.

BNF Publications. (n.d.). Retrieved from: www.bnf.org/.

Bodrogi, J., & Kaló, Z. (2010). Principles of pharmacoeconomics and their impact on strategic imperatives of pharmaceutical research and development. *British Journal of Pharmacology*; 159(7):1367–1373.

Bongers, M., Coupe, V., Jansma, E. et al. (2011). PCN93 Cost-Effectiveness of Treatment with New Agents in Advanced Non-Small-Cell Lung Cancer: A Systematic Review. *Value in Health*. 2011; 14(7): A451.

Bongers, M.L., de Ruysscher, D., Oberije, C. et al. (2016). Multistate statistical modeling: A tool to build a lung cancer microsimulation model that includes parameter uncertainty and patient heterogeneity. *Medical Decision Making*; 36(1):86–100.

Bossers, N., Van Engen, A., & Heemstra, L. (2015). Understanding key drivers of successful Hta submission — Developing a model. *Value in Health*; 18(7):A342.

Brada, M., Stenning, S., Gabe, R. et al. (2010). Temozolomide versus procarbazine, lomustine, and vincristine in recurrent high-grade glioma. *Journal of Clinical Oncology*; 28(30):4601–4608.

Bradbury, P.A., Tu, D., Seymour, L. et al. & the NCIC Clinical Trials Working Group on Economic Analysis. (2010). Economic analysis: Randomized placebo-controlled clinical trial of erlotinib in advanced non-small cell lung cancer. *Journal of the National Cancer Institute*; 102(5):298–306. Epub 2010 February 16.

Brandes, A.A., Finocchiaro, G., Zagonel, V. et al. (2016). AVAREG: A phase II, randomized, noncomparative study of fotemustine or bevacizumab for patients with recurrent glioblastoma. *Neuro-Oncology*; 18(9):1304–1312.

Bragg, R.H. & Packer, C.M. (1962). Orientation Dependence of Structure in Pyrolitic Graphite. *Nature*; 195: 1080–1082.

Brard, C., Le Teuff, G., Le Deley, M.C. et al. (2017). Bayesian survival analysis in clinical trials: What methods are used in practice? *Clinical Trials*; 14(1):78–87.

Bray, F., Ferlay, J., Soerjomataram, I. et al. (2018). Global cancer statistics 2018: GLOBOCAN estimates of incidence and mortality worldwide for 36 cancers in 185 countries. *CA: A Cancer Journal for Clinicians*; 68(6):394–424.

Brazier, J., & Longworth, L. (2011). NICE DSU Technical Support Document 8: An introduction to the measurement and valuation of health for NICE submissions. https://www.ncbi.nlm.nih.gov/books/NBK425820/pdf/Bookshelf_NBK425820.pdf

Brazier, J., & Longworth, L. (2013). Mapping to obtain EQ-5D utility values for use in NICE health technology appraisals. *Value in Health*; 16(1):202–210.

Brazier, J., Ratcliffe, J., Salomon, J. et al. (2016). *Measuring and valuing health benefits for economic evaluation*. Oxford: Oxford University Press.

Brazier, J., Rowen, D. et al. (2012). NICE DSU Technical Support Document 11: Alternatives to EQ-5D for generating health state utility values. Report by the decision support unit, March 2011. London: National Institute for Health and Care Excellence (NICE)

Brazier, J., Yang, Y., Tsuchiya, A. et al. (2009). A review of studies mapping (or cross walking) non-preference based measures of health to generic preference-based measures. *The European Journal of Health Economics*; 11(2):215–225.

Brent, R. (2014). *Cost-Benefit and Health Care Evaluations*, 2nd Edition. Edward Elgar.

Briggs, A., & Tambour, M. (2001). The design and analysis of stochastic cost-effectiveness studies for the evaluation of health care interventions. *Drug Information Journal*; 35(4):1455–1468.

Brito, M., Esteves, S., André, R. et al. (2016). Comparison of effectiveness of biosimilar filgrastim (Nivestim), reference Amgen filgrastim and pegfilgrastim in febrile neutropenia primary prevention in breast cancer patients treated with neo(adjuvant) TAC: A non-interventional cohort study. *Supportive Care in Cancer*; 24(2):597–603.

Brookhart, M.A., Wang, P.S., Solomon, D.H. et al. (2006). Evaluating short-term drug effects using a physician-specific prescribing preference as an instrumental variable. *Epidemiology*; 17(3):268–275.

Brooks, R., Rosalind, R., & de Charro, F. (2013). *The measurement and valuation of health status using EQ-5D: A European perspective: Evidence from the EuroQol BIOMED research programme*. Springer Science & Business Media.

Brown, T., Boland, A., Bagust, A. et al. (2010). Gefitinib for the first-line treatment of locally advanced or metastatic non-small cell lung cancer. *Health Technology Assessment*; 14(Suppl 2):71–79.

Bryant, J., & Day, R. (1995). Incorporating toxicity considerations into the design of two-stage phase II clinical trials. *Biometrics*; 51(4):1372–1383.

Buchholz, I., Thielker, K., Feng, Y.S. et al. (2015). Measuring changes in health over time using the EQ-5D 3L and 5L: A head-to-head comparison of measurement properties and sensitivity to change in a German inpatient rehabilitation sample. *Quality of Life Research*; 24(4):829–835.

Burau, V., & Blank, R.H. (2006). Comparing health policy: An assessment of typologies of health systems. *Journal of Comparative Policy Analysis: Research and Practice*; 8(1):63–76. Published online: 24 Jan 2007.

Calman, K.C. (1984). Quality of life in cancer patients—An hypothesis. *Journal of Medical Ethics*; 10(3):124–127.

Calvo, E., Escudier, B., Motzer, R.J. et al. (2012). Everolimus in metastatic renal cell carcinoma: Subgroup analysis of patients with 1 or 2 previous vascular endothelial growth factor receptor-tyrosine kinase inhibitor therapies enrolled in the phase III RECORD-1 study. *European Journal of Cancer*; 48(3):333–339.

Camm, A.J., & Fox, K.A.A. (2018). Strengths and weaknesses of 'real-world' studies involving non-vitamin K antagonist oral anticoagulants. *Open Heart*; 5(1):e000788.

Canadian Agency for Drugs and Technologies in Health. (n.d.). CADTH pan-Canadian oncology drug review. Retrieved from: https://cadth.ca/pcodr.

Canadian Agency for Drugs and Technologies in Health. (2004). Recommendation on reconsideration and reason for reconsideration. Retrieved from: www.cadth.ca/media/cdr/complete/cdr_complete_iressa_06-23-04.pdf.

Canadian Agency for Drugs and Technologies in Health. (2005). CEDAC final recommendation and reason for recommendation. Retrieved from: www.cadth.ca/media/cdr/complete/cdr_complete_Tarceva_Dec605.pdf.

Cancer Research UK. (n.d.). Cancer incidence for all cancers combined. Retrieved from: www.cancerresearchuk.org/health-professional/cancer-statistics/incidence/all-cancers-combined#heading-One.

Cancer Facts & Figures (2011). (2010). American cancer society report. Retrieved from: https://www.cancer.org/content/dam/cancer-org/research/cancer-facts-and-statistics/annual-cancer-facts-and-figures/2011/cancer-facts-and-figures-2011.pdf.

Cancer Patients Alliance. (n.d.). Pancreatic Cancer Prognosis & Survival. Pancreatica. Retrieved from: https://pancreatica.org/pancreatic-cancer/pancreatic-cancer-prognosis/.

Cancer Research UK. (n.d.) Cancer statistics for the UK. Retrieved from: www.cancerresearchuk.org/health-professional/cancer-statistics/statistics-by-cancer-type/lung-cancer

Cancer Research UK. (n.d). UK Lung Cancer and Smoking Statistics.

Cancer Research UK. (n.d) . World Wide Cancer Statistics. Retrieved from: www.cancerresearchuk.org/health-professional/cancer-statistics/worldwide-cancer.

Cappuzzo, F., Ciuleanu, T., Stelmakh, L., et al. (2010). Erlotinib as maintenance treatment in advanced non-small-cell lung cancer: a multicentre, randomised, placebo-controlled phase 3 study. *Lancet Oncol.*; 11(6): 521–529.

Carlson, J.J., Chen, S., & Garrison, L.P. Jr. (2017). Performance-based risk-sharing arrangements: An updated international review. *Pharmacoeconomics*; 35(10):1063–1072.

Carlson, J.J., Reyes, C., Oestreicher, N. et al. (2008). Comparative clinical and economic outcomes of treatments for refractory non-small cell lung cancer (NSCLC). *Lung Cancer*; 61(3):405–415.

Carlson, J.J., Sullivan, S.D., Garrison, L.P. et al. (2010). Linking payment to health outcomes: A taxonomy and examination of performance-based reimbursement schemes between healthcare payers and manufacturers. *Health Policy*; 96(3):179–190.

Caro, J., Möller, J., Karnon, J. et al. (2016). *Discrete event simulation for health technology assessment*. New York: Chapman and Hall/CRC.

Carpenter, J., & Kenward, M. (2013). *Multiple imputation and its application*. John Wiley Publications.

Carreon, L.Y., Berven, S.H., Djurasovic, M. et al. (2013). The discriminative properties of the SF–6D compared With the SF–36 and ODI. *Spine*; 38(1):60–64.

Center for Medical Technology Policy. (n.d.). Best practices for the design, implementation, analysis, and reporting of oncology trials with high rates of treatment switching. Resource Center. Retrieved from: www.cmtpnet.org/resource-center/view/new-guidance-for-treatment-switching-in-oncology-drug-trials/.

Collet, D. (2017). Modelling Survival Data in Medical Research, Second Edition. Chapman & Hall/CRC Texts in Statistical Science.

Cerri, K.H., Knapp, M., Fernández, J.L. (2014). Decision making by NICE: Examining the influences of evidence, process and context. *Health Econ. Policy Law*; 9(2):119–141.

Cesarec, A., & Likić, R. (2017). Budget impact analysis of biosimilar trastuzumab for the treatment of breast cancer in Croatia. *Applied Health Economics and Health Policy*; 15(2):277–286.

Chabot, I., & Rocchi, A. (2010). How do cost-effectiveness analyses inform reimbursement decisions for oncology medicines in Canada? The example of sunitinib for first-line treatment of metastatic renal cell carcinoma. *Value in Health*; 13(6):837–845.

Chamberlain, C., Collin, S.M., Hounsome, L. et al. (2015). Equity of access to treatment on the Cancer Drugs Fund: A missed opportunity for cancer research? *Journal of Cancer Policy*; 5:25–30.

Chhatwal, J., He, T., & Lopez-Olivo, M.A. (2016). Systematic review of modelling approaches for the cost effectiveness of hepatitis C treatment with direct-acting antivirals. *Pharmacoeconomics*; 34(6):551–67. doi: 10.1007/s40273-015-0373-9.

Chiou, V.L., & Burotto, M. (2015). Pseudoprogression and immune-related response in solid tumors. *Journal of Clinical Oncology*; 33(31):3541–3543.

Chouaid. (2012). Health-related quality of life in advanced non-small cell lung cancer (NSCLC) patients. *Value in Health*; 15(4):A227.

Chouaid, C., Le Caer, H., Locher, C. et al. & GFPC 0504 Team. (2012). Cost effectivenes of erlotinib versus chemotherapy for first-line treatment of non small cell lung cancer (NSCLC) in fit elderly patients participating in a prospective phase 2 study (GFPC 0504). *BMC Cancer*; 12:301.

Ciani, O., Buyse, M., Drummond, M. et al. (2016). Use of surrogate end points in healthcare policy: A proposal for adoption of a validation framework. *Nature Reviews Drug Discovery*; 15(7):516.

Ciani, O., Buyse, M., Garside, R. et al. (2013). Comparison of treatment effect sizes associated with surrogate and final patient relevant outcomes in randomised controlled trials: Meta-epidemiological study. *BMJ*; 346:f457.

Clauser, S.B. (2004). Use of cancer performance measures in population health: A macro-level perspective. *Journal of the National Cancer Institute Monographs*; (33):142–154.

Claxton, K. (2008). Exploring uncertainty in cost-effectiveness analysis. *PharmacoEconomics*; 26(9):781–798.

Claxton, K. (2011). Heterogeneity in cost-effectiveness of medical interventions: The Cochrane Review 2008; challenges of matching patients to appropriate care. 14th Annual ISPOR Congress, 1–8 November 2011.

Claxton, K., Martin, S., Soares, M., (2015). Methods for the estimation of the NICE cost effectiveness threshold. *Health Technology Assessment*; 19(14):1–503.

Claxton, K., Paulden, M., Gravelle, H. et al. (2011). Discounting and decision making in the economic evaluation of health-care technologies. *Health Economics*; 20(1):2–15.

Clement, F.M., Ghali, W.A., Donaldson, C. et al. (2009). The impact of using different costing methods on the results of an economic evaluation of cardiac care: Microcosting vs. gross-costing approaches. *Health Economics*; 18(4):377–388.

Clement, F.M., Harris, A., Li, J.J. et al. (2009). Using effectiveness and cost-effectiveness to make drug coverage decisions: A comparison of Britain, Australia, and Canada. *JAMA*; 302(13):1437–1443.

Cohen, D. (2017). Most drugs paid for by £1.27bn Cancer Drugs Fund had no "meaningful benefit". *BMJ*; 357:j2097.

Collet, D. (2014). *Modelling survival data*, 3rd Edition. Chapman & Hall.

Comabella, C.C.I., Gibbons, E., & Fitzpatrick, R. (2010). *A structured review of patient-reported outcome measures (PROMs) for lung cancer*. Oxford: University of Oxford.

Courtney, D., Huseyin, N., Evrim, G. et al. (2017). Availability of evidence of benefits on overall survival and quality of life of cancer drugs approved by European Medicines Agency: Retrospective cohort study of drug approvals 2009–13. *BMJ*; 359:j4530.

Coyle, D., & Coyle, K. (2014). The inherent bias from using partitioned survival models in economic evaluation. *Value in Health*; 17(3):A194.

Coyle, T. (2017). Sentinel system overview. Center for Drug Evaluation and Research. United States Food and Drug Administration. Retrieved from: www.fda.gov/downloads/ForPatients/About/UCM595420.pdf.

Cromwell, I., van der Hoek, K., Melosky, B. et al. (2011). Erlotinib or docetaxel for second-line treatment of non-small cell lung cancer: A real-world cost-effectiveness analysis. *Journal of Thoracic Oncology*; 6(12):2097–2103.

Cronin, A. (2016). STRMST2: Stata module to compare restricted mean survival time. Statistical software components S458154. Boston, MA, : Boston College Department of Economics.

Crott, R., & Briggs, A. (2010). Mapping the QLQ-C30 quality of life cancer questionnaire to EQ-5D patient preferences. *European Journal of Health Economics*; 11(4):427–434.

Crott, R., Versteegh, M., & Uyl-de-Groot, C. (2013). An assessment of the external validity of mapping QLQ-C30 to EQ-5D preferences. *Quality of Life Research*; 22(5):1045–1054.

Crowther, L. (2016). Multi-state survival analysis in Stata, Stata UK Meeting 8th–9th September 2016. Retrieved from: www.stata.com/meeting/uk16/slides/crowther_uk16.pdf.

Cykert, S., Kissling, G., & Hansen, C.J. (2000). Patient preferences regarding possible outcomes of lung resection: What outcomes should preoperative evaluations target? *Chest*; 117(6):1551–1559.

Dakin, H., Devlin, N., Feng, Y. et al. (2015). The influence of cost-effectiveness and other factors on NICE decisions. *Health Economics*; 24(10):1256–1271.

Dakin, H., Devlin, N.J., Odeyemi, I.A. (2006). "Yes", "No" or "Yes, but"? Multinomial modelling of NICE decision-making. *Health Policy*; 77(3): 352–367.

Damm, K., Roeske, N., & Jacob, C. (2013). Health-related quality of life questionnaires in lung cancer trials: A systematic literature review. *Health Economics Review*; 3(1):15.

Davis, C., Naci, H., Gurpinar, E., (2017). Availability of evidence of benefits on overall survival and quality of life of cancer drugs approved by European Medicines Agency: Retrospective cohort study of drug approvals 2009–13. *BMJ*; 359:j4530.

Day, S. (2002). Dictionary of Clinical Trials, First Ed. John Wiley.

de Bock, G.H., Putter, H., Bonnema, J. et al. (2009). The impact of loco-regional recurrences on metastatic progression in early-stage breast cancer: A multistate model. *Breast Cancer Research and Treatment*; 117(2):401–408.

de Glas, N.A., Kiderlen, M., Vandenbroucke, J.P. et al. (2016). Performing survival analyses in the presence of competing risks: A clinical example in older breast cancer patients. *Journal of the National Cancer Institute*; 108(5):djv366.

de WreedeL.C., & Fiocco, P. (2010). The mistate package for estimation and prediction in non- and semi-parametric multi-state and competing risks models. *Computer Methods and Programs in Biomedicine*, 261–274.

de Wreede, L.C., Fiocco, M., & Putter, H. (2011). Mstate: An R package for the analysis of competing risks and multi-state models. *Journal of Statistical Software*; 38(7):1–30.

Dehbi, H.M., Royston, P., & Hackshaw, A. (2017). Life expectancy difference and life expectancy ratio: Two measures of treatment effects in randomised trials with non-proportional hazards. *BMJ*; 357:j2250.

Del Paggio, J.C., Azariah, B., Sullivan, R. et al. (2017). Do contemporary randomized controlled trials meet ESMO thresholds for meaningful clinical benefit? *Annals of Oncology*; 28(1):157–162.

Denis, F., Lethrosne, C., Pourel, N. et al. (2017). Randomized trial comparing a web mediated follow-up with routine surveillance in lung cancer patients. *Journal of the National Cancer Institute*; 109(9).

Department of Health and Social Care. (n.d.). NHS prescription services. Retrieved from: www.nhsbsa.nhs.uk/nhs-prescription-services.

Department of Health and Social Care. (n.d.). Publications by Department of Health and Social Care. Retrieved from: www.gov.uk/government/publications?departments%5B%5D=department-of-health-and-social-care.

Department of Health and Social Care. (2011). Equity and excellence: Liberating the NHS. Retrieved from: www.gov.uk/government/news/equity-and-excellence-liberating-the-nhs.

DeVine, J., Norvell, D.C., Ecker, E. et al. (2011). Evaluating the correlation and responsiveness of patient-reported pain with function and quality-of-life outcomes after spine surgery. *Spine*; 36(21 Suppl):S69–S74.

Devlin, N., & Parkin, D. (2004). Does NICE have a cost-effectiveness threshold and what other factors influence its decisions? A binary choice analysis. *Health Economics*; 13(5):437–452.

Dewar, R., & Khan, I. (2015). A new SAS macro for flexible parametric survival modeling: Applications to clinical trials and surveillance data. *Clinical Investigation London*; 5(12):00–00.

Díaz-Ordaz, K., Kenward, M.G., & Grieve, R. (2014). Handling missing values in cost-effectiveness analyses that use data from cluster randomised trials. *Journal of the Royal Statistical Society: Series A*; 177(2):457–474.

Doble, B., & Lorgelly, P. (2016). Mapping the EORTC QLQ-C30 onto the EQ-5D-3L: Assessing the external validity of existing mapping algorithms. *Quality of Life Research*; 25(4):891–911.

Dobrez, D., Cella, D., Pickard, A.S. et al. (2007). Estimation of patient preference-based utility weights from the functional assessment of cancer therapy—general. *Value in Health*; 10(4):266–272.

Dolan, P. (1997). Modelling valuations for EuroQol health states. *Medical Care*; 35(11):1095–1108.

Dobrez, D.G., Mathes, A, Amdahl, M., et al. (2004). Paricalcitol-treated patients experience improved hospitalization outcomes compared with calcitriol-treated patients in real-world clinical settings. *Nephrology Dialysis Transplantation*; 19(5): 1174–1181.

Doyle, S., Lloyd, A., & Walker, M. (2008). Health state utility scores in advanced non-small cell lung cancer. *Lung Cancer*; 62(3):374–380.

Drummond, M., & McGuire, A. (2001). Economic evaluation in health care : merging theory with practice. Oxford University Press. Retrieved from https://books.google.fr/books?hl=en&lr=&id=_fJK15F75-EC&oi=fnd&pg=PP2&dq=drummond+McGuire&ots=JUaIBpVA-F&sig=rNq0WR4nVWcvI0q8d5ufL4s9z8s#v=onepage&q=drummond McGuire&f=false.

Drummond, M.F., & McGuire, A. (2002). *Economic evaluation in health care: Merging theory with practice*. Oxford: Oxford University Press.

Drummond, M.F., & O'Brien, B. (1993). Clinical importance, statistical significance and the assessment of economic and quality-of-life outcomes. *Health Economics*; 2(3):205–212.

Drummond, M.F., Sculpher, M.J., Torrance, G.W. et al. (2005). *Methods for the economic evaluation of health care programmes*, 3rd Edition. Oxford: Oxford University Press.

Drummond, M.F., Sculpher, M.J., Torrance, G.W. et al. (2015). *Methods for the economic evaluation of health care programmes*, 4th Edition. Oxford University Press.

Dukes, O., Vansteelandt, S. (2018). A note of G-estimation of causal risk ratios. *American Journal of Epidemiology*; 187(5): 1079–1084.

Duan, N. (1983). Smearing estimate: A nonparametric retransformation method. *Journal of the American Statistical Association*; 78(383):605–610.

Dukhovny, D., Lorch, S.A., Schmidt, B. et al. & Caffeine for Apnea of Prematurity Trial Group. (2011). Economic evaluation of caffeine for apnea of prematurity. *Pediatrics*; 127(1):e146–e155.

Dunlop, W., Iqbal, I., Khan, I. et al. (2013). Cost-effectiveness of modified-release prednisone in the treatment of moderate to severe rheumatoid arthritis with morning stiffness based on directly elicited public preference values. *ClinicoEconomics and Outcomes Research*; 5:555–564.

Dukhobny, D., Lorch, S.A., Schmidt, B. (2012). Economic evaluation of caffeine for apnea of prematurity; caffeine for apnea of prematurity trial group. *Pediatrics*; 127(1): e146–155.

Dunlop, W., Uhl, R., Khan, I. et al. (2012). Quality of life benefits and cost impact of prolonged release oxycodone/naloxone versus prolonged release oxycodone in patients with moderate-to-severe non-malignant pain and opioid-induced constipation: A UK cost-utility analysis. *Journal of Medical Economics*; 15(3):564–575.

Dunn, A., Grosse, S.D., & Zuvekas, S.H. (2018). Adjusting health expenditures for inflation: A review of measures for health services research in the United States. *Health Services Research*; 53(1):175–196.

Dvortsin, E., Gout-Zwart, J., Eijssen, E. L. M., Van Brussel, J., & Postma, M. J. (2016). Comparative cost-effectiveness of drugs in early versus late stages of cancer; Review of the literature and a case study in breast cancer. *PLoS ONE*. https://doi.org/10.1371/journal.pone.0146551

Eddy, D.M., Hollingworth, W., Caro, J.J. et al., & ISPOR-SMDM Modeling Good Research Practices Task Force. (2012). Model transparency and validation: A report of the ISPOR-SMDM Modeling Good Research Practices Task Force-7. *Medical Decision Making*; 32(5):733–743.

Eisenhauer, E.A., Therasse, P., Bogaerts, J. et al. (2009). New response evaluation criteria in solid tumours: Revised recist guideline (Version 1.1). *European Journal of Cancer*; 45(1):228–247.

Ekelund, R.B. Jr., & Hébert, R.F. (1999). *Secret origins of modern microeconomics: Dupuit and the engineers*. Chicago: University of Chicago Press.

Elbasha, E.H., & Chhatwal, J. (2016). Myths and misconceptions of within-cycle correction: A guide for modelers and decision makers. *Pharmacoeconomics*; 34(1):13–22.

EMA (2012). Methodological consideration for using progression-free survival (PFS) or disease-free survival (DFS) in confirmatory trials; https://www.ema.europa.eu/en/appendix-1-guideline-evaluation-anticancer-medicinal-products-man-methodological-consideration-using.

Etzioni, R.D., Feuer, E.J., Sullivan, S.D. et al. (1999). On the use of survival analysis techniques to estimate medical care costs. *Journal of Health Economics*; 18(3):365–380.

EUnetHTA (2018). European Network for Health Technology Assessment. Retrieved from: www.eunethta.eu.

European Medicines Agency. (2017). ICH E9 (R1) addendum on estimates and sensitivity analysis in clinical trials to the guideline on statistical principles for clinical trials. Retrieved from: www.ema.europa.eu/documents/scientific-guideline/draft-ich-e9-r1-addendum-estimands-sensitivity-analysis-clinical-trials-guideline-statistical_en.pdf.

European Organisation for Research and Treatment of Cancer. (n.d.). Manuals. EORCT Quality of Life. Retrieved from: http://groups.eortc.be/qol/manuals.

European Society for Medical Oncology. (2015). ESMO Press release: ESMO announces a scale to stratify the magnitude of clinical benefit of anti-cancer medicines. Retrieved from: www.esmo.org/Press-Office/Press-Releases/ESMO-Announces-a-Scale-to-Stratify-the-Magnitude-of-Clinical-Benefit-of-Anti-Cancer-Medicines.

European Union. (n.d.). The EU general data protection regulation. Retrieved from: https://eugdpr.org/.

Evidence Review Group. (2008). The clinical- and cost-effectiveness of lenalidomide for multiple myeloma in people who have received at least one prior therapy: An evidence review of the submission from celgene. PenTAG on behalf of NICE. Retrieved from: www.nice.org.uk/guidance/ta171/resources/multiple-myeloma-lenalidomide-evidence-review-group-report2

Fabrini, M.G., Silvano, G., Lolli, I. et al. (2009). A multi-institutional phase II study on second-line fotemustine chemotherapy in recurrent glioblastoma. *Journal of Neuro-Oncology*; 92(1):79–86.

FACIT. (n.d.). Questionnaires. FACIT measurement system. Retrieved from: www.facit.org/facitorg/questionnaires.

Fairclough, L.D. (2010). *Design and analysis of quality of life studies in clinical trials*, 2nd Edition. London: Chapman & Hall/CRC Interdisciplinary Statistics.

Fan, M.Y., & Zhou, X.H. (2007). A simulation study to compare methods for constructing confidence intervals for the incremental cost-effectiveness ratio. *Health Services and Outcomes Research Methodology*; 7(1–2):57–77.

Fan, X. Sivo, S., Keenan, S. (2002). *SAS for Monte Carlo Studies: A guide for Quantitative Researchers*. Cary, NC: SAS Institute.

Faria, R., Gomes, M., Epstein, D. et al. (2014). A Guide to handling missing data in cost-effectiveness analysis conducted within randomised controlled trials. *PharmacoEconomics*; 32(12):1157–1170.

Faries, D.E., Leon, A.C., Haro, J.M. et al. (2010). *Analsis of observational health care data using SAS*. SAS Publications.

Fayers, P.M., Aaronson, N.K., Bjordal, K. et al. (2001). *The EORTC QLQ-C30 scoring manual*, 3rd Edition. Brussels: European Organisation for Research and Treatment of Cancer.

FDA (2018). Guidance to Industry. Retrieved from https://www.fda.gov/downloads/Drugs/Guidances/ucm071590.pdf.

Federal Ministry of Health (Germany). (n.d.). German System of Healthcare. Retrieved from: www.bundesgesundheitsministerium.de/

Fenwick, E., Claxton, K., & Sculpher, M. (2008). The value of implementation and the value of information: Combined and uneven development. *Medical Decision Making*; 28(1):21–32.

Ferlay, J., Shin, H.R., Bray, F. et al. (2010). Estimates of worldwide burden of cancer in 2008: GLOBOCAN 2008. *International Journal of Cancer*; 127(12):2893–2917.

Ferver, K., Burton, B., & Jesilow, P. (2009).The use of claims data in healthcare research. *Open Public Health Journal*; 2(1):11–24.

Fiteni, F., Westeel, V., Pivot, X. et al. (2014). Endpoints in cancer clinical trials. *Journal Visceral Surgeon*; 151(1):17–22.

Fleishman, A.I. (1978). A method for simulating non-normal distributions. *Psychometrika*; 43(4):521–532.

Fojo, T., Mailankody, S., & Lo, A. (2014). Unintended consequences of expensive cancer therapeutics—The pursuit of marginal indications and a me-too mentality that stifles innovation and creativity: The John Conley Lecture. *JAMA Otolaryngology Head and Neck Surgery*; 140(12):1225–1236.

Folland, S., Goodman, A.C., & Stano, M. (2012). *The economics of health and health care*, 7th Edition. Boston, MA.Prentice Hall.

Food and Drug Administration. (2017) Sentinel System Overview. Retrieved from: https://www.fda.gov/downloads/ForPatients/About/UCM595420.pdf.

Food and Drug Administration. (2018). Information Exchange and Data Transformation (INFORMED). Retrieved from: https://www.fda.gov/aboutfda/centersoffices/officeofmedicalproductsandtobacco/oce/ucm543768.htm.

Fragoulakis, V., Pallis, A., & Georgoulias, M. (2014). Economic evaluation of pemetrexed versus erlotinib as second-line treatment of patients with advanced/metastatic non-small cell lung cancer in Greece: A cost minimization analysis. *Lung Cancer: Targets and Therapy*;21(7) 43–51.

Friedman, H.S., Prados, M.D., Wen, P.Y. et al. (2009). Bevacizumab alone and in combination with irinotecan in recurrent glioblastoma. *Journal of Clinical Oncology*; 27(28):4733–4740.

Fukuoka, M., Wu, Y.L., Thongprasert, S. et al. (2011). Biomarker analyses and final overall survival results from a phase III, randomized, open-label, first-line study of gefitinib versus carboplatin/paclitaxel in clinically selected patients with advanced non-small-cell lung cancer in Asia (IPASS). *Journal of Clinical Oncology*; 29(21):2866–2874.

Fundamental Finance. (n.d.). Marginal Cost (MC) & Average Total Cost (ATC). Retrieved from: http://economics.fundamentalfinance.com/micro_atc_mc.php.

Gaafar, R.M., Surmont, V.F., Van Klaveren, R.J., et al. (2011). A double-blind, randomised, placebo-controlled phase III intergroup study of gefitinib in patients with advanced NSCLC, non-progressing after first line platinum-based chemotherapy (EORTC 08021/ILCP 01/03). *Eur. J Cancer*; 47(15): 2331–2340.

Gansen, F.M. (2018). Health economic evaluations based on routine data in Germany: A systematic review. *BMC Health Services Research*; 18(1):268.

Garber, A.M., & Phelps, C.E. (1997). Economic foundations of cost-effectiveness analysis. *Journal of Health Economics*; 16(1):1–31.

Gardiner, J.C. (2010). Survival Analysis: Overview of parametric, nonparametric and semiparametric approaches and new developments, Paper 252-2010, SAS Global Forum 2010, Seattle, WA, April 11–14. Retrieved from: https://support.sas.com/resources/papers/proceedings10/252-2010.pdf.

Gazdar, A.F. (2009). Activating and resistance mutations of EGFR in non-small-cell lung cancer: Role in clinical response to EGFR tyrosine kinase inhibitors. *Oncogene*; 28(Suppl 1):S24–S31.

Gelber, R.D., Goldhirsch, A., Cole, B.F. et al. (1996). A quality-adjusted time without symptoms or toxicity (Q-TWiST) analysis of adjuvant radiation therapy and chemotherapy for resectable rectal cancer. *Journal of the National Cancer Institute*; 88(15):1039–1045.

Gerard, K., Ryan, M., & Amaya-Amaya, M. (2008). Introduction. In: M. Ryan, K. Gerard, & M. Amaya-Amaya (Eds.). *Using discrete choice experiments to value health and health care*. Dordrecht, Netherlands: Springer, 1–10.

Gerkens, S., Neyt, M., San Miguel, L. et al. (2017). KCE report 288. Health Service Research: How to improve the Belgian process for Managed Entry Agreements? An analysis of the Belgian and international experience. Brussels: Belgian Health Care Knowledge Centre (KCE). see: https://kce.fgov.be/sites/default/files/atoms/files/KCE_288_Improve_Belgian_process_managed_entry_agreements_Report.pdf

Gheorghe, A., Roberts, T., Hemming, K. et al. (2015). Evaluating the generalisability of trial results: Introducing a centre- and trial-level generalisability index. *Pharmacoeconomics*; 33(11):1195–1214.

Gibbons, E.C., Casañas i Comabella, C., & Fitzpatrick, R. (2013). A structured review of patient-reported outcome measures for patients with skin cancer, 2013. *British Journal of Dermatology* (2013); 168(6):1176–1186.

Gilbert, M.R., Dignam, J.J., Armstrong, T.S. et al. (2014). A randomized trial of bevacizumab for newly diagnosed glioblastoma. *New England Journal of Medicine*; 370(8):699–708.

Gilbert, M.R., Wang, M., Aldape, K.D. et al. (2013). Dose-dense temozolomide for newly diagnosed glioblastoma: A randomized phase III clinical trial. *Journal of Clinical Oncology*; 31(32):4085–4091.

Gilberto de Lima, L.G., Segel, J., Tan, D. et al. (2011). Cost-effectiveness of epidermal growth factor receptor mutation testing and first-line treatment with gefitinib for patients with advanced adenocarcinoma of the lung. *Cancer*; 118(4):1032–1039.

Glasziou, P.P., Simes, R.J., & Gelber, R.D. (1990). Quality adjusted survival analysis. *Statistics in Medicine*; 9(11):1259–1276.

Glick, H.A. (2011). Sample size and power for cost-effectiveness analysis (Part 1). *Pharmacoeconomics*; 29(3):189–198.

Glick, H.A., Doshi, J.A., Sonnad, S.S., & Polsky, D. (2014). *Economic evaluation in clinical trials*. Oxford University Press.

Goldberg, S.B., Supko, J.G., Neal, J.W. et al. (2012). A phase I study of erlotinib and hydroxychloroquine in advanced non-small-cell lung cancer. *Journal of Thoracic Oncology*; 7(10):1602–1608.

Goldhirsch, A., Gelber, R.D., Simes, R.J. et al. (1989). Costs and benefits of adjuvant therapy in breast cancer: A quality-adjusted survival analysis. *Journal of Clinical Oncology*; 7(1):36–44.

Gonçalves, F.R., Santos, S., Silva, C. et al. (2018). Risk-sharing agreements, present and future. *Ecancermedicalscience*; 12:823.

Goodwin, P.J., Black, J.T., Bordeleau, L.J. et al. (2003). Health-related quality-of-life measurement in randomized clinical trials in breast cancer—Taking stock. *Journal of the National Cancer Institute*; 95(4):263–281.

Goozner, M. (2012). Drug approvals 2011: Focus on companion diagnostics. *Journal of the National Cancer Institute*; 104(2):84–86.

Goulart, B., & Ramsey, S. (2011). A trial-based assessment of the cost-utility of bevacizumab and chemotherapy versus chemotherapy alone for advanced non-small cell lung cancer. *Value in Health*; 14(6):836–845.

Government of UK. Medicines and Healthcare products Regulatory Agency. (2014). Apply for the early access to medicines scheme (EAMS). Retrieved from: www.gov.uk/guidance/apply-for-the-early-access-to-medicines-scheme-eams.

Graham, C.N., Hechmati, G., & Hjelmgren, J. (2014). Cost-effectiveness analysis of panitumumab plus mFOLFOX6 compared with bevacizumab plus mFOLFOX6 for first-line treatment of patients with wild-type *RAS* metastatic colorectal cancer. *Journal of Cancer*; 50(16):2791–2801.

Gray, A.M., Clarke, P.M., Wolstenholme, J.L. et al. (2011). *Applied methods of cost-effectiveness in health care*. Oxford: Oxford University Press.

Green Park Collaborative. (2016). Retrieved from: http://www.cmtpnet.org/resource-center/view/new-guidance-for-treatment-switching-in-oncology-drug-trials/.

Greenhalgh, J., McLeod, C., Bagust, A. et al. (2010). Pemetrexed for the maintenance treatment of locally advanced or metastatic non-small cell lung cancer. *Health Technology Assessment*; 14(Suppl 2):33–39.

Greenland, S., Lanes, S., & Jara, M. (2008). Estimating effects from randomized trials with discontinuations: The need for intent-to-treat design and G-estimation. *Clinical Trials*; 5(1):5–13.

Gridelli, C., Ciardiello, F., Gallo, C. et al. (2012). First-line erlotinib followed by second-line cisplatin-gemcitabine chemotherapy in advanced non-small-cell lung cancer: The TORCH randomized trial. *Journal of Clinical Oncology*; 30(24):3002–3011.

Grieve, R., Nixon, R., Thompson, S.G. et al. (2005). Using multilevel models for assessing the variability of multinational resource use and cost data.*Health Economics*; 14(2):185–196.

Grieve, R., Nixon, R., Thompson, S.G. et al. (2007). Multilevel models for estimating incremental net benefits in multinational studies. *Health Economics*; 16(8):815–826.

Grieve, R., Nixon, R., & Thompson, S.G. (2014). Bayesian hierarchical models for cost-effectiveness analyses that use data from cluster randomized trials; healthcare: A review of principles and applications. *Journal of Medical Economics*; 20(2): 163–175.

Guo, S., & Fraser, M.E. (2014). *Propensity score analysis: Statistical methods and applications*. Sage Publications.

Hall, A.E., & Highfill, T. (2013). Calculating disease-based medical care expenditure indexes for Medicare beneficiaries: A comparison of method and data choices. nber.org.

Hao, Y., Wolfram, V., & Cook, J.S. (2016). A structured review of health utility measures and elicitation in advanced/metastatic breast cancer. *ClinicoEconomics and outcomes research*.

Harris, A.H., Hill, S.R., Chin, G., et al. (2008). The role of value for money in public insurance coverage decisions for drugs in Australia: a retrospective analysis 1994-2004. *Decis. Making*; 28(5): 713–722.

Hashim, D., Boffetta, P., La Vecchia, C. et al. (2016). The global decrease in cancer mortality: trends and disparities*Annals of Oncology*; 27(5):926–933.

Haycox, A., Drummond, M., & Walley, T. (1997). Pharmacoeconomics: Integrating economic evaluation into clinical trials. *British Journal of Clinical Pharmacology*; 43(6):559–562.

Henry, J., & Kaise Family Foundation. (2018). Public opinion on prescription drugs and their prices. KFF health tracking poll. Retrieved from: www.kff.org/slideshow/public-opinion-on-prescription-drugs-and-their-prices/.

Herbst, R.S., Prager, D., Hermann, R.L. et al. (2005). Tribute: A phase III trial of erlotinib hydrochloride (OSI-774) combined with carboplatin and paclitaxel chometherapy in advanced non-small-cell lung cancer. *Journal of Clinical Oncology*; 23(25):5892–5899. Epub 2005 July 25.

Herdman, M., Gudex, C., Lloyd, A. et al. (2011). Development and preliminary testing of the new five-level version of EQ-5D (EQ-5D-5L). *Quality of Life Research*; 20(10):1727–1736. Epub 2011 April 9.

Hernández, M.A., Vázquez-Polo, F.J., González-Torre, F.J. et al. (2009). Complementing the net benefit approach: A new framework for Bayesian cost-effectiveness analysis. *International Journal of Technology Assessment in Health Care*; 25(4):537–545.

Herrlinger, U., Schäfer, N., Steinbach, J.P. et al. (2016). Bevacizumab plus irinotecan versus temozolomide in newly diagnosed O6-Methylguanine-DNA methyltransferase nonmethylated glioblastoma: The randomized GLARIUS trial. *Journal of Clinical Oncology*; 34(14):1611–1619.

Hettle, R., Posnett, J., & Borrill, J. (2015). Challenges in economic modeling of anticancer therapies: An example of modeling the survival benefit of olaparib maintenance therapy for patients with BRCA-mutated platinum-sensitive relapsed ovarian cancer. *Journal of Medical Economics*; 18(7):516–524.

Hlatky, M.A., Boothroyd, D.B., & Johnstone, I.M. (2002). Economic evaluation in long-term clinical trials. *Statistics in Medicine*; 21(19):2879–2888.

Hoaglin, D.C., Hawkins, N., Jansen, J.P. et al. (2011). Conducting indirect-treatment-comparison and network-meta-analysis studies: Report of the ISPOR Task Force on indirect treatment comparisons good research practices: Part 2. *Value in Health*; 14(4):429–437.

Hoch, J.S., & Dewa, C.S. (2014). Advantages of the net benefit regression framework for economic evaluations of interventions in the workplace: A case study of the cost-effectiveness of a collaborative mental health care program for people receiving short-term disability benefits for psychiatric disorders. *Journal of Occupational and Environmental Medicine*; 56(4):441–445.

Hodi, F.S., Ribas, A., Daud, A. et al. (2014). Evaluation of immune-related response criteria (irRC) in patients (pts) with advanced melanoma (MEL) treated with the anti-PD-1 monoclonal antibody MK-3475. *Journal of Clinical Oncology*; 32(suppl 15s; abstr3006):10.

Hoefman, R.J., van Exel, J., & Brouwer, W. (2013). How to include informal care in economic evaluations. *Pharmacoeconomics*; 31(12):1105–1119.

Hollen, P.J., Gralla, R.J., Cox, C. et al. (1997). A dilemma in analysis: Issues in the serial measurement of quality of life in patients with advanced lung cancer. *Lung Cancer*; 18(2):119–136.

Holmes, J., Dunlop, D., Hemmett, L. et al. (2004). A cost-effectiveness analysis of docetaxel in the second-line treatment of non-small cell lung cancer. *Pharmacoeconomics*; 22(9):581–589.

Howard, D.H., Bach, P.B., Berndt, E.R. et al. (2015.) Pricing in the market for anticancer drugs. *Journal of Economic Perspectives*; 29(1):139–162.

Huang, Y. (2009). Cost analysis with censored data. *Medical Care*; 47(7 Suppl 1): S115–S119.

Hughes, D.A., Bagust, A., Haycox, A. et al. (2001). The impact of non-compliance on the cost-effectiveness of pharmaceuticals: A review of the literature. *Health Economics*; 10(7):601–615.

Hurst, N.P. (1997). Re: Quality of life measures. *Rheumatology*; 36(1):147–148.

Husereau, D., Drummond, M.F., Petrou, S. et al. (2013). Consolidated health economic evaluation reporting standards (CHEERS)—Explanation and elaboration: A report of the ISPOR health economic evaluations publication guidelines good reporting practices task force. *Value in Health*; 16(2):231–250.

Husson, O., Steenbergen, L.N., Koldewijn, E.L. et al. (2014). Excess mortality in patients with prostate cancer. *BJU International*; 114:691–697.

Hutchinson, C.L., Menck, H.R., Burch, M. et al. (2004). *Cancer Registry Management Principles & Practice*, 2nd Edition. Kendall & Hunt Publishing.

Institute for Clinical and Economic Review. (n.d.). Methodology. Retrieved from: https://icer-review.org/methodology/.

Institute for Quality and Efficiency in Healthcare. (n.d.). Retrieved from: www.iqwig.de/en/home.2724.html.

Irwin, J.O. (1949). The standard error of an estimate of expectation of life, with special reference to expectation of tumourless life in experiments with mice. *Journal of Hygiene*; 47(2):188.

Ishak, K.J., Proskorovsky, I., Korytowsky, B. et al. (2014). Methods for adjusting for bias due to crossover in oncology trials. *Pharmacoeconomics*; 32(6):533–546.

Janne, P.A., Ramalingam, S.S., Yang, J.C. et al. (2014). Clinical activity of the mutant-selective EGFR inhibitor AZD9291 in patients (pts) with EGFR inhibitor–resistant non-small cell lung cancer (NSCLC). [ASCO abstract 8009]. *Journal of Clinical Oncology*; 32(5_suppl): 8009.

Jansen, J.P., Fleurence, R., Devine, B. et al. (2011). Interpreting indirect treatment comparisons and network meta-analysis for health-care decision making: Report of the ISPOR task force on indirect treatment comparisons good research practices: Part 1. *Value Health*; 14(4):417–428.

Jemal, A., Bray, F., Center, M.M. et al. (2011). Global cancer statistics. *CA: A Cancer Journal for Clinicians*; 61(2):69–90.

Jiaqi, L. (2016). Modeling approaches for cost and cost-effectiveness estimation using observational data. Publicly accessible Penn dissertations. 1858. Retrieved from: http://repository.upenn.edu/edissertations/1858.

Jones, B., & Kenward, M.G. (2014). *Design and analysis of cross-over trials*, 3rd Edition. Chapman and Hall/CRC.

Jönsson, B., Ramsey, S., & Wilking, N. (2014). Cost effectiveness in practice and its effect on clinical outcomes. *Journal of Cancer Policy*; 2(1):12–21.

Jönsson, L., Sandin, R., Ekman, M. et al. (2014). Analyzing overall survival in randomized controlled trials with crossover and implications for economic evaluation. *Value in Health*; 17(6):707–713.

Kaplan, E.L., & Meier, P. (1958). Nonparametric estimation from incomplete observations. *Journal of the American Statistical Association*; 53(282):457–481.

Karrison, T. (1987). Restricted mean life with adjustment for covariates. *Journal of the American Statistical Association*; 82(400):1169–1176.

Katakami, N., Atagi, S., Goto, K. et al. (2013). LUX-Lung 4: A phase II trial of afatinib in patients with advanced non-small-cell lung cancer who progressed during prior treatment with erlotinib, gefitinib, or both. *Journal of Clinical Oncology*; 31(27):3335–3341.

Keeble, G.R.L., Barber, S., & Baxter, P.D. (2015). Choosing a method to reduce selection bias: A tool for researchers. *Open Journal of Epidemiology*; 5:155–162.

Kenneth, C., Park, B.S., Schwimmer, J.E. et al. (2001). Decision analysis for the cost-effective management of recurrent colorectal cancer. *Annals of Surgery*; 233(3):310–319.

Khan, I. (2015). *Design & analysis of clinical trials for economic evaluation & reimbursement: An applied approach using SAS & STATA*. Chapman & Hall.

Khan, I. (2019). Modelling and extrapolating post progression utility in NSCLC patients; a modelling approach (Medical Decision Making), [in press].

Khan, I., Bashir, Z., & Forster, M. (2015). Interpreting small treatment differences from quality of life data in cancer trials: An alternative measure of treatment benefit and effect size for the EORTC-QLQ-C30. *Health and Quality of Life Outcomes*; 13(1):180.

Khan, I., Morris, S., Pashayan, N. et al. (2016). Comparing the mapping between EQ-5D-5L, EQ-5D-3L and the EORTC-QLQ-C30 in non-small cell lung cancer patient. *Health and Quality of Life Outcomes*; 14:60.

Khan, I., Sarker, S.J., & Hackshaw, A. (2012). Smaller sample sizes for phase II trials based on exact tests with actual error rates by trading-off their nominal levels of significance and power. *British Journal of Cancer*; 107(11):1801–1809.

Khan, I., Stavros, P., Khan, K. et al. (2018). Does exercise improve cognitive impairment in people with mild to moderate dementia? A cost-effectiveness analysis from a confirmatory randomised controlled trial *(DAPA Trial). PharmacoEconomics*; [in Press].

Khozin, S., Blumenthal, G.M., & Pazdur, R. (2017). Real-world data for clinical evidence generation in oncology. *JNCI: Journal of the National Cancer Institute*; 109(11).

Kim, C., & Prasad, V. (2015). Cancer drugs approved on the basis of a surrogate end point and subsequent overall survival: An analysis of 5 years of US Food and Drug Administration approvals. *JAMA Internal Medicine*; 175(12):1992–1994.

Kim, C., & Prasad, V. (2016). Strength of validation for surrogate end points used in the US Food and Drug Administration's approval of oncology drugs. *Mayo Clinic Proceedings*; 91(6):713–725.

King, M.T. (1996). The interpretation of scores from the EORTC quality of life questionnaire QLQ-C30. *Quality of Life Research*; 5(6):555–567.

Kish, J.K., Ward, M.A., Garofalo, D. et al. (2018). Real-world evidence analysis of palbociclib prescribing patterns for patients with advanced/ metastatic breast cancer treated in community oncology practice in the USA one year post approval. *Breast Cancer Research*; 20(3):1–8.

Klaxton, C. (1999). The irrelevance of inference: A decision-making approach to the stochastic evaluation of health care technologies. *Journal of Health Economics*; 18(3):341–364.

Klein, J.P., & Moeschberger, M. (2005). *Survival analysis: Techniques for censored and truncated data*, 2nd Edition. New York: Springer.

Klein, J.P., Gerster, M., Andersen, P.K. et al. (2008). SAS and R functions to compute pseudo-values for censored data regression. *Computer Methods and Programs in Biomedicine*; 89(3):289–300.

Klein, R., Muehlenbein, C., Liepa, A.M. et al. (2009). Cost-effectiveness of pemetrexed plus cisplatin as first-line therapy for advanced nonsquamous non-small cell lung cancer. *Journal of Thoracic Oncology*; 4(11):1404–1414.

Kong, D.S., Lee, J.I., Kim, J.H. et al. (2010). Phase II trial of low-dose continuous (metronomic) treatment of temozolomide for recurrent glioblastoma. *Neuro-Oncology*; 12(3):289–296.

Konnerup, M. & Kongsted, H.C., (2012). Are more observational studies being included in Cochrane Reviews? *BMC Research Notes*; 5:570.

Krahn, M., Bremner, K.E., Tomlinson, G. et al. (2007). Responsiveness of disease-specific and generic utility instruments in prostate cancer patients. *Quality of Life Research*; 16(3):509–522.

Kruger, C.J.C. (2004). Constrained cubic spline interpolation for chemical engineering applications. Retrieved from: www.korf.co.uk/spline.pdf.

Kumar, H., Fojo, T., & Mailankody, S. (2016). An appraisal of clinically meaningful outcomes guidelines for oncology clinical trials. *JAMA Oncology*; 2(9):1238–1240.

Kuntz, K.M., & Weinstein, M.C. (2001). Modeling in economic evaluation. In: M. Drummond, & A. McGuire (Eds.). *Economic evaluation in health care: Merging theory with practice*. New York: Oxford University Press, 141–171.

Kunz, R., Vist, G., & Oxman, A.D. (2007). Randomisation to protect against selection bias in healthcare trials. *Cochrane Database of Systematic Reviews*; 2(2):MR000012.

Lai, X., & Zee, B.C.Y. (2015). Mixed response and time-to-event endpoints for multistage single-arm phase II design. *Trials*; 16:250.

Landrum, M.B., & Ayanian, J.Z. (2001). Causal effect of ambulatory specialty care on mortality following myocardial infarction: A comparison of propensity score and instrumental variable analyses. *Health Services and Outcomes Research Methodology*; 2(3–4):221–245.

Latimer, N.R., Siebert, U., Henshall, C. et al. Treatment switching: Statistical and decision-making challenges and approaches. *International Journal of Technology Assessment in Health Care*; 32(2): 160–166.

Latimer, N.R. (2011). NICE DSU Technical Support Document 14: Survival analysis for economic evaluations alongside clinical trials – Extrapolation with patient-level data. Report by the Decision Support Unit, June 2011 (last updated March 2013). Retrieved from: http://nicedsu.org.uk/wp-content/uploads/2016/03/NICE-DSU-TSD-Survival-analysis.updated-March-2013.v2.pdf.

Latimer, N.R. (2015) Treatment switching in oncology trials and the acceptability of adjustment methods. *Expert Review of Pharmacoeconomics & Outcomes Research*; 15(4): 561–564.

Latimer, N.R., & Abrams, K.R. (2014). NICE DSU Technical Support Document 16: Adjusting survival time estimates in the presence of treatment switching. Retrieved from: http://nicedsu.org.uk/wp-content/uploads/2016/03/TSD16_Treatment_Switching.pdf.

Latimer, N.R., Abrams, K.R., Lambert, P.C. et al. (2017). Adjusting for treatment switching in randomised controlled trials – A simulation study and a simplified two-stage method. *Statistical Methods in Medical Research*; 26(2):724–751.

Latimer, N.R., White, I.R., Abrams, K.R. et al. (2018). Causal inference for long-term survival in randomised trials with treatment switching: Should re-censoring be applied when estimating counterfactual survival times? *Statistical Methods in Medical Research*. Retrieved from: www.sheffield.ac.uk/scharr/sections/heds/staff/latimer_n_publications.

Ledermann, J.A., Embleton, A.C., Perren, T. et al. (2017). Overall survival results of ICON6: A trial of chemotherapy and cediranib in relapsed ovarian cancer. *Journal of Clinical Oncology*; 35(15_suppl):5506–5506. Retrieved from: www.icon6.org/media/1390/asco_2017.pdf.

Lee, C.F., Luo, N., Ng, R. et al. (2013). Comparison of the measurement properties between a short and generic instrument, the 5-level EuroQoL Group's 5-dimension (EQ-5D-5L) questionnaire, and a longer and disease-specific instrument, the Functional Assessment of Cancer Therapy—Breast (FACT-B), in Asian breast cancer patients. *Quality of Life Research*; 22(7):1745–1751.

Lee, L., Wang, L., & Crump, M. (2011). Identification of potential surrogate endpoints in randomized clinical trials of aggressive and indolent non-Hodgkin's lymphoma: Correlation of complete response, time-to-even and overall survival endpoints. *Annals of Oncology*; 22(6):1392–1403.

Lee, S.M., Khan, I., Upadhyay, S. et al. (2012). First-line erlotinib in patients with advanced non-small-cell lung cancer unsuitable for chemotherapy (TOPICAL): A double-blind, placebo-controlled, phase 3 trial. *Lancet Oncology*; 13(11):1161–1170.

Lewis, G., Peake, M., Aultman, R. et al. (2010). Cost-effectiveness of erlotinib versus docetaxel for second-Line treatment of advanced non-small-cell lung cancer in the United Kingdom. *Journal of International Medical Research*; 38(1):9–21.

Li, H., Han, D., Hou, Y. et al. (2015). Statistical interference methods for two crossing survival curves: A comparison of methods. *PLoS One*; 10(1):1–18.

Lin, D.Y. (2000). Proportional means regression for censored medical costs. *Biometrics;* 56(3):775–778.

Lin, D.Y., Feuer, E.J., Etzioni, R. et al. (1997). Estimating medical costs from incomplete follow-up data. *Biometrics;* 53(2):419–434.

Linley, W.G., Hughes, D.A. (2012). Reimbursement decisions of the All Wales Medicines Strategy Group: influence of policy and clinical and economic factors. *Pharmacoeconomics;* 30(9): 779–794.

Littlejohns, P., & Rawlins, M. (2009). *Patients, the public and priorities in healthcare,* 1st Edition. CRC Press.

Long, E.R. (1928). *A history of pathology*. London: Baillière, Tindall & Cox.

Lorgelly, P.K., Doble,B., Rowen, D. et al., & Cancer 2015 Investigators. (2017). Condition-specific or generic preference-based measures in oncology? A comparison of the EORTC-8D and the EQ-5D-3L. *Quality of Life Research;* 26(5):1163–1176.

Maeso, S., Callejo, D., Hernández, R. et al. (2011). Esophageal Doppler monitoring during colorectal resection offers cost-effective improvement of hemodynamic control. *Value in Health;* 14(6):818–826.

Maguire, J., Khan, I., McMenemin, R. et al. (2014). SOCCAR: A randomised phase II trial comparing sequential versus concurrent chemotherapy and radical hypofractionated radiotherapy in patients with inoperable stage III non-small cell lung cancer and good performance status. *European Journal of Cancer;* 50(17):2939–2949.

Maisonneuve, H., & Floret, D. (2012). Wakefield's affair: 12 years of uncertainty whereas no link between autism and mmr vaccine has been proved. *Presse Medicale;* 41(9 Pt 1):827–834.

Maiwenn, J., & Van Hout, B. (2000). A Bayesian approach to economic analyses of clinical trials: The case of stenting versus balloon angioplasty. *Health Economics;* 9(7):599–609.

Malkin, A.G., Goldstein, J.E., Perlmutter, M.S. et al. (2013). Responsiveness of the EQ-5D to the effects of low vision rehabilitation. *Optometry and Vision Science;* 90(8):799–805.

Manca, A., Rice, N., Sculpher, M.J. et al. (2005). Assessing generalisability by location in trial-based cost-effectiveness analysis: The use of multilevel models. *Health Economics;* 14(5):471–485; Erratum in: *Health Economics;* 14(5):486.

Maniadakis, N., Fragoulakis, V., Pallis, A.G. et al. (2010). Economic evaluation of docetaxel-gemcitabine versus vinorelbine-cisplatin combination as front-line treatment of patients with advanced/metastatic non-small-cell lung cancer in Greece: A cost-minimization analysis. *Annals of Oncology;* 21(7):1462–1467.

Manzini, G., Ettrich, T.J., Kremer, M. et al. (2018). Advantages of a multi-state approach in surgical research: How intermediate events and risk factor profile affect the prognosis of a patient with locally advanced rectal cancer. *BMC Medical Research Methodology;* 18(1):23.

Maringwa, J., Quinten, C., King, M. et al. (2011). Minimal clinically meaningful differences for the EORTC QLQ-C30 and EORTC QLQ-BN20 scales in brain cancer patients. *Annals of Oncology;* 22(9):2107–2112.

Martell, R.E., Sermer, D., Getz, K. et al. (2013). Oncology drug development and approval of systemic anticancer therapy by the U.S. Food and Drug Administration. *Oncologist;* 18(1):104–111.

Matulonis, U.A., Oza, A., Ho, M. et al. (2015). Intermediate clinical endpoints: A bridge between progression-free survival and overall survival in ovarian cancer trials. *Cancer;* 121(11):1737–1746.

McCabe, C., Claxton, K., & Culyer, A.J. (2008). The NICE cost-effectiveness threshold: What it is and what that means. *Pharmacoeconomics*; 26(9):733–744.

McIntosh, E., Louviere, J.J., Frew, E. et al. (2010). *Applied methods of cost–benefit analysis in health care*. Oxford University Press.

Meads, D.M., Marshall, A., Hulme, C.T. et al. (2016). The cost effectiveness of docetaxel and active symptom control versus active symptom control alone for refractory oesophagogastric adenocarcinoma: Economic analysis of the COUGAR-02 trial. *Pharmacoeconomics*; 34(1):33–42.

Meier-Hirmer, C., & Schumacher, M. (2013). Multi-state model for studying an intermediate event using time-dependent covariates: Application to breast cancer. *BMC Medical Research Methodology*; 13:80.

Menon, U., McGuire, A.J., Raikou, M. et al. (2017). The cost-effectiveness of screening for ovarian cancer: Results from the UK Collaborative Trial of Ovarian Cancer Screening (UKCTOCS). *British Journal of Cancer*; 117(5):619–627.

Messori, A., & Trippoli, S. (2017). The results of a pharmacoeconomic study: Incrementalcost-effectiveness ratio versus net monetary benefit. *Heart*; 103(21):1746.

Messori, A., & Trippoli, S. (2018). Incremental cost-effectiveness ratio and net monetary benefit, promoting the application of value-based pricing to medical devices. *Therapeutic Innovation & Regulatory Science*; 52(6):755–756.

Miller, R.G. (1981). *Survival Analysis*. New York: Wiley.

Miller, V.A., Hirsh, V., Cadranel, J. et al. (2012). Afatinib versus placebo for patients with advanced, metastatic non-small-cell lung cancer after failure of erlotinib, gefitinib, or both, and one or two lines of chemotherapy (LUX-Lung 1): A phase 2b/3 randomised trial. *Lancet. Oncology*; 13(5):528–538.

Miller, J.D., Foley, K.A., Russel,l M.W. (2014).; Current challenges in health economic modeling of cancer therapies: a research inquiry. *Am. Health Drug Benefits*; 7(3): 153–162.

Montazeri, A., Harirchi, I., Vahdani, M. et al. (2000). The EORTC breast cancer-specific quality of life questionnaire (EORTC QLQ-BR23): Translation and validation study of the Iranian version. *Quality of Life Research*; 9(2):177–184.

Montazeri, A., Milroy, R., Hole, D. et al. (2001). Quality of life in lung cancer patients: As an important prognostic factor. *Lung Cancer*; 31(2–3):233–240.

Morden, J.P., Lambert, P.C., Latimer, N. et al. (2011). Assessing methods for dealing with treatment switching in randomised controlled trials: A simulation study. *BMC Medical Research Methodology*; 11(1): 4.

Moreno, E., Girón, F.J., Martínez, M.L. et al. (2013). Optimal treatments in cost-effectiveness analysis in the presence of covariates: Improving patient subgroup definition. *European Journal of Operational Research*; 226(1):173–182.

Morris, S., Devlin, N., & Spencer, A. (Eds.). *Economic analysis in health care*, 2nd Edition. Chichester, UK: John Wiley & Sons.

Msheilla, I., White, R., & Mukku, S.R. An Investigation into the Key Drivers Influencing the Decision Making of the Scottish Medicines Consortium. *Value in Health*; 16(3): A264.

Mullins, C.D., Montgomery, R., & Tunis, S. (2010). Uncertainty in assessing value of oncology treatments. *Oncologist*; 15:58–64.

Murray, T.A., Thall, P.F., Yuan, Y. et al. (2017). Robust treatment comparison based on utilities of semi-competing risks in non-small-cell lung cancer. *Journal of the American Statistical Association*; 112:11–23.

Nafees, B., Stafford, M., Gavriel, S. et al. (2008). Health state utilities for non-small cell lung cancer. *Health and Quality of Life Outcomes*; 6(1):84.

National Cancer Institute. (n.d.). Dictionary of cancer terms. Retrieved from: www.cancer.gov/publications/dictionaries.

National Comprehensive Care Network. (2015). NCCN guidelines & clinical resources. NCCN clinical practice guidelines in oncology: Non-small cell lung cancer. National Comprehensive Cancer Network. Retrieved from: https://improvement.nhs.uk/resources/reference-costs/#rc1718.

National Health Service. (n.d.). Reference costs. NHS improvement. Retrieved from: https://improvement.nhs.uk/resources/reference-costs/.

National Health Service. (n.d.). Technology appraisal data. NHS improvement. Retrieved from: www.nice.org.uk/about/what-we-do/our-programmes/nice-guidance/nice-technology-appraisal-guidance/data.

National Health Service England. (n.d.). Cancer Drugs Fund. Retrieved from: www.england.nhs.uk/cancer/cdf/.

National Health Service England. (2013). Appraisal and funding of cancer drugs from July 2016 (including the new Cancer Drugs Fund). A new deal for patients, taxpayers and industry. Retrieved from: www.england.nhs.uk/wp-content/uploads/2013/04/cdf-sop.pdf.

National Health Service England. (2015). NHS increases budget for cancer drugs fund from £280 million in 2014/15 to an expected £340 million in 2015/16. Retrieved from: www.england.nhs.uk/2015/01/12/cancer-drug-budget/.

National Health Service (NHS). (2015). Statistics. Retrieved from: https://www.england.nhs.uk/2015/01/cancer-drug-budget/.

National Institute for Health and Care Excellence. (n.d.). How we work. Retrieved from: www.nice.org.uk/aboutnice/howwework/devnicetech/technologyappraisalprocessguides/GuideToMethodsTA201112.jsp.

NIH National Cancer Institute. (n.d). NCI dictionary of cancer terms. Retrieved from: www.cancer.gov/publications/dictionaries/cancer-terms?cdrid=45333.

NIH National Cancer Institute. (n.d.) Retrieved from: www.cancer.gov/about-cancer/understanding/what-is-cancer.

National Institutes of Health (2001). Considerations in the evaluation of surrogate endpoints in clinical trials. Summary of a National Institutes of Health workshop. *Control Clin Trials*. 2001 Oct; 22(5): 485–502.

National Institute for Health and Care Excellence. (n.d.). NICE TA269. Retrieved from: https://www.nice.org.uk/Guidance/TA269.

National Institute for Health and Care Excellence. (n.d.). Search results. Retrieved from: www.nice.org.uk/Guidance/TA202.

National Institute for Health and Care Excellence. (n.d.). Utilities TSD series. Retrieved from: http://nicedsu.org.uk/technical-support-documents/utilities-tsd-series/.

National Institute for Health and Care Excellence. (2007a). Bortezomib monotherapy for relapsed multiple myeloma. Technology appraisal guidance [TA129]. Retrieved from: www.nice.org.uk/guidance/ta129.

National Institute for Health and Care Excellence. (2007b). Pemetrexed for the treatment of non-small-cell lung cancer. Technology appraisal guidance [TA124]. Retrieved from: www.nice.org.uk/guidance/ta124.

National Institute for Health and Care Excellence. (2008a). Erlotinib for the treatment of non-small-cell lung cancer. Technology appraisal guidance [TA162]. Retrieved from: www.nice.org.uk/guidance/ta162.

National Institute for Health and Care Excellence. (2008b). TA171. Retrieved from: https://www.nice.org.uk/guidance/ta171/resources/multiple-myeloma-lenalidomide-evidence-review-group-report2.

National Institute for Health and Care Excellence. (2008c). TA162: Erlotinib for the treatment of non-small-cell lung cancer. Retrieved from: http://www.nice.org.uk/guidance/TA162.

National Institute for Health and Care Excellence. (2009a). Pemetrexed for the first-line treatment of non-small-cell lung cancer. Technology appraisal guidance [TA181]. Retrieved from: www.nice.org.uk/guidance/ta181.

National Institute for Health and Care Excellence. (2009b). Rituximab for the first-line treatment of chronic lymphocytic leukaemia. Technology appraisal guidance [TA174]. Retrieved from: www.nice.org.uk/guidance/ta174.

National Institute for Health and Care Excellence. (2010a). Gefitinib for the first-line treatment of locally advanced or metastatic non-small-cell lung cancer. Technology appraisal guidance [TA192]. Retrieved from: www.nice.org.uk/guidance/TA192.

National Institute of Health and Care Excellence. (2009c). Sunitinib for the treatment of gastrointestinal stromal tumours - guidance (TA179). HTA TA179. Retrieved from: https://www.nice.org.uk/guidance/ta179.

National Institute for Health and Care Excellence. (2010b). Ofatumumab (Arzerra®) for the treatment of chronic lymphocytic leukaemia in patients who are refractory to fludarabine and alemtuzumab. National Institute for Health and Clinical Excellence. Retrieved from: www.nice.org.uk/guidance/ta202/documents/chronic-lymphocytic-leukaemia-ofatumumab-manufacturers-submission2.

National Institute for Health and Care Excellence. (2010c). Pemetrexed for the maintenance treatment of non-small-cell lung cancer. Technology appraisal guidance [TA190]. Retrieved from: www.nice.org.uk/guidance/TA190.

National Institute for Health and Care Excellence. (2010d). Sorafenib for the treatment of advanced hepatocellular carcinoma. Technology appraisal guidance [TA189]. Retrieved from: www.nice.org.uk/guidance/TA189.

National Institute for Health and Care Excellence. (2010e). HTA TA189. Retrieved from: https://www.nice.org.uk/guidance/ta189.

National Institutes for Health and Care Excellence. (2010f). TA189. Retrieved from: https://www.nice.org.uk/guidance/ta189.

National Institute for Health and Care Excellence. (2010g). HTA TA202. Retrieved from: https://www.nice.org.uk/guidance/ta202/documents/chronic-lymphocytic-leukaemia-ofatumumab-manufacturers-submission2.

National Institute for Health and Care Excellence. (2011a). Erlotinib monotherapy for maintenance treatment of non-small-cell lung cancer. Technology appraisal guidance [TA227]. Retrieved from: www.nice.org.uk/guidance/TA227.

National Institute for Health and Care Excellence. (2011b). Lung cancer: Diagnosis and management. Retrieved from: www.nice.org.uk/guidance/cg121.000.

National Institute for Health and Care Excellence. (2011c). Advanced or metastatic NSCLC treatment pathway based on NICE guidance CG121 23. Retrieved from: www.nice.org.uk/guidance/cg121.

National Institute for Health and Care Excellence. (2011d). TA227: Erlotinib monotherapy for maintenance treatment of non-small-cell lung cancer. Retrieved from: http://www.nice.org.uk/guidance/TA227.
National Institute for Health and Care Excellence. (2012a). Erlotinib for the first-line treatment of locally advanced or metastatic EGFR-TK mutation-positive non-small-cell lung cancer. Technology appraisal guidance [TA258]. Retrieved from: www.nice.org.uk/guidance/TA258.
National Institute for Health and Care Excellence. (2012b). Erlotinib for the first-line treatment of locally advanced or metastatic EGFR-TK mutation-positive non-small-cell lung cancer. Retrieved from: http://www.nice.org.uk/guidance/TA258.
National Institute for Health and Care Excellence. (2013a). Bosutinib for previously treated chronic myeloid leukaemia. Technology appraisal guidance [TA299]. Retrieved from: www.nice.org.uk/guidance/TA299.
National Institute for Health and Care Excellence. (2013b). Pertuzumab for the neoadjuvant treatment of HER2-positive breast cancer. Technology appraisal guidance [TA424]. Retrieved from: www.nice.org.uk/guidance/TA424.
National Institute for Health and Care Excellence. (2013c). Olaparib for maintenance treatment of relapsed, platinum-sensitive, BRCA mutation-positive ovarian, fallopian tube and peritoneal cancer after response to second-line or subsequent platinum-based chemotherapy. Technology appraisal guidance [TA381]. Retrieved from: www.nice.org.uk/guidance/TA381.
National Institute for Health and Care Excellence. (2013d). Crizotinib for previously treated non-small-cell lung cancer associated with an anaplastic lymphoma kinase fusion gene. Technology appraisal guidance [TA296]. Retrieved from: www.nice.org.uk/guidance/TA296.
National Institute for Health and Care Excellence. (2013e). How NICE measures value for money in relation to public health interventions. Local government briefing. Retrieved from: www.nice.org.uk/media/default/guidance/lgb10-briefing-20150126.pdf.
National Institute for Health and Care Excellence. (2014a). Afatinib for treating epidermal growth factor receptor mutation-positive locally advanced or metastatic non-small-cell lung cancer. Technology appraisal guidance [TA310]. Retrieved from: www.nice.org.uk/guidance/TA310.
National Institute for Health and Care Excellence (2014b). Pemetrexed maintenance treatment following induction therapy with pemetrexed and cisplatin for non-squamous non-small-cell lung cancer. Technology appraisal guidance [TA309]. Retrieved from: www.nice.org.uk/guidance/TA309.
National Institute for Health and Care Excellence. (2017a). Pembrolizumab for treating PD-L1-positive non-small-cell lung cancer after chemotherapy. Technology appraisal guidance [TA447]. Retrieved from: www.nice.org.uk/guidance/TA447.
National Institute for Health and Care Excellence. (2017b). Pembrolizumab for untreated PD-L1-positive metastatic non-small-cell lung cancer. Technology appraisal guidance [TA428]. Retrieved from: www.nice.org.uk/guidance/TA428.
National Institute for Health and Care Excellence. (2017c). Nivolumab for previously treated squamous non-small-cell lung cancer. Technology appraisal guidance [TA483]. Retrieved from: www.nice.org.uk/guidance/TA483.

National Institute for Health and Care Excellence. (2017d). Venetoclax for treating chronic lymphocytic leukaemia. Technology appraisal guidance [TA487]. Retrieved from: www.nice.org.uk/guidance/ta487.

National Institute for Health and Care Excellence. (2017e). TA487. Retrieved from: https://www.nice.org.uk/guidance/ta487.

National Institute for Health and Care Excellence. (2018a). Atezolizumab for treating locally advanced or metastatic non-small-cell lung cancer after chemotherapy. Technology appraisal guidance [TA520]. Retrieved from: www.nice.org.uk/guidance/TA520.

National Institute for Health and Care Excellence. (2018b). Cabozantinib for treating medullary thyroid cancer. Technology appraisal guidance [TA516]. Retrieved from: www.nice.org.uk/guidance/TA516.

National Institute for Health and Care Excellence. (2018c). TA516. Retrieved from: https://www.nice.org.uk/guidance/ta516.

National Institute for Health and Care Excellence. (2019). NICE Technology Appraisal Data. Retrievede from: https://www.nice.org.uk/about/what-we-do/our-programmes/nice-guidance/nice-technology-appraisal-guidance/data/cancer-appraisal-recommendations.

National Institute for Sickness and Disability Insurance. (n.d.). INAMI home page. Retrieved from: www.inami.fgov.be/fr/Pages/default.aspx.

Neumann, P.J., Kim, D.D., Trikalinos, T.A. et al. (2018). Future directions for cost-effectiveness analyses in health and medicine. *Medical Decision Making*; 38(7):767–777.

Ng, R., Kornas, K., Sutradhar, R. et al. (2018). The current application of the Royston-Parmar model for prognostic modeling in health research: A scoping review. *Diagnostic and Prognostic Research*; 2(1):4.

Nguyen, V.T., & Dupuy, J.F. (2018). Zero-inflated Poisson regression with right-censored data. Retrieved from: https://hal.archives-ouvertes.fr/hal-01811949.

Nishino, M., Jagannathan, J.P., Krajewski, K.M. et al. (2012). Personalized tumor response assessment in the era of molecular medicine: Cancer-specific and therapy-specific response criteria to complement pitfalls of RECIST. *American Journal of Roentgenology*; 198(4):737–745.

Noble, S.M., Hollingworth, W., & Tilling, K. (2012). Missing data in trial-based cost-effectiveness analysis: The current state of play. *Health Economics*; 21(2):187–200.

Norden, A.D., Lesser, G.J., Drappatz, J. et al. (2013). Phase 2 study of dose-intense temozolomide in recurrent glioblastoma. *Neuro-Oncology*; 15(7):930–935.

Oaknin, A. (2015). XVII Simposio de Revisiones en Cancer. Madrid 11–13 February 2015; accessed March 2018.

O'Brien, B.J., & Briggs, A.H. (2002). Analysis of uncertainty in health care cost-effectiveness studies: An introduction to statistical issues and methods. *Statistical Methods in Medical Research*; 11(6):455–468.

O'Connor, R.D., O'Donnell, J.C., Pinto, L.A. et al. (2002). Two-year retrospective economic evaluation of three dual-controller therapies used in the treatment of asthma. *Chest*; 121(4):1028–1035.

Olchanski, N., Zhong, Y., Cohen, J.T. et al. (2015). The peculiar economics of life-extending therapies: A review of costing methods in health economic evaluations in oncology. *Expert Review of Pharmacoeconomics and Outcomes Research*; 15(6):931–940.

O'Mahony, J.F., Newall, A.T., & van Rosmalen, J. (2015). Dealing with time in health economic evaluation: Methodological issues and recommendations for practice. *PharmacoEconomics*; 33(12):1255–1268.

Omuro, A., Chan, T.A., Abrey, L.E. et al. (2013). Phase II trial of continuous low-dose temozolomide for patients with recurrent malignant glioma. *Neuro-Oncology*; 15(2):242–250.

Oppe, M., Devlin, N.J., van Hout, B. et al. (2014). A program of methodological research to arrive at the new international EQ-5D-5L valuation protocol. *Value in Health*; 17(4):445–453.

Osoba, D. (2007). Translating the science of patient-reported outcomes assessment into clinical practice. *Journal of the National Cancer Institute Monographs*; 37(37):5–11.

O'Sullivan, A.K., Thompson, D., & Drummond, M.F. (2005). Collection of health-economic data alongside clinical trials: Is there a future for piggyback evaluations? *Value in Health*; 8(1):67–79.

Oxnard, G.R., Morris, M.J., Hodi, F.S. et al. (2012). When progressive disease does not mean treatment failure: Reconsidering the criteria for progression. *JNCI Journal of the National Cancer Institute*; 104(20):1534–1541.

Pan, W., & Bai, H. (2015). Propensity score interval matching: Using bootstrap confidence intervals for accommodating estimation errors of propensity scores. *BMC Medical Research Methodology*; 15:53.

Papaioannou, D., Brazier, J., & Paisley, S. (2013). Systematic searching and selection of health state utility values from the literature. *Value in Health*; 16(4):686–695.

Parikh, R.C., Du, X.L., Morgan, R.O. et al. (2016). Patterns of treatment sequences in chemotherapy and targeted biologics for metastatic colorectal cancer: Findings from a large community-based cohort of elderly patients. *Drugs Real World Outcomes*; 3(1):69–82.

Parikh, R.C., Du, X.L., Robert, M.O. et al. (2017). Cost-effectiveness of treatment sequences of chemotherapies and targeted biologics for elderly metastatic colorectal cancer patients. *Journal of Managed Care and Specialty Pharmacy*; 23(1):64–73.

Parkin, M. (2016). Opportunity cost: A re-examination. *Journal of Economic Education*; 47(1):12–22.

Parner, E.T., & Andersen, P.K. (2010). Regression analysis of censored data using pseudo-observations. *The STATA Journal*; 10(3):408–422.

pBAC. (2013c). 07-2013: Gefitinib, tablet, 250 mg, Iressa®. Retrieved from: http://www.pbs.gov.au/info/industry/listing/elements/pbac-meetings/psd/2013-07/gefitinib.

pCODR. (2013a). Crizotinib (Xalkori) Resubmission for Advanced Non-Small Cell Lung Cancer. Retrieved from: www.pcodr.ca/wcpc/portal/Home/FindaReview/XalkoriAdvNSCLCResub?_afrLoop=457986569182000&_afrWindowMode=0&_adf.ctrl-state=17jia3apey_276.

pCODR. (2013b). Pemetrexed (Alimta) for Non-Squamous Non-Small Cell Lung Cancer. Retrieved from: http://www.pcodr.ca/wcpc/portal/Home/FindaReview/AlimtaNS-NSCLC?_afrLoop=458044314492000&_afrWindowMode=0&_adf.ctrl-state=17jia3apey_347.

Peng, Y., & Taylor, J.M.G. (2014). Chapter 6: Cure models. In: J. Klein, H. van Houwelingen, J.G. Ibrahim, T.H. Scheike (Eds.). *Handbooks of modern statistical methods series: Handbook of survival analysis*, Boca Raton, FL: Chapman & Hall, 113–134.

Penn. Medicine. (n.d.). Division of general internal medicine research. Retrieved from: www.pennmedicine.org/departments-and-centers/department-of-medicine/divisions/general-internal-medicine/research.

Petrou, S.A.G., & Gray, A. (2011a). Economic evaluation alongside randomised controlled trials: Design, conduct, analysis, and reporting. *BMJ*; 342:d1548.

Petrou, S.A.G., & Gray, A. (2011b). Economic evaluation using decision analytical modelling: Design, conduct, analysis, and reporting. *BMJ*; 342:d1766.

Pickard, A.S., Neary, M.P., & Cella, D. (2007). Estimation of minimally important differences in EQ-5D utility and VAS scores in cancer. *Health and Quality of Life Outcomes*; 5(1):70.

Pocock, S.J. (1983). *Clinical trials: A practical approach*. New York: Wiley.

Polley, W.J. (2015). The rhetoric of opportunity cost. *American Economist*; 60(1):9–19.

Popat, R., Khan, I., Dickson, J. et al. (2015). An alternative dosing strategy of lenalidomide for patients with relapsed multiple myeloma. *British Journal of Haematology*; 168(1):148–151.

Porter, M.E. (2010). What is value in health care? *New England Journal of Medicine*; 363(26):2477–2481.

Public health France. (n.d.). Epidemiological surveillance of cancers in France. Institute for Public Health Surveillance (InVS). Retrieved from: http://invs.santepubliquefrance.fr/surveillance/cancers/acteurs.htm.

Putter, H., Fiocco, M., & Geskus, R.B. (2007). Tutorial in biostatistics: Competing risks and multi-state models. *Statistics in Medicine*; 26(11):2389–2430.

Putter, H., van der Hage, J., de Bock, G.H. et al. (2006). Estimation and prediction in a multi-state model for breast cancer. *Biometrical Journal. Biometrische Zeitschrift*; 48(3):366–380.

Rabin, R., & de Charro, Fd (2001). EQ-5D: A measure of health status from the EuroQol Group. *Annals of Medicine*; 33(5):337–343.

Ramsey, S.D, Willke, R.J, Briggs, A. et al. (2005). Good research practices for cost-effectiveness analysis alongside clinical trials: The ISPOR RCT-CEA task force report. *Value in Health*; 8(5):521–533.

Ramsey, S.D., Willke, R.J., Glick, H. et al. (2015). Cost-effectiveness analysis alongside clinical trials II—An ISPOR good research practices task force report. *Value in Health*; 18(2):161–172.

Rappange, D.R., van Baal, P.H., van Exel, N.J. et al. (2008). Unrelated medical costs in life-years gained: Should they be included in economic evaluations of healthcare interventions? *Pharmacoeconomics*; 26(10):815–830.

Rascati, K.L. (2009). *Essentials of Pharmacoeconomics*. Philadelphia, PA: Lippincott Williams & Wilkins.

Ratowsky D. & Ratkowsky, A. (1989). *Handbook of nonlinear regression models*, New York : M. Dekker.

Rawlins, M., Barnett, D., & Stevens, A. (2010). Pharmacoeconomics: NICE's approach to decision-making. *British Journal of Clinical Pharmacology*; 70(3):346–349.

Richardson, J., Khan, M.A., Iezzi, A. et al. (2015). Comparing and explaining differences in the magnitude, content, and sensitivity of utilities predicted by the EQ-5D, SF–6D, HUI 3, 15D, QWB, and AQoL-8D multi-attribute utility instruments. *Medical Decision Making*; 35(3):276–291.

Rivera, F., Valladares, M., Gea, S. et al. (2017). Cost-effectiveness analysis in the Spanish setting of the PEAK trial of panitumumab plus mFOLFOX6 compared with bevacizumab plus mFOLFOX6 for first-line treatment of patients with wild-type RAS metastatic colorectal cancer. *Journal of Medical Economics*; 20(6):574–584.

Robert J. Brent; A Simple Method for Converting a Cost-Effectiveness Analysis into a Cost-Benefit Analysis with an Application to State Mental Health Expenditures First Published March 1, 2002 Research Article; https://doi.org/10.1177/109114210203000204 https://journals.sagepub.com/doi/abs/10.1177/109114210203000204

Robins, J.M. (1986). A new approach to causal inference in mortality studies with sustained exposure periods –Application to control the healthy worker survivor effect. *Mathematical Modelling*; 7:1392–1512.

Robins, J.M., & Finkelstein, D.M. (2000). Correcting for noncompliance and dependent censoring in an AIDS Clinical Trial with inverse probability of censoring weighted (IPCW) log-rank tests. *Biometrics*; 56(3):779–788.

Robins, J.M., Rotnitzky, A., & Zhao, L.P. (1994). Estimation of regression coefficients when some regressors are not always observed. *Journal of the American Statistical Association*; 89(427): 846–866.

Rodriguez, G. (2010). Parametric survival models. Retrieved from: ata.princeton.edu/pop509/ParametricSurvival.pdf.

Rowen, D., Brazier, J., & Van Hout, B. (2015). A comparison of methods for converting DCE values onto the full health-dead QALY scale. *Medical Decision Making*; 35(3):328–340.

Rowen, D., Brazier, J., Young, T. et al. (2011). Deriving a preference-based measure for cancer using the EORTC QLQ-C30. *Value Health*; 14(5):721–731.

Royal College of Physicians. (n.d.). Organising an audit or quality improvement project: Tips for beginners. Student and foundation doctor network. Retrieved from: www.rcplondon.ac.uk/projects/outputs/organising-audit-or-quality-improvement-project-tips-beginners.

Royston, P. (2015). Restricted mean survival time: Calculation and some applications in trials and prognostic studies. Flexible parametric survival models workshop. Stockholm, November 2011.

Royston, P., & Lambert, P.C. (2011). *Flexible parametric survival analysis using Stata: Beyond the Cox Model*. College Station, TX: Stata Press.

Royston, P., & Parmar, M.K.B. (2002). Flexible proportional-hazards and proportional odds models for censored survival data, with application to prognostic modelling and estimation of treatment effects. *Statistics in Medicine*; 21(15):2175–2197.

Royston, P., & Parmar, M.K.B. (2013). Restricted mean survival time: An alternative to the hazard ratio for the design and analysis of randomized trials with a time-to-event outcome. *BMC Medical Research Methodology*; 13(1):15.

Royston, P., Parmar, M.K.B., & Qian, W. (2003). Novel designs for multi-arm clinical trials with survival outcomes with an application in ovarian cancer. *Statistics in Medicine*; 22(14):2239–2256.

Rubin, D.B. (2004). *Multiple imputation for nonresponse in surveys*. Hoboken, NJ: Wiley.

Saad, E.D., Zalcberg, J.R., Péron, J. et al. (2018). Understanding and communicating measures of treatment effect on survival: Can we do better? *Journal of the National Cancer Institute*; 110(3):232–240.

Sacco, E., Tienforti, D., D'Addessi, A. et al. (2010). Social, economic, and health utility considerations in the treatment of overactive bladder. *Open Access. Journal of Urology*; 2:11–24.

Sacher, A.G., Le, L.W., Lau, A. et al. (2015). Real-world chemotherapy treatment patterns in metastatic non-small cell lung cancer: Are patients undertreated? *Cancer*; 121(15):2562–2569.

Saint-Pierre, P. (2016). Multi-state models and cost-effectiveness analysis. *Journal de Gestion et d'Économie Médicales*; 34(2):133–144.

Salleh, S., Thokala, P., Brennan, A. et al. (2017). Discrete event simulation-based resource modelling in health technology assessment. *Pharmacoeconomics*; 35(10):989–1006.

Sandmann, F.G., Robotham, J.V., Deeny, S.R. et al. (2018). Estimating the opportunity costs of bed-days. *Health Economics*; 27(3):592–605.

Santerre, R.E., & Neun, S.P. (2000). *Health economics: Theories, insights, and industry studies*. Fort Worth, TX: Dryden Press.

Sartor, O., & Halabi, U. (2015). Independent data monitoring committees: An update and overview. *Urologic Oncology*; 33(3):143–148.

Schnipper, L.E., Davidson, N.E., Wollins, D.S. et al. (2015). American Society of Clinical Oncology statement: A conceptual framework to assess the value of cancer treatment options. *Journal of Clinical Oncology*; 33(23):2563–2577. Retrieved from: http://ascopubs.org/doi/abs/10.1200/jco.2015.61.6706.

Scuffham, P.A., Whitty, J.A., Mitchell, A. et al. (2008). The use of QALY weights for QALY calculations. *Pharmacoeconomics*; 26(4):297–310.

Sculpher, M.J., Claxton, K., Drummond, M. et al. (2006). Whither trial-based economic evaluation for health care decision making? *Health Economics*; 15(7):677–687.

Seruga, B., Pond, G.R., Hertz, P.C. et al. (2012). Comparison of absolute benefits of anticancer therapies determined by snapshot and area methods. *Annals of Oncology*; 23(11):2977–2982.

Shaw, J.W., Johnson, J.A., & Coons, S.J. (2005). US valuation of the EQ-5D health states: Development and testing of the D1 valuation model. *Medical Care*; 43(3):203–220.

Shepherd, F.A., Rodrigues Pereira, J.R., Ciuleanu, T. et al. (2005). Erlotinib in previously treated non-small-cell lung cancer. *New England Journal of Medicine*; 353(2):123–132.

Simes, R.J., & Coates, A.S. (2001). Patient preferences for adjuvant chemotherapy of early breast cancer: How much benefit is needed? *Journal of the National Cancer Institute Monographs*; 30(30):146–152.

Sleeper, L.A., & Harrington, D.P. (1990). Regression splines in the Cox Model with application to covariate effects in liver disease. *Journal of the American Statistical Association*; 85(412):941–949.

Slevin, M.L., Plant, H., Lynch, D. et al. (1988). Who should measure quality of life, the doctor or the patient? *British Journal of Cancer*; 57(1):109–112.

SMC (2006). 220/05: Erlotinib (Tarceva®) re-submission. Retrieved from: https://www.scottishmedicines.org.uk/SMC_Advice/Advice/Erlotinib__Tarceva__Resubmission/Erlotinib__Tarceva__.

SMC (2012). 749/11: erlotinib (Tarceva). Retrieved from: https://www.scottishmedicines.org.uk/SMC_Advice/Advice/749_11_erlotinib_Tarceva/erlotinib_Tarceva.

SMC (2013). Crizotinib (Xalkori). Retrieved from: http://www.scottishmedicines.org.uk/SMC_Advice/Advice/865_13_crizotinib_Xalkori/crizotinib_Xalkori_Resubmission.

SMC (2014). SMC. 920/13: afatinib (Giotrif). Retrieved from: https://www.scottishmedicines.org.uk/SMC_Advice/Advice/920_13_afatinib_Giotrif/afatinib_Giotrif.

Sorenson, C., Kanavos, P., & Drummond, M. (2008). *Ensuring value for money in health care: The role of HTA in the European Union*. Copenhagen: European Observatory on Health Systems and Policies, World Health Organisation.

Spiegelhalter, D.J., & Best, N.G. (2003). Bayesian approaches to multiple sources of evidence and uncertainty in complex cost-effectiveness modelling. *Statistics in Medicine*; 22(23):3687–3709.

Spruance, S.L., Reid, J.E., Grace, M. et al. (2004). Hazard ratio in clinical trials. *Antimicrobial Agents and Chemotherapy*; 48(8):2787–2792.

Stadtmauer, E., Weber, D., Dimopolous, M. et al. (2006). Lenalidomide in combination with dexamethasone is more effective Than dexamethasone at first relapse in relapsed multiple myeloma. *ASH Annual Meeting Abstracts*; 108(11):3552.

Stafinski, T., Menon, D., Davis, C. et al. (2011). Role of centralized review processes for making reimbursement decisions on new health technologies in Europe; *ClinicoEconomics and Outcomes Research*; 3:117–186.

Stare, J., & Boulch, D.M. (2016). Odds ratio, hazard ratio and relative risk. *Metodoloski Zvezki*; 13(1):59–67. Retrieved from: www.stat-d.si/mz/mz13.1/p4.pdf.

Steckler, A., & McLeroy, K.R. (2008). The importance of external validity. *American Journal of Public Health*; 98(1):9–10.

Stinnett, A.A., & Mullahy, J. (1998). Net health benefits. *Medical Decision Making*; 18 (2 Suppl):S68–S80.

Sullivan, S.D., Mauskopf, J.A., Augustovski, F. et al. (2015). Budget impact analysis: Principles of good practice. Report of the ISPOR working group on good practices for budget impact analysis II, 2012. *Kachestvennaya Klinicheskaya Praktika*; 2:104–118.

Susarla, V., & Van Rizyn, J. (1980). Large sample theory for an estimator of the mean survival time from censored samples. *The Annals of Statistics*; 8(5):1002–1016.

Susarla, V., & Van Rizyn, J. (1984). A Buckley-James-type estimator for the mean with censored data. *Biometrika*; 71(3):624–629.

Sydes, M.R., Parmar, M.K.B., James, N.D. et al. (2009). Issues in applying multi-arm multi-stage methodology to a clinical trial in prostate cancer: The MRC STAMPEDE trial. *Trials*; 10:39.

Tai, B.C., Wee, J., & Machin, D. (2011). Analysis and design of randomised clinical trials involving competing risks outcomes. *Trials*; 12:127.

Taphoorn, M.J.B., Henriksson, R., Bottomley, A. et al. (2015). Health-related quality of life in a randomized phase III study of bevacizumab, temozolomide, and radiotherapy in newly diagnosed glioblastoma. *Journal of Clinical Oncology*; 33:2166–2175.

Tappenden, P., Brazier, J., Ratcliffe, J., Chilcott, J. (2007). A stated preference binary choice experiment to explore NICE decision making. *Pharmacoeconomics*; 25(8): 685–693.

Temel, J.S., Greer, J.A., Muzikansky, A. et al. (2010). Early palliative care for patients with metastatic non–small-cell lung cancer. *New England Journal of Medicine*; 363(8):733–742.

Thatcher, N., Chang, A., Parikh, P. et al. (2005). Gefitinib plus best supportive care in previously treated patients with re-fractory advanced non-small-cell lung cancer: Results from a randomised, placebo-controlled, multicentre study (Iressa Survival Evaluation in Lung Cancer). *Lancet*; 366(9496):1527–1537.

The Professional Society for Health Economics and Outcomes Research. (2009). Germany: Pharmaceutical. Global health technology assessment road map. Retrieved from: https://tools.ispor.org/htaroadmaps/Germany.asp.

The World Bank. (n.d.). Current health expenditure (% of GDP). Retrieved from: https://data.worldbank.org/indicator/SH.XPD.CHEX.GD.ZS.

Thein, H.H., Isaranuwatchai, W., Qiao, Y. et al. (2017). Cost-effectiveness analysis of potentially curative and combination treatments for hepatocellular carcinoma with person-level data in a Canadian setting. *Cancer Medicine*; 6(9):2017–2033.

Thompson, S.G., Nixon, R.M., & Grieve, R. (2006). Addressing the issues that arise in analysing multicentre cost data, with application to a multinational study. *Journal of Health Economics*; 25(6):1015–1028.

Thongprasert, S., Tinmanee, S., & Permsuwan, U. (2012). Cost-utility and budget impact analyses of gefitinib in second-line treatment for advanced non-small cell lung cancer from Thai payer perspective. *Asia-Pacific Journal of Clinical Oncology*; 8(1):53–61.

Timmins, N., Rawlins, M., & Appleby, J. (2016). A terrible beauty. A short history of NICE, the National Institute for Health and Care Excellence. Retrieved from: www.idsihealth.org/wp-content/uploads/2016/02/A-TERRIBLE-BEAUTY_resize.pdf.

Titman, A. (2016). Multi-state models: An overview. Presentation. Retrieved from: www.maths.lancs.ac.uk/~titman/leeds_seminar.pdf.

Toms, J.R. (2004). *CancerStats monograph 2004: Cancer incidence, survival and mortality in the UK and EU*. London: Cancer Research UK.

Trinquart, L., Jacot, J., Conner, S.C. et al. (2016). Comparison of treatment effects measured by the hazard ratio and by the ratio of restricted mean survival times in oncology randomized controlled trials. *Journal of Clinical Oncology*; 34(15):1813–1819.

Truven https://truvenhealth.com/Portals/1/.../INTL_12543_0413_RedbookPS_WEB1.pdf, accessed 31 Jan 2018.

Tuffaha, H.W., Gordon, L.G., & Scuffham, P.A. (2016). Efficient value of information calculation using a nonparametric regression approach: An applied perspective. *Value Health*; 19(4):505–509. Epub 2016.

Tuffaha, H.W., Reynolds, H., Gordon, L.G. et al. (2014). Value of information analysis optimizing future trial design from a pilot study on catheter securement devices. *Society for Clinical Trials*; 11(6):648–656.

Uhry, Z., Hédelin, G., Colonna, M. et al. (2010). Multi-state Markov models in cancer screening evaluation: A brief review and case study. *Statistical Methods in Medical Research*; 19(5):463–486.

Ulmeanu, R., Antohe, I., Anisie, E. et al. (2016). Nivolumab for advanced non-small cell lung cancer: An evaluation of a phase III study. *Expert Review of Anticancer Therapy*; 16(2)165–167.

U.S. Department of Health and Human Services. Food and Drug Administration. (2018). Clinical trial endpoints for the approval of cancer drugs and biologics: Guidance for industry. Retrieved from: www.fda.gov/downloads/Drugs/Guidances/ucm071590.pdf.

University of Kent. (n.d.). Unit costs of health and social care. Personal social services reesearch unit. Retrieved from: www.pssru.ac.uk/project-pages/unit-costs/.

University of Texas at Dallas. (n.d.). Markov chains. Retrieved from: www.utdallas.edu/~jjue/cs6352/markov/markov.html.

U.S. Department of Health and Human Services. Food and Drug Administration. (2007). Clinical trial endpoints for the approval of cancer drugs and biologics: Guidance for industry. Center for Drug Evaluation and Research (CDER), Center for Biologics Evaluation and Research (CBER). Retrieved from: www.fda.gov/downloads/Drugs/Guidances/ucm071590.pdf.

U.S. Food and Drug Administration. (n.d.). Information exchange and data transformation (INFORMED). Retrieved from: www.fda.gov/aboutfda/centersoffices/officeofmedicalproductsandtobacco/oce/ucm543768.htm.

U.S. Food and Drug Administration. (n.d.). 21st century cures act. Retrieved from: www.fda.gov/regulatoryinformation/lawsenforcedbyfda/significantamendmentstothefdcact/21stcenturycuresact/default.htm.

van Agt, H.M.E., Essink-Bot, M., Krabbe, P.F.M. et al. (1994). Test-retest reliability of health state valuations collected with the EuroQol questionnaire. *Social Science and Medicine*; 39(11):1537–1544.

van Agt, H.M.E., van der Stege, H.A., de Ridder-Sluiter, H.A. et al. (2005). Quality of life of children with language delays. *Qual Life Res.* 2005 Jun; 14(5): 1345–55.

Vale, C.D., Maurelli, V.A. (1983). Simulating multivariate nonnormal distributions. *Psychometrika*; 48: 465–471.

van Baal, P.H., Feenstra, T.L., Polder, J.J. et al. (2011). Economic evaluation and the postponement of health care costs. *Health Economics*; 20(4):432–445.

van Baal, P.H., Morton, A., Brouwer, W. et al. (2017). Should cost effectiveness analyses for NICE always consider future unrelated medical costs? *BMJ*; 359:j5096.

Van Buuren, S. (2018). *Flexible imputation of missing data*, 2nd Edition. Chapman & Hall.

van Erning, F.N., van Steenbergen, L.N., Lemmens, V.E.P.P. et al. (2014). Conditional survival for long-term colorectal cancer survivors in the Netherlands: Who do best? *European Journal of Cancer*; 50(10):1731–1739.

Van Harten, W., & IJzerman, M.J. (2017). Responsible pricing in value-based assessment of cancer drugs: Real-world data are an inevitable addition to select meaningful new cancer treatments. *Ecancermedicalscience*; 11:ed71.

Van Hout, B., Janssen, M.F., Feng, Y.S. et al. (2012). Interim scoring for the EQ-5D-5L: Mapping the EQ-5D-5L to EQ-5D-3L value sets. *Value in Health*; 15(5):708–715.

Van Houwelingen, H., & Putter, H. (2012). *Dynamic prediction in clinical survival analysis*. Boca Raton, FL: CRC Press, Taylor & Francis.

Vázquez, G.H., Holtzman, J.N., Lolich, M. et al. (2015). Recurrence rates in bipolar disorder: Systematic comparison of long-term prospective, naturalistic studies versus randomized controlled trials. *European Neuropsychopharmacology*; 25(10):1501–1512.

Vergnenegre, A., Corre, R., Berard, H. et al. (2011). Cost-effectiveness of second-line chemotherapy for non-small cell lung cancer: An economic, randomized, prospective, multicenter Phase III trial comparing docetaxel and pemetrexed: The GFPC 05–06 study. *Journal of Thoracic Oncology*; 6(1):161–168.

Versteegh, M., Knies, S., & Brouwer, W. (2016). From good to better: New Dutch guidelines for economic evaluations in healthcare. *Pharmacoeconomics*; 34(11):1071–1074.

Vredenburgh, J.J., Desjardins, A., Reardon, D.A. et al. (2010). Bevacizumab (BEV) in combination with temozolomide (TMZ) and radiation therapy (XRT) followed by BEV, TMZ, and irinotecan for newly diagnosed glioblastoma multiforme (GBM). *Journal of Clinical Oncology*; 28(15_suppl):2023–2023.

Wailoo, A., Alava, M.H., Grimm, S. et al. (2017). Comparing the EQ-5D-3L and 5L versions. What are the implications for cost effectiveness estimates? Report by the Decision Support Unit.Retrieved from: http://scharr.dept.shef.ac.uk/nicedsu/wp-content/uploads/sites/7/2017/05/DSU_3L-to-5L-FINAL.pdf.

Walker, A.S., White, I.R., & Babiker, A.G. (2004). Parametric randomization-based methods for correcting for treatment changes in the assessment of the causal effect of treatment. *Statistics in Medicine*; 23(4):571–590.

Wang, Y.-W. & Li, N. (2010). Statistical Analysis for Treatment Crossover or Nonsynchronized Interval-Censoring Data in a Mortality Trial. *Statistics in Biopharmaceutical Research*; 2(2): 175–181.

Wang, S., Peng, L., Li, J. et al. (2013). A trial-based cost-effectiveness analysis of erlotinib alone versus platinum-based doublet chemotherapy as first-line therapy for eastern asian nonsquamous non–small-cell lung cancer. *PLoS One*; 8(3).

Weinstein, M.C., Fineberg, H.V., Elstein, A.S. et al. (1980). *Clinical decision analysis*. Philadelphia, PA: W. B. Saunders.

Weinstein, M.C., & Manning, W.G. Jr. (1997). Theoretical issues in cost-effectiveness analysis. *Journal of Health Economics*; 16(1):121–128.

Weintraub, W.S., Daniels, S.R., Burke, L.E. et al. (2011). Value of primordial and primary prevention for cardiovascular disease: A policy statement from the American Heart Association. *Circulation*; 124(8):967–990. Retrieved from: http://circ.ahajournals.org/content/124/8/967/F2.

Wendt, C., Frisina, L., & Rothgang, H. (2009). Social policy & healthcare system types: A conceptual framework for comparison. *Administration*; 43(1):70–90.

White, I.R., Babiker, A.G., Walker, S. et al. (1999). Randomization-based methods for correcting for treatment changes: Examples from the Concorde trial. *Statistics in Medicine*; 18(19):2617–2634.

Wijeysundera, H.C., Wang, X., Tomlinson, G. et al. (2012). Techniques for estimating health care costs with censored data: An overview for the health services researcher. *ClinicoEconomics and Outcomes Research*; 4:145–155.

Willan, A.R., & Briggs, A.H. (2006). *Statistical analysis of cost-effectiveness data*. New York: John Wiley Publications.

Willan, A.R., Briggs, A.H., & Hoch, J.S. (2004). Regression methods for covariate adjustment and subgroup analysis for non-censored cost-effectiveness data. *Health Economics*; 13(5):461–475.

Willekens, F.J., & Putter, H. (2014). Software for multistate analysis. *Demographic Research*; 31:381–420.

Williams, C., Lewsey, J.D., Briggs, A.H. et al. (2017). Cost-effectiveness analysis in R using a multi-state modeling survival analysis framework: A tutorial. *Medical Decision Making*; 37(4):340–352.

Williams, C., Lewsey, J.D., Mackay, D.F. et al. (2017). Estimation of survival probabilities for use in cost-effectiveness analyses: A comparison of a multi-state modeling survival analysis approach with partitioned survival and Markov decision-analytic modeling. *Medical Decision Making*; 37(4):427–439.

Willke, R.J., Glick, H.A., Polsky, D. et al. (1998). Estimating country-specific cost-effectiveness from multinational clinical trials. *Health Economics*; 7(6):481–493.

Wilson, A., Grimshaw, G., Baker, R. et al. (1999). Differentiating between audit and research: Postal survey of health authorities' views. *BMJ*; 319(7219):1235.

Wilson, E.C. (2015). A practical guide to value of information analysis. *Pharmacoeconomics*; 33(2):105–121.

Wilson, E.C., Mugford, M., Barton, G. et al. (2016). Efficient research design: Using; value-of-information analysis to estimate the optimal mix of top-down and bottom-up costing approaches in an economic evaluation alongside a clinical trial. *Medical Decision Making*; 36(3):335–348.

Winsor, S., Smith, A., Vanstone, M. et al. (2013). Experiences of patient-centredness with specialized community-based care: A systematic review and qualitative meta-synthesis. *Ontario Health Technology Assessment Series;* 13(17):1–33.

Wolchok, J.D., Hoos, A., O'Day, S. et al. (2009). Guidelines for the evaluation of immune therapy activity in solid tumors: Immune-related response criteria. *Clinical Cancer Research;* 15(23):7412–7420.

Woods, B., Sideris, E., Palmer, S. et al. (2017). NICE DSU document 19: Partitioned survival analysis for decision modelling in health care: A critical review report by the decision support unit. ScHARR, University of Sheffield.Retrieved from: http://scharr.dept.shef.ac.uk/nicedsu/wp-content/uploads/sites/7/2017/06/Partitioned-Survival-Analysis-final-report.pdf.

World Health Organization. (1947). The constitution of the World Health Organization. *WHO Chronicle;* 1:29.

World Health Organization (2014). Who we are. Retrieved from: www.who.int/about/who-we-are/constitution.

Yamaguchi, T., & Ohashi, Y. (2004). Adjusting for differential proportions of second-line treatment in cancer clinical trials. Part I: Structural nested models and marginal structural models to test and estimate treatment arm effects. *Statistics in Medicine;* 23(13):1991–2003.

Yanni, H., Wolfram, V., & Cook, J.S. (2016). A structured review of health utility measures and elicitation in advanced/metastatic breast cancer. *ClinicoEconomics and Outcomes Research;* 8(1):293–303.

Yap, C., Pettitt, A., & Billingham, K. (2013). Screened selection design for randomised phase II oncology trials: An example in chronic lymphocytic leukaemia. *BMC Medical Research Methodology;* 13(1):87.

Zahid, K.F., Burney, I., Ahmed, T. et al. (2015). Clinicopathological features and treatment outcomes of breast cancer patients with brain metastases. *Annals of Oncology;* 26(Suppl 9):22–23.

Zeng, X., Li, J., Peng, L. et al. (2014). Economic outcomes of maintenance gefitinib for locally advanced/metastatic non-small-cell lung cancer with unknown EGFR mutations: A semi-Markov model analysis. *PLoS One;* 9(2):e88881. eCollection 2014.

Zhang, L., Ma, S., Song, X. et al. (2012). Gefitinib versus placebo as maintenance therapy in patients with locally advanced or metastatic non-small-cell lung cancer (INFORM; C-Tong 0804): A multi-centre, double-blind randomised phase 3 trial. *Lancet;* 13(5):466–475.

Zhao, H., & Bang, H. (2012). *Pharmacoeconomics.* 2015 February; 33(2):105–121. doi: 10.1007/s40273-014-0219-x. PubMed PMID: 24194511.

Zhao, H., Zuo, C., Chen, S. et al. (2012). Nonparametric inference for median costs with censored data. *Biometrics;* 68(3):717–725.

Zhao, Y., Li, S.P., Liu, L. et al. (2017). Does the choice of tariff matter?: A comparison of EQ-5D-5L utility scores using Chinese, UK, and Japanese tariffs on patients with psoriasis vulgaris in Central South China Chinese. *Medicine (Baltimore);* 96(34):e7840.

Zhu, J., Li, T., Wang, X. et al. (2013). Gene-guided gefitinib switch maintenance therapy for patients with advanced EGFR mutation-positive non-small cell lung cancer: An economic analysis. *BMC Cancer;* 13(1):39.

Zuur, A.F., Ieno, E.N., & Saveliev, A.A. (2017). *Beginner's guide to spatial, temporal and spatial-temporal ecological data analysis with R-INLA.* Newburgh, UK: Highland Statistics.

Additional Bibliography

Chapter 1

Araújo, A., Parente, B., Sotto-Mayor, R. et al. (2008). An economic analysis of erlotinib, docetaxel, pemetrexed and best supportive care as second or third line treatment of non-small cell lung cancer. *Revista Portuguesa de Pneumologia (English Edition)*; 14(6):803–827.

Asukai, Y., Valladares, A., Camps, C. et al. (2010). Cost-effectiveness analysis of pemetrexed versus docetaxel in the second-line treatment of non-small cell lung cancer in Spain: Results for the non-squamous histology population. *BMC Cancer*; 10(1):26.

Berthelot, J.M., Will, B.P., Evans, W.K. et al. (2000). Decision framework for chemotherapeutic interventions for metastatic non-small-cell lung cancer. *Journal of the National Cancer Institute*; 92(16):1321–1329.

Bradbury, P.A., Tu, D., Seymour, L. et al. (2010). Economic analysis: Randomized placebo-controlled clinical trial of erlotinib in advanced non-small cell lung cancer. *Journal of the National Cancer Institute*; 102(5):298–306. Epub 2010 February.

Brown, T., Boland, A., Bagust, A. et al. (2010). Gefitinib for the first-line treatment of locally advanced or metastatic non-small cell lung cancer. *Health Technology Assessment*; 14(Suppl 2):71–79.

Carlson, J.J., Reyes, C., Oestreicher, N. et al. (2008). Comparative clinical and economic outcomes of treatments for refractory non-small cell lung cancer (NSCLC). *Lung Cancer*; 61(3):405–415.

Chouaid, C., Le Caer, H., Locher, C. et al., & GFPC 0504 Team. (2012). Cost effectivenes of erlotinib versus chemotherapy for first-line treatment of non small cell lung cancer (NSCLC) in fit elderly patients participating in a prospective phase 2 study (GFPC 0504). *BMC Cancer*; 12:301.

Cromwell, I., van der Hoek, K., Melosky, B. et al. (2011). Erlotinib or docetaxel for second-line treatment of non-small cell lung cancer: A real-world cost-effectiveness analysis. *Journal of Thoracic Oncology*; 6(12):2097–2103.

Fragoulakis, V., Pallis, A., & Georgoulias, M. (2014). Economic evaluation of pemetrexed versus erlotinib as second-line treatment of patients with advanced/metastatic non-small cell lung cancer in Greece: A cost minimization analysis. *Lung Cancer: Targets and Therapy*; 3:43–51.

Gilberto de Lima, L.G., Segel, J., Tan, D. et al. (2011). Cost-effectiveness of epidermal growth factor receptor mutation testing and first-line treatment with gefitinib for patients with advanced adenocarcinoma of the lung. *Cancer*; 118(4):1032–1039.

Goulart, B., & Ramsey, S. (2011). A trial-based assessment of the cost-utility of bevacizumab and chemotherapy versus chemotherapy alone for advanced non-small cell lung cancer. *Value in Health*; 14(6):836–845.

Greenhalgh, J., McLeod, C., Bagust, A. et al. (2010). Pemetrexed for the maintenance treatment of locally advanced or metastatic non-small cell lung cancer. *Health Technology Assessment*; 14(Suppl 2):33–39.

Maniadakis, N., Fragoulakis, V., Pallis, A.G. et al. (2010). Economic evaluation of docetaxel-gemcitabine versus vinorelbine-cisplatin combination as front-line treatment of patients with advanced/metastatic non-small-cell lung cancer in Greece: A cost-minimization analysis. *Annals of Oncology*; 21(7):1462–1467.

Thongprasert, S., Tinmanee, S., & Permsuwan, U. (2012). Cost-utility and budget impact analyses of gefitinib in second-line treatment for advanced non-small cell lung cancer from Thai payer perspective. *Asia-Pacific Journal of Clinical Oncology*; 8(1):53–61.

Vergnenegre, A., Corre, R., Berard, H. et al., & GFPC 0506 Team. (2011). Cost-effectiveness of second-line chemotherapy for non-small cell lung cancer: An economic, randomized, prospective, multicenter phase III trial comparing docetaxel and pemetrexed: The GFPC 05–06 study. *Journal of Thoracic Oncology*; 6(1):161–168.

Wang, S., Peng, L., Li, J. et al. (2013). A trial-based cost-effectiveness analysis of erlotinib alone versus platinum-based doublet chemotherapy as first-line therapy for Eastern Asian nonsquamous non–small-cell lung cancer. *PLoS One*; 8(3):e55917.

Winsor, S., Smith, A., Vanstone, M. et al. (2013). Experiences of patient-centredness With specialized community-based care: A systematic review and qualitative meta-synthesis. *Ontario Health Technology Assessment Series*; 13(17):1–33.

Zhu, J., Li, T., Wang, X. et al. (2013). Gene-guided gefitinib switch maintenance therapy for patients with advanced EGFR mutation-positive Non-small cell lung cancer: An economic analysis. *BMC Cancer*; 13(1):39.

Chapter 3

Brooks, R., Rosalind, R., & de Charro, F. (Eds.) (2013). *The measurement and valuation of health status using EQ-5D: A European perspective: Evidence from the EuroQol BIOMED research programme*. Dordrecht, Netherlands: Springer Science & Business Media.

Cella, D.F., Wiklund, I., Shumaker, S.A. et al. (1993). Integrating health-related quality of life into cross-national clinical trials. *Quality of Life Research*; 2(6):433–440.

European Organisation for Research and Treatment of Cancer. (n.d.). Manuals. EORCT Quality of Life. Retrieved from: http://groups.eortc.be/qol/manuals.

Hollen, P.J., Gralla, R.J., Cox, C. et al. (1997). A dilemma in analysis: Issues in the serial measurement of quality of life in patients with advanced lung cancer. *Lung Cancer*; 18(2):119–136.

Chapter 4

A'Hern, R.P. (2016). Restricted mean survival time: An obligatory end point for time-to-event analysis in cancer trials? *Journal of Clinical Oncology*; 34(28):3474–3476.

Ajani, J.A. (2007). The area between the curves gets no respect: Is it because of the median madness? *Journal of Clinical Oncology*; 25(34):5531.

Albertsen, P.C., Hanley, J.A., Gleason, D.F. et al. (1998). Competing risk analysis of men aged 55 to 74 years at diagnosis managed conservatively for clinically localized prostate cancer. *JAMA*; 280(11):975–980.

Amdahl, J., Manson, S.C., Isbell, R. et al. (2014). Cost-effectiveness of pazopanib in advanced soft tissue sarcoma in the United Kingdom. *Sarcoma*; 2014:481071.

American Cancer Society. (2018). Breast cancer survival rates. Retrieved from: www.cancer.org/cancer/breast-cancer/understanding-a-breast-cancer-diagnosis/breast-cancer-survival-rates.html.

Amico, M., & Van Keilegom, I. (2018). Cure models in survival analysis. *Annual Review of Statistics and Its Application*; 5(1):311–342.

Andersen, P.K., Esbjerg, S., & Sorensen, T.I. (2000). Multi-state models for bleeding episodes and mortality in liver cirrhosis. *Statistics in Medicine*; 19(4):587–599.

Andersen, P.K., & Keiding, N. (2002). Multi-state models for event history analysis. *Statistical Methods in Medical Research*; 11(2):91–115.

Armero, C., Cabras, S., Castellanos, M.E., et al. (2016). Bayesian analysis of a disability model for lung cancer survival. *Statistical Methods in Medical Research*; 25(1):336–351.

Bongers, M.L., de Ruysscher, D., Oberije, C., et al. (2016). Multistate statistical modeling: A tool to build a lung cancer microsimulation model that includes parameter uncertainty and patient heterogeneity. *Medical Decision Making*; 36(1):86–100.

Cancer Patients Alliance. (n.d.). Pancreatic cancer prognosis & survival. Pancreatica. Retrieved from: https://pancreatica.org/pancreatic-cancer/pancreatic-cancer-prognosis/.

Coyle, D., & Coyle, K. (2014). The inherent bias from using partitioned survival models in economic evaluation. *Value in Health*; 17(3):A194.

Cronin, A. (2016). STRMST2: Stata module to compare restricted mean survival time. Statistical software components S458154. Boston, MA: Boston College Department of Economics.

de Bock, G.H., Putter, H., Bonnema, J. et al. (2009). The impact of loco-regional recurrences on metastatic progression in early-stage breast cancer: A multistate model. *Breast Cancer Research and Treatment*; 117(2):401–408.

de Glas, N.A., Kiderlen, M., Vandenbroucke, J.P. et al. (2016). Performing survival analyses in the presence of competing risks: A clinical example in older breast cancer patients. *Journal of the National Cancer Institute*; 108(5):djv366.

de Wreede, L.C., & Fiocco, M.,(2010). The mstate package for estimation and prediction in non- and semi-parametric multi-state and competing risks models. *Computers Methods and Programs in Biomedicine*, 261–274.

de Wreede, L.C., Fiocco, M., & Putter, H. (2011). Mstate: An R package for the analysis of competing risks and multi-state Models. *Journal of Statistical Software*; 38(7).

Elgalta, R., Putter, H., van der Hage, J. et al. (2006). Estimation and prediction in a multi-state model for breast cancer. *Biomedical Journal*; 48:366–380.

Gardiner, J.C. (2010). Survival analysis: Overview of parametric, nonparametric and semiparametric approachesand new developments, Paper 252-2010, SAS Global Forum 2010, Seattle WA, April 11–14. Retrieved from: https://support.sas.com/resources/papers/proceedings10/252-2010.pdf.

Gelber, R.D., Goldhirsch, A., Cole, B.F. et al. (1996). A quality-adjusted time without symptoms or toxicity (Q-TWiST) analysis of adjuvant radiation therapy and chemotherapy for resectable rectal cancer. *Journal of the National Cancer Institute*; 88(15):1039–1045.

Glasziou, P.P., Simes, R.J., & Gelber, R.D. (1990). Quality adjusted survival analysis. *Statistics in Medicine*; 9(11):1259–1276.

Goldhirsch, A., Gelber, R.D., Simes, R.J. et al. (1989). Costs and benefits of adjuvant therapy in breast cancer: A quality-adjusted survival analysis. *Journal of Clinical Oncology*; 7(1):36–44.

Hansen, L.S., Andersen, P.K., & Keiding, N. (1991). Assessing the influence of reversible disease indicators on survival. *Statistics in Medicine*; 10(7):1061–1067.

Husson, O., Steenbergen, L.N., Koldewijn, E.L. et al. (2014). Excess mortality in patients with prostate cancer. *BJU International*; 114:691–697.

Irwin, J.O. (1949). The standard error of an estimate of expectation of life, with special reference to expectation of tumourless life in experiments with mice. *Journal of Hygiene*; 47(2):188.

Karrison, T. (1987). Restricted mean life with adjustment for covariates. *Journal of the American Statistical Association*; 82(400):1169–1176.

Lai, X., & Zee, B.C.Y. (2015). Mixed response and time-to-event endpoints for multistage single-arm phase II design. *Trials*; 16:250.

Ledermann, J.A. (2013). Ecco 2013. Retrieved from: ww.cancernetwork.com/conference.../slide-show-2013-european-cancer-congress.

Ledermann, J.A., Embleton, A.C., Perren, T. et al. (2017). Overall survival results of ICON6: A trial of chemotherapy and cediranib in relapsed ovarian cancer. *Journal of Clinical Oncology*; 35(15_suppl):5506–5506. Retrieved from: www.icon6.org/media/1390/asco_2017.pdf.

Lewsey, J.D., Williams, C., Mackay, D.F. et al. (2017). Estimation of survival probabilities for use in cost-effectiveness analyses: A comparison of a multi-state modeling survival analysis approach with partitioned survival and Markov decision-analytic modeling. *Medical Decision Making*; 37(4):427–439.

Manzini, G., Ettrich, T.J., Kremer, M. et al. (2018). Advantages of a multi-state approach in surgical research: How intermediate events and risk factor profile affect the prognosis of a patient with locally advanced rectal cancer. *BMC Medical Research Methodology*; 18(1):23.

Meier-Hirmer, C., & Schumacher, M. (2013). Multi-state model for studying an intermediate event using time-dependent covariates: Application to breast cancer. *BMC Medical Research Methodology*; 13:80.

Murray, T.A., Thall, P.F., Yuan, Y. et al. (2017). Robust treatment comparison based on utilities of semi-competing risks in non-small-cell lung cancer. *Journal of the American Statistical Association*; 112:11–23.

National Cancer Institute. (n.d.). Dictionary of cancer terms. Retrieved from: www.cancer.gov/publications/dictionaries/cancer-terms/.

National Institute for Health and Care Excellence. (2009b). Rituximab for the first-line treatment of chronic lymphocytic leukaemia. Technology appraisal guidance [TA174]. Retrieved from: www.nice.org.uk/guidance/TA174.

Ng, R., Kornas, K., Sutradhar, R. et al. (2018). The current application of the Royston-Parmar model for prognostic modeling in health research: A scoping review. *Diagnostic and Prognostic Research*; 2(1):4.

Nishino, M., Jagannathan, J.P., Krajewski, K.M. et al. (2012). Personalized tumor response assessment in the era of molecular medicine: Cancer-specific and therapy-specific response criteria to complement pitfalls of RECIST. *AJR. American Journal of Roentgenology*; 198(4):737–745.

Oaknin, A. (2015). XVII Simposio de Revisiones en Cancer. Madrid 11–13 February 2015; accessed March 2018.https://seom.org/agenda2/106803-xxi-simposio-de-revisiones-en-cancer-2019.

Oxnard, G.R., Morris, M.J., Hodi, F.S. et al. (2012). When progressive disease does not mean treatment failure: Reconsidering the criteria for progression. *JNCI Journal of the National Cancer Institute*; 104(20):1534–1541.

Parikh, R.C., Du, X.L., Morgan, R.O. et al. (2016). Patterns of treatment sequences in chemotherapy and targeted biologics for metastatic colorectal cancer: Findings from a large community-based cohort of elderly patients. *Drugs Real World Outcomes*; 3(1):69–82.

Parmar, M.K.B., & Royston, P. (2013). Restricted mean survival time: An alternative to the hazard ratio for the design and analysis of randomized trials with a time-to-event outcome. *BMC Medical Research Methodology*; 13(1):15.

Parner, E.T., & Andersen, P.K. (2010). Regression analysis of censored data using pseudo-observations. *The STATA Journal*; 10(3):408–422.

Peng, Y., & Taylor, J.M.G. (2014). Chapter 6: Cure models. In: J. Klein, H. van Houwelingen, J.G. Ibrahim, T.H. Scheike (Eds.). *Handbooks of modern statistical methods series: Handbook of survival analysis*. Boca Raton, FL: Chapman & Hall.

Putter, H., Fiocco, M., & Geskus, R.B. (2007). Tutorial in biostatistics: Competing risks and multi-state models. *Statistics in Medicine*; 26(11):2389–2430.

Ratkowsky, D.A. (1989). *Handbook of nonlinear regression models*. New York: Marcel Dekker.

Rodriguez, G. (2010). Parametric survival models. Retrieved from: ata.princeton.edu/pop509/ParametricSurvival.pdf.

Royston, P. (2015). Restricted mean survival time: Calculation and some applications in trials and prognostic studies. Flexible parametric survival models workshop. Stockholm 10 November 2011. Retrieved from: www2.le.ac.uk/Members/pl4/workshop2011-1/Royston-Stockholm-10nov2011b.pdf.

Seruga, B., Pond, G.R., Hertz, P.C. et al. (2012). Comparison of absolute benefits of anticancer therapies determined by snapshot and area methods. *Annals of Oncology*; 23(11):2977–2982.

Tai, B.C., Wee, J., & Machin, D. (2011). Analysis and design of randomised clinical trials involving competing risks outcomes. *Trials*; 12:127.

Titman, A. (2016). Multi-state models: An overview. Presentation. Retrieved from: www.maths.lancs.ac.uk/~titman/leeds_seminar.pdf.

Trinquart, L., Jacot, J., Conner, S.C. et al. (2016). Comparison of treatment effects measured by the hazard ratio and by the ratio of restricted mean survival times in oncology randomized controlled trials. *Journal of Clinical Oncology*; 34(15):1813–1819.

Uhry, Z., Hédelin, G., Colonna, M. et al. (2010). Multi-state Markov models in cancer screening evaluation: A brief review and case study. *Statistical Methods in Medical Research*; 19(5):463–486.

University of Texas at Dallas. (n.d.). Markov chains. Retrieved from: www.utdallas.edu/~jjue/cs6352/markov/markov.html.

U.S. Department of Health and Human Services. Food and Drug Administration. (2007). Clinical trial endpoints for the approval of cancer drugs and biologics: Guidance for industry. Center for Drug Evaluation and Research (CDER), Center for Biologics Evaluation and Research (CBER). Retrieved from: www.fda.gov/downloads/Drugs/Guidances/ucm071590.pdf.

Van Erning, F.N., van Steenbergen, L.N., Lemmens, V.E.P.P. et al. (2014). Conditional survival for long-term colorectal cancer survivors in the Netherlands: Who do best? *European Journal of Cancer*; 50(10):1731–1739.

Van Houwelingen, H., & Putter, H. (2012). *Dynamic prediction in clinical survival analysis*. Boca Raton, FL: CRC Press, Taylor & Francis.

Willekens, F.J., & Putter, H. (2014). Software for multistate analysis. *Demographic Research*; 31:381–420.

Williams, C., Lewsey, J.D., Briggs, A.H. et al. (2017). Cost-effectiveness analysis in R using a multi-state modeling survival analysis framework: A tutorial. *Medical Decision Making*; 37(4):340–352.

Chapter 5

Department of Health and Social Care. (n.d.). NHS prescription services. Retrieved from: www.nhsbsa.nhs.uk/nhs-prescription-services.

Fundamental Finance. (n.d.). Marginal Cost (MC) & Average Total Cost (ATC). Retrieved from: http://economics.fundamentalfinance.com/micro_atc_mc.php.

National Institute for Sickness and Disability Insurance. (n.d.). INAMI home page. Retrieved from: www.inami.fgov.be/fr/Pages/default.aspx.

Chapter 7

Anderson, D.F., & Kurtz, T. (2015). *Stochastic analysis of biochemical systems*, Stochastics in Biological Systems Series, Volume 1.2. Springer International Publishing.

Caro, J., Möller, J., Karnon, J. et al. (2016). *Discrete event simulation for health technology assessment*. New York: Chapman and Hall/CRC.

Parikh, R.C., Du, X.L., Robert, M.O. et al. (2017). Cost-effectiveness of treatment sequences of chemotherapies and targeted biologics for elderly metastatic colorectal cancer patients. *Journal of Managed Care and Specialty Pharmacy*; 23(1):64.

Saint-Pierre, P. (2016). Multi-state models and cost-effectiveness analysis. *Journal de Gestion et d'Économie Médicales*; 34(2):133.

Salleh, S., Thokala, P., Brennan, A. et al. (2017). Discrete event simulation-based resource modelling in health technology assessment. *Pharmacoeconomics*; 35(10):989.

Zeng, X., Li, J., Peng, L. et al. (2014). Economic outcomes of maintenance gefitinib for locally advanced/metastatic non-small-cell lung cancer with unknown EGFR mutations: A semi-Markov model analysis. *PLoS One*; 9(2):e88881. eCollection 2014.

Chapter 9

Bang, H., & Zhao, H. (2014). Cost-effectiveness analysis: A proposal of new reporting standards in statistical analysis. *Journal of Biopharmaceutical Statistics*. Taylor & Francis.

Bang, H., & Zhao, H. (2016). Median-based incremental cost-effectiveness ratios with censored data. *Journal of Biopharmaceutical Statistics*; 26(3):552–564.

Bebu, I., Luta, G., Mathew, T. et al. (2016). Parametric cost-effectiveness inference with skewed data. *Computational Statistics and Data Analysis*; 94(February):210–220.

Brard, C., Le Teuff, G., Le Deley, M.C. et al. (2017). Bayesian survival analysis in clinical trials: What methods are used in practice? *Clinical Trials*; 14(1):78–87.

Fan, M.Y., & Zhou, X.H. (2007). A simulation study to compare methods for constructing confidence intervals for the incremental cost-effectiveness ratio. *Health Services and Outcomes Research Methodology*; 7(1–2):57–77.

Gordon, L.G., Tuffaha, H.W., & Scuffham, P.A. (2016). Efficient value of information calculation using a nonparametric regression approach: An applied perspective. *Value Health*; 19(4):505–509. Epub 2016.

Grieve, R., Nixon, R., & Thompson, S.G. (2014). Bayesian hierarchical models for cost-effectiveness analyses that use data from cluster randomized trials; healthcare: A review of principles and applications. *Journal of Medical Economics*.

Hoch, J.S., & Dewa, C.S. (2014). Advantages of the net benefit regression framework for economic evaluations of interventions in the workplace: A case study of the cost-effectiveness of a collaborative mental health care program for people receiving short-term disability benefits for psychiatric disorders. *Journal of Occupational and Environmental Medicine*; 56(4):441–445.

Meads, D.M., Marshall, A., Hulme, C.T. et al. (2016). The cost effectiveness of docetaxel and active symptom control versus active symptom control alone for refractory oesophagogastric adenocarcinoma: Economic analysis of the COUGAR-02 trial. *Pharmacoeconomics*; 34(1):33–42.

Stinnett, A.A., & Mullahy, J. (1998). Net health benefits. *Medical Decision Making*; 18(2 Suppl):S68–80.

Tuffaha, H.W., Reynolds, H., Gordon, L.G. et al. (2014). Value of information analysis optimizing future trial design from a pilot study on catheter securement devices. *Society for Clinical Trials*.11(6):648–658

Weintraub, W.S., Daniels, S.R., Burke, L.E. et al. (2011). Value of primordial and primary prevention for cardiovascular disease: A policy statement from the American Heart Association. *Circulation*; 124(8):967–990; originally published online. Retrieved from: http://circ.ahajournals.org/content/124/8/967/F2.

Wilson, E.C. (2015). A practical guide to value of information analysis. *Pharmacoeconomics*; 33(2):105–121.

Wilson, E.C., Mugford, M., Barton, G. et al. (2016). Efficient research design: Using; value-of-information analysis to estimate the optimal mix of top-down and bottom-up costing approaches in an economic evaluation alongside a clinical trial. *Medical Decision Making*; 36(3):335–348.

Zhao, H., & Bang, H. (2012). *Pharmacoeconomics*. 2015 February; 33(2):105–121. doi: 10.1007/s40273-014-0219-x. PubMed PMID: 24194511. PMID: 25336432. PubMed PMID: 24650041.

Zhao, H., Zuo, C., Chen, S., & Bang, H. (2012). Nonparametric inference for median costs with censored data. *Biometrics*; 68(3):717–725.

Index